CAMBRIDGE LIBRARY COLLECTION

Books of enduring scholarly value

Archaeology

The discovery of material remains from the recent or the ancient past has always been a source of fascination, but the development of archaeology as an academic discipline which interpreted such finds is relatively recent. It was the work of Winckelmann at Pompeii in the 1760s which first revealed the potential of systematic excavation to scholars and the wider public. Pioneering figures of the nineteenth century such as Schliemann, Layard and Petrie transformed archaeology from a search for ancient artifacts, by means as crude as using gunpowder to break into a tomb, to a science which drew from a wide range of disciplines - ancient languages and literature, geology, chemistry, social history - to increase our understanding of human life and society in the remote past.

Life of Thomas Young

Admired long after his death by the likes of Lord Rayleigh and Einstein, Thomas Young (1773–1829) was the definition of a polymath. By the age of fourteen he was proficient in thirteen languages, including Greek, Hebrew and Persian. After studies in Edinburgh, London, Göttingen and Cambridge he established himself as a physician in London, and over the course of his life made contributions to science, linguistics and music. He was the first to prove that light is a wave rather than molecular, his three-colour theory of vision was confirmed in the twentieth century, and his work in deciphering the Rosetta Stone laid the foundations for its eventual translation. Published in 1855, this engaging biography drew on letters, journals and private papers, taking the mathematician George Peacock (1791–1858) twenty years to complete. It stands as a valuable and affectionate portrait of 'the last man who knew everything'.

T0188061

Life of
Thomas Young

GEORGE PEACOCK

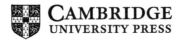

CAMBRIDGE UNIVERSITY PRESS

Cambridge, New York, Melbourne, Madrid, Cape Town,
Singapore, São Paolo, Delhi, Mexico City

Published in the United States of America by Cambridge University Press, New York

www.cambridge.org
Information on this title: www.cambridge.org/9781108057363

© in this compilation Cambridge University Press 2013

This edition first published 1855
This digitally printed version 2013

ISBN 978-1-108-05736-3 Paperback

LIFE

OF

THOMAS YOUNG, M.D., F.R.S., &c.

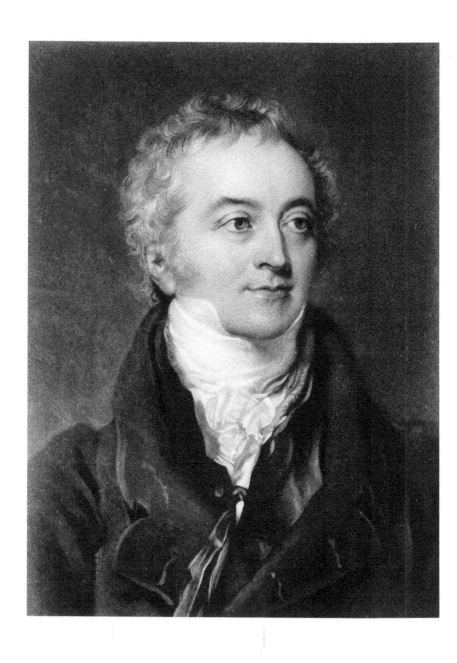

THOMAS YOUNG, M.D., F.R.S.

Engraved by G. R. Ward, from a Picture by Sir Thomas Lawrence, P.R.A.

LIFE

OF

THOMAS YOUNG, M.D., F.R.S., &c.,

AND ONE OF THE EIGHT FOREIGN ASSOCIATES OF THE NATIONAL INSTITUTE OF FRANCE.

BY GEORGE PEACOCK, D.D.,

F.R.S., F.G.S., F R.A.S., F.C.P.S., ETC.,

DEAN OF ELY,

LOWNDEAN PROFESSOR OF ASTRONOMY IN THE UNIVERSITY OF CAMBRIDGE, AND FORMERLY FELLOW AND TUTOR OF TRINITY COLLEGE.

LONDON:

JOHN MURRAY, ALBEMARLE STREET.

1855.

LONDON : PRINTED BY W. CLOWES AND SONS, STAMFORD STREET,
AND CHARING CROSS.

TO

HUDSON GURNEY, ESQ.,

THE OLDEST AND ONE OF THE MOST VALUED OF THE FRIENDS

OF

DR. YOUNG,

THIS MEMOIR OF HIS LIFE

IS INSCRIBED

WITH EVERY SENTIMENT OF RESPECT AND REGARD

BY

THE AUTHOR,

PREFACE.

It is now more than twenty years since I somewhat rashly undertook to write the Life of Dr. Young. For many years, however, after making this engagement, I found myself so much occupied by the duties of a very laborious college office, that I had no leisure to commence the work; and when the possession of leisure would have enabled me to have done so, my health became so seriously deranged that I felt myself unequal to any continued and severe literary labour. The undertaking was consequently abandoned, and it was proposed to transfer it to other hands; but it was not found easy to secure the services of a person who possessed sufficient scientific knowledge to enable him to write the life of an author whose works were so various in their character and not unfrequently so difficult to understand and analyse, as those of Dr. Young.

It had always been the opinion of Mr. Gurney, one of the most intimate of Dr. Young's friends, that the best monument which could be dedicated to his memory would be a complete edition of his Miscellaneous Works, the greatest part of which had been published anonymously, in scientific journals and elsewhere, in a form not easily accessible to literary or scientific students. In consequence of this opinion, in which I entirely concurred, an arrangement was made by Mrs. Young, somewhat more than three years ago, in virtue of which I undertook to edit the scientific portion of Dr. Young's Works, whilst his Hieroglyphical Memoirs and Correspondence were entrusted to Mr. Leitch. As it was in the first instance intended to prefix to this edition of Dr. Young's Works a short introductory notice only and not a formal memoir, of his life and writings, such explanatory notes and selections from his correspondence were added as were deemed necessary for the general illustration of his literary life and labours. The notes and letters which were added with this view to the volume edited by Mr. Leitch, were of very considerable extent and importance.

When this work was completed—and a great delay had been occasioned by the destruction of the greatest part of the impression, first struck off, by a fire in the warehouse in which it was deposited—Mrs. Young resumed her original design—to which she had always adhered with affectionate constancy and which she had never altogether abandoned—of doing honour to the memory of her husband by a Memoir which should combine a detailed narrative of his personal history with a review of his various publications. She urged her wishes with so much earnestness, that I was at last persuaded—under a sense of the responsibility which I had incurred by disappointing her hopes for so many years—to undertake the task, subject to the condition, however, that I should be at liberty to transfer the materials which I had collected and the portions of the work which in the mean time I might have finished, to other hands, in case of being again disabled by the recurrence of those serious attacks of illness from which I had previously suffered. It is now about fifteen months since my labours were resumed, and they have been continued ever since with few and not very considerable interruptions; and I gratefully acknowledge the goodness of God for granting me the renewed enjoyment of the blessings of health and strength, which has enabled me to complete my task, imperfectly it is true, but I trust not so much so as altogether to defeat the pious views in which it originated.

The materials which I have employed in editing Dr. Young's Works, and in the preparation of his Life, have been chiefly—in addition to the information supplied by his Works, his Journals, and Letters to his uncle, Dr. Brocklesby, in early life—a short autobiographical sketch of his life, written for one of the sisters of Mrs. Young, headed *An Article intended for a Future Edition of the Encyclopædia Britannica*, the greatest part of which is included in Mr. Gurney's very pleasing Memoir—and a large collection of letters addressed to him by Arago, Fresnel, Humboldt, Sir David Brewster, Dr. Brinkley, Mr. George Ellis, Mr. Gifford, Captain Kater, Schumacher, Bessel, Mr. Macvey Napier, Sir William Gell, and many other correspondents. Mr. Gurney furnished me with a nearly unbroken series of confidential letters addressed to him by Dr. Young, from the year 1804 to the end of his life, which have been of the greatest service to

me, as recording without disguise his thoughts and
opinions upon almost every subject upon which he
was engaged, or about which he was interested. The
late lamented M. Arago placed in my hands several
letters from Dr. Young, which have become important
documents in the history of the progress of the undulatory theory of light. An equally liberal course was
followed by Sir David Brewster, though some of the
letters thus furnished were in opposition to views of
his own. The late Mr. Macvey Napier sent me the
letters relating to Dr. Young's contributions to the
Supplement of the Encyclopædia Britannica, of which
he was the editor; and the Astronomer Royal some
others relating to proposed alterations in the Nautical
Almanac and other astronomical questions. Other
letters were forwarded to me by Mr. Shepherd, of
Frome, the late Dr. Bostock, and other correspondents.
Dr. Young, in his letters to Sir William Gell, would
appear to have occasionally imitated the *plaisanteries*
of his lively and ingenious correspondent, and to have
been somewhat less guarded in his expressions than
was usual with him in his other letters, which are remarkable for the fairness and temperance with which
he speaks of men and of things, even when writing to
his most intimate friends. Finally, I beg to return
my best thanks to the family of the late Mrs. Chambers,
Mrs. Earle, and the Countess of Buchan, the sisters of
Mrs. Young, who have placed at my disposal a series
of letters, written with all the affectionate freedom and
confidence of a brother to his sisters, and which present
the most lively and agreeable references to the society

in which he was moving, and to the various subjects of interest which arose out of the events of the day.

It is hardly necessary for me to add that, throughout the whole progress of the work, I have received the most important information and assistance from Mr. Gurney.

From various members of Dr. Young's family, and more especially from his nephew, Mr. Thomas Young, of Sackville Street, I have received very valuable information, with respect to the events of his early life.

I have also to express my thanks to Mr. De Morgan, Dr. J. A. Wilson of Dover Street, London, Dr. Clarke of Cambridge, the Astronomer Royal, and others, who have furnished me with information.

I have elsewhere expressed my obligations to Mr. Leitch, which have been further increased by the assistance which he has given me in the progress of this work.

Deanery, Ely,
December 13th, 1854.

CONTENTS.

MEMOIR

OF

DR. THOMAS YOUNG.

CHAPTER I.

EARLY EDUCATION.

DR. THOMAS YOUNG, the subject of the following Memoir, was born at Milverton, in Somersetshire, on the 13th of June, 1773. He was the eldest of ten children of Thomas and Sarah Young; his mother—whose maiden name was Davis—was the niece of Dr. Richard Brocklesby, a physician of great eminence in London. His parents were both members of the Society of Friends, occupying a respectable station in the middle ranks of life. They were strict observers of the principles of their sect, in which their children were very carefully educated; and their eldest son appears to have adopted in his earlier years, all the characteristic observances and tenets of this society, though he afterwards abandoned it. Some of those principles which recognise the immediate influence of a supreme intelligence as a guide in the ordinary conduct of life, are not a little calculated, when not properly regulated, to encourage feelings of self-confidence and pride in the achievement of intellectual as well as moral triumphs; and it was to the operation of these early impressions that Dr. Young was accustomed in after-life, to attribute, in no slight degree, the formation of those habits of perseverance in labouring to conquer every difficulty, however formidable it might appear to be, by which he was so remarkably distinguished, and which enabled him, even from his boyhood, to work out his own education with little comparative assistance or direction from others.

The details of this education—which made him at an early period of life an accurate classical scholar; perfectly familiar with the principal European languages; well acquainted with mathematics, and with almost every department of natural philosophy and natural history; profoundly versed in medical and anatomical knowledge, and in possession of more than ordinary personal and ornamental accomplishments—must necessarily possess no common interest and value; not merely as explaining the formation of his own intellectual habits and character, but as illustrating the progress of the human mind in one of the most remarkable examples of its development; and it may be considered fortunate, that the materials for a very minute history of his early studies and occupations exist, in his very ample journals, in his letters to his relatives and others, and in the notes which he has left behind him, upon most of the books which he read for the first twenty years or more of his life.[a]

---

[a] Amongst these are two thick volumes, entitled *Studia Quotidiana*, containing an account—in many cases with copious extracts—of every book which he read from the year 1789 to the summer of 1794; with notices of his botanical and entomological observations, the greatest part of which is written in Latin. There are also, in three smaller volumes, ample notes of all the medical and anatomical lectures which he attended in London in 1793 and 1794: to these may be added minute and very carefully written journals of his studies at Edinburgh and at Göttingen, and of his journeys in Scotland and Germany in 1795, 1796, and 1797: and also a nearly unbroken series of letters to his uncle Dr. Brocklesby during the greatest part of this period.

The following fragment of an autobiography is nearly a literal translation from a short account written in Latin, as a record of his studies as far as the end of his fourteenth year, with the addition of a few explanatory particulars which have been derived from other sources :—

" For the greatest part of the first seven years of my life, I was an inmate in the house of my maternal grandfather, Mr. Robert Davis, a merchant of great respectability, who lived at Minehead in Somersetshire. At two years of age I had learnt to read with considerable fluency, and I subsequently used to attend the school of a village schoolmistress, besides being taught at home by my aunt Mary Davis. Under their instructions I read the Bible twice through, and also Watts's Hymns, before I was four years of age. Being naturally fond of reading, I was supplied with the usual run of children's books, and I well recollect the effect produced on my mind by the first perusal of Gulliver's Travels. From my earliest years I was in the habit of committing pieces of poetry to memory, such as Pope's Messiah, his Universal Prayer, Parnell's Hermit, Rack's Lavinia, and many others. When six years old I learnt by heart the whole of Goldsmith's Deserted Village, which was the work of six weeks during the hours of my absence from school.ᵃ At a later period, I was taught to repeat some Latin verses, which I found no difficulty in remembering, though I did not, at the time, understand the meaning of the words. When not quite six years of age, I began to learn the rudiments of the Latin grammar, in Lilly's Grammar, under the instruction of a dissenting clergyman of the name of Knyfton, who possessed, however, neither talents nor temper to teach anything well : at the same time I read with him Gay's Fables and Goadby's Weekly Miscellany, and he also began to teach me writing. I always look back with pleasure to this period of my life, and to the affectionate care and instructions of my aunt

ᵃ In a quarto edition of this poem in possession of his family, his grandfather had inserted the following memorandum :—" *This poem was repeated by Thomas Young to me, with the exception of a word or two, before the age of five.*"

Mary Davis, a most admirable woman, who is now no more, and also of one of her most intimate friends and relatives, an inmate of the same house, and who afterwards married a Mr. Thompson, at whose school I was subsequently placed. My grandfather—with whom I was a great favourite—was fond of classical learning, and encouraged my taste for study by every means in his power. I well recollect the distich which he used constantly to repeat to me,

> " A little learning is a dangerous thing,—
> Drink deep, or taste not the Pierian spring."

The principles which I imbibed, and the habits which I formed under the guidance of these dear and excellent relatives, have more or less determined my character in future life, whatever it may be,

> " Quo semel est imbuta recens, servabit odorem
> Testa diu."

" I now entered upon a totally new scene of life. In March 1780, when not quite seven years of age, I was placed by my father at a miserable boarding-school kept by a person of the name of King, first at Stapleton near Bristol, and afterwards at Downend near Kingswood. At this school I remained for a year and a half. I here was taught arithmetic, but even at this age I began to be my own teacher; for I had mastered the last rules of Walkinghame's Tutor's Assistant before I had reached the middle of it under my master's inspection. He was a good writing-master, but quite ignorant of Greek and Latin, which were taught, however, by his step-son on two days of the week. During the first two months, I was very ill employed in learning Fisher's English Grammar, and not much better in learning the Syntax of Lilly: I afterwards began to read, at the same time, Loggan's Corderius, and Clarke's Introduction; having finished Corderius, I read through two books of Phædrus's Fables. I at last gladly quitted a master, who was extremely morose and severe, under whom I had made very little progress, and whose manners and character were little calculated to gain the confidence and affection of his scholars. His school was shortly afterwards broken up.

" During this period, I had read Robinson Crusoe, Gesner's Death of Abel, Stories on Shakspeare, the Seven Stages of Life,

Needham's Select Lessons, and Tom Telescope's Newtonian Philosophy.

"The next half-year, I spent almost entirely at home. My father had a neighbour of the name of Kingdon, a man of great ingenuity, who, though originally a tailor, had raised himself by his talents and good conduct to a respectable situation in life—being at that time a land-surveyor and also land-steward to several gentlemen in the neighbourhood. His daughters had always treated me, when a child, with great kindness, and I was in consequence very fond of going to his house, where I found many books relating to science, and particularly a Dictionary of Arts and Sciences, in three volumes, folio, which I began to read with the most intense interest and delight; at his house I also found several mathematical and philosophical instruments, the use of many of which I learnt with the assistance of his daughters and his nephew.

"In March 1782, when nearly nine years of age, I was sent to the school of Mr. T. Thompson, at Compton in Dorsetshire, where I continued for nearly four years, having only left it for six months, during the year 1784. Mr. Thompson was a man of liberal and enlarged mind, who possessed a tolerable collection of English and classical books, which his pupils were allowed to make use of. It was his custom likewise to allow them a certain degree of discretion in the employment of their time :—the following is the list of books which I read with Mr. Thompson in the school.

"The remaining part of Phædrus's Fables and of Clarke's Introduction, Cornelius Nepos, Selecta e Scriptoribus Romanis, Virgil, Horace expurgated by Knox, the Eton Selections from Cicero, the Westminster Greek Grammar (the greater part of which I committed to memory), the whole of Beza's Greek and Latin Testament, the Cyropædia of Xenophon by Hutchinson ; the First Seven Books of the Iliad, which I began in 1786.

"I also translated into Latin the whole of Garretson's and Ellis's Exercises. In Mathematics I read Walkinghame's Tutor's Assistant, Ewing's Mathematics, omitting gunnery, and Dilworth's Book-keeping.—The usher of the school was a very ingenious young man of the name of Josiah Jeffrey, who was in the habit of lending me books, and amongst them Benjamin Martin's Lectures on Natural Philosophy, and Ryland's Intro-

duction to the Newtonian Philosophy. I was particularly
delighted with the optical part of Martin's book, which contains
many detailed rules for the practical construction of optical
instruments; I also learnt the first elements of Algebra from
Vyse and Ward.

"Mr. Jeffrey was a good mechanic, and it was from him
that I acquired my fondness for turning and for making telescopes. He had made also an electrical machine, which I very
frequently used. I was in the habit of grinding and preparing
various kinds of colours for him, which he used to sell to the
boys and to others; from him likewise I learnt the first principles of drawing, and copied under his directions several specimens from the copper-plates of a book entitled The Principles
of Design. He was also a bookbinder, an occupation in which
I assisted him. After he left the school, I succeeded to some
of his employments and perquisites, and I used to sell paper,
copper-plates, copy-books, and colours to my schoolfellows, by
which means I contrived to collect in 1786, as much as 5s.,
which, added to 10s. 6d. given me by my parents, enabled
me to buy some Greek and Latin books, which were sold to me
by Mr. Thompson at extremely low prices, and likewise Mon-
tanus's Hebrew Bible, for which I gave 5s.; for I was at that
time enamoured of Oriental literature, and I had already
read through Buxtorf's Compendium, and Taylor's Tract at
the end of his Concordance; and before I left Compton School,
I had succeeded in getting through six chapters of the Hebrew
Bible.[a]

"In the intervals of my residence at this school, during my
occasional visits to my grandfather at Minehead, I became
acquainted with a saddler of the name of Atkins, a person of
considerable mechanical skill and ingenuity, whose journal of

---

[a] Some of his letters, written in very rude Latin, and addressed to a
young friend at Milverton, have been preserved, in which he gives an
account of his occupations, very similar to that in the text. In answer
to some observations against studying Hebrew, he says : — "Ne puta
linguam Hebraicam inutilem fore mihi vel iniquam alio. Nonne eâ
linguâ oracula edita sunt divina? Nonne est mater omnium prope lin-
guarum? Nonnulli dicunt esse linguam ' quâ locutus est Deus,' sed hoc
audaciam existimo. Biblia emi Hebraica cum Montani versione pro 5s."
This is sufficiently remarkable for a very young schoolboy nearly self-
taught.

the heights of the barometer and thermometer, of the state of the weather, and direction of the wind for three times a day during the whole of the year 1782, is published in the Philosophical Transactions for 1784. Amongst many other instruments which he possessed was a quadrant, which became the constant companion of my walks, and with which I attempted to measure the heights of the principal eminences in the neighbourhood. I had imbibed also a wish to study botany, from a conversation with Morris Birkbeck; and in order to enable me to examine the minute organs of plants, I was anxious to construct a microscope from the description of Benjamin Martin. For this purpose I procured a lathe, and I succeeded in getting the requisite materials by the assistance of my grandfather and one of my father's clerks. My zeal for botany during these operations was replaced by my fondness for optics, and subsequently by that for turning. I well recollect likewise, that, having seen a demonstration in Martin which exhibited, though unnecessarily, some fluxional symbols, I never felt satisfied until I had read, a year or two afterwards, a Short Introduction to the Method of Fluxions.

"My father had purchased at an auction, a volume of Priestley on Air, the reading of which delighted me greatly, and first turned my attention to making chemical experiments.

"I was in the habit of rising an hour sooner than my schoolfellows in summer, and of going to bed an hour or two later in winter, for the purpose of mastering my lesson for the day; my school business was thus soon finished. I was at that time however perfectly ignorant of prosody, as well as my master, and I possessed no very accurate grammatical knowledge of the Greek and Latin languages.

"One of my schoolfellows, of the name of Fox, had made himself master of the Italian language: with his assistance and that of Veneroni's Italian and French Grammar, I was enabled to read *Lettere d' una Peruviana*, and some other works. I had before acquired some slight knowledge of French.

"I read through Penn's Reflections and Maxims.

"Upon my return home, after finally leaving Compton School, I devoted myself almost entirely to the study of Hebrew and to the practice of turning and telescope-making. I read through thirty chapters of the Book of Genesis without points.

That most excellent man, Mr. Toulmin, who had heard of the nature of my studies, though perfectly unknown to me, lent me Masclef's Hebrew, Chaldee, Syriac, and Samaritan grammars, and also some works of Gregory Sharp[a] and Mr. Bayley,[b] which I studied with great diligence. Mr. John Fry lent me Robertson on Reading Hebrew without Points. Mr. Toulmin also lent me The Lord's Prayer in more than 100 Languages, the examination of which gave me extraordinary pleasure. I had also read through the greatest part of Sir William Jones's Persian Grammar."

Amongst the many accounts which have been published of the premature acquirements of extraordinary boys, it might be very possible to find some which are even more remarkable than that which is given in the preceding narrative. In most cases, however, the vigour of the plant seems to have been somewhat exhausted by the unnatural excitement of its early growth, and the instances are very rare where the mature fruits have fully corresponded to the expectations which had been formed. In the subsequent history of Young's education, we shall discover no symptoms of decay, either in the desire or power of acquiring knowledge; and the firmness of purpose with which he persevered in mastering the most difficult and repulsive studies, seems to have advanced with his increase of years. It was, perhaps, a fortunate circumstance for him that the modest station in life of his parents and connexions, and the severe habits of the sect to which they belonged, saved him in some degree at least from the misfortune of being paraded as a prodigy; a fate to

[a] Upon the original powers of letters, wherein it is proved, from the analogy of alphabets and the proportion of letters, that the Hebrew ought to be used without points.—1750.

[b] An Entrance into the Sacred Language, containing the necessary Rules of Hebrew Grammar in English, by the Rev. C. Bayley. Trinity College, 1782.

which wonderful boys have been more or less commonly exposed, in order to gratify the impatient vanity and ostentation of their friends. As it was, however, his acquirements and his talents had already begun to excite considerable attention, not merely amongst his relatives, but also amongst other persons to whom they were made known; and his parents had already begun to think seriously of the line of life which might be most advantageously taken by a youth of such uncommon promise.

It was about this time that a young lady, Priscilla Gurney, a niece of Mr. David Barclay, of Youngsbury, near Ware, in Hertfordshire, was ordered by her medical attendants to spend a few years in a quiet part of the country, for the benefit of her health, and she went to reside with a sister of Mrs. Young, who had long been her intimate friend. The acquirements and industry of her friend's nephew, at that time absorbed in the study of the Oriental languages, were noticed by this lady, and she joined Sir William Watson, who had married her mother, and to whom also Young's family were well known, in strongly recommending him to Mr. Barclay, who was then making arrangements for the domestic education of his grandson, Hudson Gurney, and looking out for a proper companion of his studies, under a private tutor who was to be engaged for that purpose. It so happened that the private tutor first engaged found a situation of a more permanent nature, and never came; so that the two boys being left together, whose ages differed only by a year and a half, Young, who was then little more than fourteen, took upon himself provisionally the office of preceptor. They were afterwards joined by Mr. Hodgkin, who has since become known to the

public as the author of the Calligraphia Græca, and
of some other extremely useful publications connected
with the business of classical education.   To this
gentleman, though himself young, and engaged in the
completion of his own education, Mr. Barclay entrusted,
in connexion with other duties, the general superintendence of the studies and conduct of his grandson,
though Young continued to retain the direction of
his classical studies during the whole period of his
residence at Youngsbury.[a]

[a] Mr. Hodgkin has communicated to me the following statement of his
relation to the two- students at Youngsbury, with a view of correcting a
somewhat erroneous impression which might be conveyed by a short
printed Memoir of Dr. Young, published in 1832, which is founded upon
an autobiographical sketch which was found amongst his papers :—"From
Dr. Young's narrative it might be inferred that John Hodgkin had undertaken the office of tutor to both Dr. Young and Hudson Gurney, but
ultimately relinquished the classical department to Dr. Young, from whom
he was glad to receive instruction ; whereas Mr. Hodgkin never undertook
to be Dr. Young's tutor,—but the person who, previously to Mr. Hodgkin's
being applied to, had been engaged to fill the post of tutor to both, having
afterwards declined it, Dr. Young undertook, provisionally, the instruction
of his young friend in Latin and Greek, in which he acquitted himself so
much to David Barclay's satisfaction that he did not consider it necessary
to look for further aid in that respect, though he did not think it desirable
to subject him to the sole direction of a youth of little more than his own
age—the one being about thirteen and the other about fourteen : he therefore invited Mr. Hodgkin (whom he knew to be at that time intending to
place himself under the instruction of Dr. Knox) to relinquish his plan
of going to Tunbridge, and to undertake in part the office of tutor to
Hudson Gurney, a situation which would afford Mr. Hodgkin an opportunity of pursuing his own classical studies, and of deriving some advice and
assistance in them, from the extraordinary youth, whose stability of
conduct and intensity of application seemed to place every desirable
object of literary or scientific pursuit within the reach of his astonishing
mental powers.   Mr. Hodgkin's wish to have the error, which he has
mentioned, obviated, does not proceed from any desire to underrate his
obligations to Dr. Young : he has always been sensible of them, and would
have rejoiced in having an opportunity of repaying the Doctor in a similar
way ; but his just reliance upon his own resources rendered him independent of the aid of others.   An example will illustrate this :—Soon after
Mr. Hodgkin went to Youngsbury, Dr. Young once asked him how to
solve an algebraical problem ; but he had scarcely proposed it before he

The five years which he spent at Youngsbury, from 1787 to 1792, were considered by himself as the most profitable in his life, with respect both to mental and moral cultivation and improvement. The greatest part of the year he remained in Hertfordshire, in the bosom of a singularly quiet and regular family. A few of the winter months only were spent in London, which was, however, in no other respect London to him than as giving him access to a few booksellers' shops and occasional lectures, and as supplying the materials for his studies.

He sometimes, though rarely, visited his family in Somersetshire, and he was brought by his occasional residence in London, and by other causes, under the more immediate notice of his uncle, Dr. Brocklesby, a circumstance which exercised, as will be seen hereafter, the most important influence upon his future life and fortunes.

The first entry which appears in his Journal, after the commencement of his residence in Hertfordshire, contains a statement of his having written out specimens of the Bible in thirteen different languages.[a] He had

said he could make it out himself, and wished for no assistance. A very few hints from Mr. Hodgkin on the subject of penmanship were sufficient to regulate his ordinary writing; and by Mr. Hodgkin's introducing to his notice Ambrose Serle's little treatise on the subject, Dr. Young not only improved his own mode of forming the Greek characters, but produced that beautiful system which he has exhibited in the Calligraphia Græca."

Though Mr. Hodgkin, with great modesty, disclaims all share in Dr. Young's education and the formation of his character, it would be unjust to him not to add that Dr. Young considered himself under great obligations to him for his advice and assistance.

Mr. Barclay, in writing to Young's father with reference to these arrangements, complains of the difficulty of finding suitable tutors amongst the members of the Society to which they belonged, more especially for a boy somewhat advanced in his studies, in consequence of the little encouragement given to men of learning and science among them.

[a] The copy-book, which contains them, is now before me : it contains

already acquired much of that accuracy and beauty of penmanship for which he was afterwards so remarkable ; and it is recorded of him as an anecdote, that when he was once requested by a friend of 'Dr. Brocklesby, who perhaps presumed somewhat upon his very youthful appearance, to exhibit a specimen of his handwriting, he very delicately rebuked the inquiry by writing a sentence, in his best style, in fourteen different languages.

The new duties which he had now undertaken, recalled his attention from his Oriental studies to the close and accurate study of the Greek and Latin languages, and he appears from this time to have devoted himself with singular determination to the acquisition of a thorough knowledge of their syntax and grammatical construction. He read over, with his fellow student, the principal Greek and Latin books which he had formerly read at Compton ; he also recommenced the study of the Iliad of Homer, the whole of which he read through, referring in the first instance to Clarke's Latin Translation and Notes and Pope's version, and subsequently, on a second perusal, using his Lexicon and the Greek Scholia alone ; and he continued to follow a similar method generally, as far as he was able, in his earlier Greek studies, until he had so far mastered the principles of construction of the language, as to be able to rely entirely upon his Lexicon. In this manner, he read through the Olympic Odes of Pindar, the Enchiridion of Epictetus, and Toup's Longinus,[a]

extracts in English, French, Italian, Latin, Greek, Hebrew, Chaldee, Syriac, Samaritan, Arabic, Persian, Turkish, and Æthiopic. Those in the Greek and Oriental languages are accompanied with a Latin translation and a homophone transcript in the characters of the English alphabet. His Greek characters were yet not well formed, but the specimens from the Eastern languages are beautifully written.

[a] It was formerly the custom in most schools to make the study of Longinus succeed to that of Homer, as if with a view to comprehend at

at the same time studying, with great care, the Port Royal Greek Grammar and practising daily Greek prose composition in Huntingford's Exercises.[a] To these authors succeeded Wharton's Theocritus and Mounteney's Demosthenes, upon both of which he wrote a very enlarged commentary.

It would be easy to give a similar enumeration of the authors which he read in Latin, French, Italian, Mathematics, Natural Philosophy, Botany, Entomology, and English Literature; but it may be more interesting to the reader to possess these details, not in the order of subjects, but of time—as far as they can be collected from his own journals and from other sources. The number of books which he read was very small, but he adhered strictly through life to the principle of doing nothing by halves. Whatever book he began to read he read completely and deliberately through; whatever study he commenced he never abandoned; and it was by steadily keeping to this principle, a most important one in education, that he was accustomed, in after-life, to attribute a great part of his success, both as a scholar and a man of science.

The following is a list of nearly all the books which he read, chiefly at Youngsbury, between the years 1787 and 1790, when he was not yet seventeen years of age. The more regular and ample notes of his studies commence at the end of this period.

once the extreme points of Greek literature : in later times the more rational practice has prevailed of confining the elementary studies of boys to Homer, and the best classical authors of the best ages.

[a] His MS. copy of these Greek exercises still exists; it is beautifully written, everywhere showing the most minute attention to accentuation and grammatical accuracy. It exhibits the usual abbreviations of the early printed Greek books, which are finished with the most elaborate correctness. These exercises were finished in two years.

Besides Homer, Pindar, Epictetus, and Longinus, he read the Hecuba and Orestes, in King's Euripides; the Œdipus Tyrannus and Coloneus and Antigone of Sophocles, the Phœnissæ of Euripides and the Septem contra Thebas of Æschylus, in Burton's Pentalogia; the Heroides and Metamorphoses of Ovid, the Satires of Juvenal and Persius, the Georgics of Virgil, the Plays of Terence, the whole of Cæsar and Sallust, the First Book of Martial, and some of the Orations of Cicero, with Scheller's Præcepta styli bene Latini,[a] as introductory to the practice of Latin prose composition.

Several French books, such as Marmontel's Bélisaire, Fenelon's Télémaque, the Numa Pompilius of Florian, with Chambord's French Exercises. In these studies he had the occasional assistance of a French master.

Simpson's Euclid, begun in February, 1788, and finished in April, 1789. Simpson's Conic Sections and Algebra, Bonnycastle's Algebra, and Popular Astronomy, and Nicholson's Introduction to Natural Philosophy. Trimmer's Introduction to Natural History, and Lee's Introduction to Botany.

Barclay's Apology, Gough's History of the Quakers, Clarke and Wormal's Heraldry, Goldsmith's Rome, Rollin's Ancient History, Sir Joshua Reynolds' Discourses, and three or four other very trifling school books.

When little more than sixteen years of age, Young's

---

[a] A very useful book, which Young appears to have studied with great effect : it gave him a very nice and even critical perception of the principles of the Latin language. His subsequent Latin translations and remarks, though greatly deficient in ease and elegance, are generally remarkable, considering the age and circumstances of the writer, for their grammatical accuracy.

studies were seriously interrupted by an illness of an alarming nature, which seemed to threaten consumption. The maternal care of Mrs. Barclay, aided by the medical advice of Baron Dimsdale,ᵃ who resided in the neighbourhood, and also of his uncle Dr. Brocklesby, succeeded in restoring him to health, though he was for a long time subjected to a rigorous diet. The following letter from his uncle, alluding to this illness and the abstemious habits which were prescribed to him in consequence of it, is a proof of the interest which he had already begun to feel in the extraordinary progress of his studies, and the somewhat peculiar development of his character.

" London, 13th October, 1789.

" DEAR THOMAS YOUNG,

"I RECEIVED your letter from Youngsbury in due time, and am glad your state of health continues mending ; however severe your abstemious habits of self-denial may seem to the inexperienced, yet, as your strength increases and your spirits keep up, why should you have a wish to alter or run a risque of a dangerous relapse? not that I am of opinion eating a little fish twice or thrice a week would hurt you, but you must make the trial cautiously and follow that which seems on experience not to be prejudicial. Be not deceived ; I argue not for any singularity, but could wish your bodily constitution and the frame of your mind did not exact so many peculiarities, which for your own case you actually do, or at least think incumbent on you to practise. Recollect that the least slip (as who can be secure against error?) would in you, who seem in all things to set yourself above ordinary humanity, seem more

ᵃ He had been physician to the Empress Catherine the Second of Russia, by whom he was ennobled : he was well known to Young, and much interested by his great attainments. In his Treatise on Consumptive Diseases, Young has described the treatment of his own case : he was twice bled, and strictly confined, for two years, to a diet of milk, buttermilk, eggs, vegetables, and very weak broth.

monstrous or reprehensible than it might be in the generality of mankind. Your prudery about abstaining from the use of sugar on account of the Negro Trade, in any one else would be altogether ridiculous, but as long as the whole of your mind keeps free from spiritual pride or too much presumption in your facility of acquiring language, which is no more than the dross of knowledge, you may be indulged in such whims, till your mind becomes enlightened with more reason. My late excellent friend, Mr. Day, the author of Sandford and Merton, abhorred the base traffic in Negroes' lives as much as you can do, and even Mr. Granville Sharp, one of the earliest writers on the subject, has not done half as much service in the business as Mr. Day in the above work. And yet Mr. Day devoured daily as much sugar as I do ; for he reasonably concluded, that so great a system as the sugar culture in the West Indies, where 60 millions of British property are employed, could never be affected either way by one or one hundred in the nation debarring themselves the reasonable use of it. Reformation must take its rise elsewhere, if ever there is a general mass of public virtue sufficient to resist such private interests. Read Locke with care, for he opens the avenues of knowledge, though he gives too little himself. I beg to present my kind respects to the worthy family where you are, and I conclude, wishing you very well,

" Dear Tommy, your loving Uncle,

" RICHARD BROCKLESBY."

The practice of abstaining from the use of sugar, which is so happily exposed in this very sensible letter, was adopted by many persons at that period, rather as a testimony of their hatred of the slave-trade, than with a view to its abolition by making the further continuance of it unprofitable.

His classical studies, between 1790 and the autumn of 1792, when he finally quitted Youngsbury, comprehended—besides the remaining books of the Iliad and Odyssey of Homer—the Hymns and Batrachomachia which pass under his name, and the works of

Hesiod, Apollonius Rhodius, and Lycophron, the whole of the Greek Tragedians and the Comedies of Aristophanes, together with the Æneid of Virgil and some portion of the works of Cicero. He likewise read through Simpson's Fluxions and the whole of the Principia and Optics of Newton, the great work of Bacon De Augmentis Scientiarum, the Philosophia Botanica, Systema Vegetabilium, Genera and Species Plantarum of Linnæus, the Methodus Studii Medici of Boerhaave, the Mineralogy of Cronstedt, the Systems of Chēmistry by Lavoisier and Nicholson, with the Præ-lections of Higgins, Walker and Black.[a] He collected and described, and sometimes figured, the principal plants in his neighbourhood, and recorded in his journal their distinctive botanical characters. The same system was subsequently extended to the science of entomology, which he studied in Fabricius with no inconsiderable success. He also read, during the same period, the principal tragedies of Corneille and Racine,[b] some of the plays of Shakspeare, the Paradise Lost of Milton, Blackstone's Commentaries on the Laws of England, Mr. Burke's Reflections on the French Revolution, and his Treatise on the Sublime and Beautiful; with three or four other works, and not more, of an occasional interest. In conformity with the severe system which he had adopted, he made few or no sacrifices to the pleasures of the imagination, and was contented to rest in almost entire ignorance of the popular literature of the day.

He had now acquired a very considerable mastery of

<hr>

[a] The Prælections of Black were in MS.; they were not published until a much later period.

[b] His remarks on French authors are written in French.

LIFE.   C the Greek language, and of all the refinements of its complicated syntax and grammar under the very various forms which they assume in the writers of different countries and ages.

He appears to have read nothing hastily or cursorily. His memory, both of facts and of words, was singularly tenacious, and whatever he had once mastered he never forgot. He was repelled by no difficulty, but relied boldly upon his clear knowledge of the principles and construction of the language to guide him to its right interpretation. The effects of this system are fully manifested in his Annotations on the Greek Tragedians and Aristophanes, which are given in his Journal, proving that he was already prepared to scrutinize a corrupt or difficult passage with the security and confidence of one whose judgment was fortified by a full knowledge of his subject.

It was his invariable habit to write exercises, or to compose, in the languages which he studied, with a view to test the accuracy of his knowledge of their idiom and syntax—a practice which no student can safely dispense with. It was with this view that he wrote his journals in Latin, and his criticisms on the French and Italian authors which he read, in French and Italian. We have already had occasion to notice the exemplary care with which he went through the whole of Huntingford's Exercises in Greek Prose Composition; and it was the Monostrophics of the same author, a collection of translations into Greek verse, which first called his attention to compositions in the Iambic metres of the Tragedians, for which his long study of the Greek poets had fully prepared him.

The first exercise of this kind, which he would ap-

pear to have finished with much care, was Wolsey's
address to Cromwell—

> " Cromwell, I did not think to shed a tear
> In all my miseries," &c ,

ending with

> " Thou fall'st a blessed martyr."

This exercise was written out, on vellum, in his best
style of penmanship, and forwarded to his uncle,
whose letter, in acknowledging it, will best show the
deep interest which he had already begun to take in
his education and fortunes.

" DEAR THOMAS YOUNG, JUN.,

 " I DULY received a pleasing letter from you with a
beautiful manuscript on vellum, a paraphrastic translation of
Wolsey's farewell to Cromwell ; better judges than I am
give it much praise for the spirit of Euripides, which they say
it breathes, but it is much to be lamented that you have not
essayed to translate—

> ' Had I but served my God with half the zeal
> I serv'd my king, he would not in mine age
> Have left me naked to mine enemies.'

" But Mr. Burke has taken the Greek manuscript from me,
and means to show it to divers learned men of his acquaintance
for their philological criticism. I should be glad to have a
copy of the same on vellum, as neatly written, with the addition
of your essay to the above : but do it at your leisure, con
amore, con studio, e diligenza. Mr. Burke wishes you to try
what you can make of Lear's horrid imprecations on his barbarous daughters, beginning with this solemn invocation :—

> ' Nature, hear ! dear goddess, hear a father ! '

If you can give the Greek the like compass of energetic expression as my favourite Shakspeare has done in his native
tongue, Mr. Burke will laud you and judge most favourably of
your performance. He advises you to study Aristotle's Logic,
his Poetics, and above all books, Cicero's moral and philosophic

works. Your mind is not yet strained to any false principles, and he thinks you should be reared and cultivated in the best manner, so as to form your views, to emulate a Bacon or a Newton in the maturity and fullness of time; for he thinks it worth while for a comprehensive mind to be disregardful of any pecuniary emoluments of a profession, if you can but be satisfied with a small competence, and feel your mind prone to and satisfied with enlarged and useful speculations. I talk to you now as if you were strong in the manhood of your mind, but I advise nothing, only to try the powers of your faculties and follow the bias that may lead you to the best for yourself and the world, if you have talents that by being properly cultivated may adorn your country and benefit mankind.

"Have a care, however, that my frankness towards you may not puff you up with vanity, which has been the rock that many others have split on, and I hope you will steer clear from.

"I wished to have seen you, but finding Mr. Barclay has not brought you, I write, unrestrained, my thoughts to you.

"Write frequent moral essays and keep them for my perusal and for the sight of Mr. Burke, who has taken a great fancy to you, and will be glad to aid you with his best advice in all your ways: read his last Appeal. I leave this at Red Lion Square, where I am going to inquire how Hudson is, and I hope well.

"Dr. Ingenhousen would be willing to aid your inquiries whether physical, moral, or philological. I hope you availed yourself of the opportunity whilst he was at Youngsbury.

"I had a fever since I last saw you, which has left exceeding weakness in my knees, so that I can hardly walk one hundred yards together, but I must learn to be satisfied in what is past. Pray God to have you under his immediate care, and that no imprudence of yours hereafter may frustrate the work that in you, with care, may be wrought. Farewell from

"RICHARD BROCKLESBY."

The exercise, alluded to in this letter, was the occasion of introducing Young to Dr. Charles Burney, who had written a very elaborate critique on the Monostrophics of Huntingford in the 68th volume of the Monthly

Review, and which produced from their author an Apology which also became the subject of a further critique from the same pen, not less minute and laborious than the former. The same eminent scholar had also criticised, in the same Review, Dr. Glasse's Translation of the Samson Agonistes of Milton, a work exhibiting no small amount of classical taste and culture, but furnishing, like other attempts of the same kind, abundant matter for objection and comment. Young would appear, from his Journal, to have very carefully studied these examples of Greek versification and the critiques upon them, and to have added not a few to the long list of errors or improprieties in grammar, syntax, or in the use of words and phrases, which had escaped the more experienced scholarship of the Reviewer ; and we find that it was one of the first uses which he made of his improved knowledge of the Greek tragic metres, to execute the task recommended to him by Mr. Burke in translating Lear's imprecations upon his daughter.

> "Hear, Nature, hear! dear goddess, hear a father!
> Suspend thy purpose, if thou didst intend
> To make this creature fruitful.
> Into her womb convey sterility,—
> Dry up in her the organs of increase,
> And from her derogate body never spring
> A babe to honour her! If she must teem,
> Create her child of spleen, that it may live,
> And be a thwart disnatured torment to her :
> Let it stamp wrinkles on her brow of youth,
> With conduit tears fret channels in her cheeks,
> Turn all her mother's pains and benefits
> To laughter and contempt, that she may find
> How sharper than a serpent's tooth it is
> To have a thankless child."

The translation, which follows, is correct and scholarlike, but rather remarkable for the peculiar circumstances under which it was produced, than as adequately expressing the terrible energy of the original.

ΛΕΑΡΟΥ ΑΡΑΙ.

'Αλλ' ὦ νέμουσα τῶν βροτῶν κράτη Φύσις,
'Άκουε δὴ νῦν τάσδε πατρῴας ἄρας·
'Ὦ δαῖμον, εἴγε προυτίθου βλάστας ποτὲ
'Εκ τοῦδε τέρατος ἐξαναστήσειν τόκον,
Γνώμην μεταγνῶθ', ἐπεσάγουσ' ἀπαιδίαν·
Αὔαινε κῶλα τεκνοποιὰ νηδύος,
'Έχοι δὲ μήποτ' ἐξ ἀπευκτοῦ σώματος
Τέκνον πεφυκὸς γηροβοσκὸν εἰσιδεῖν·
Εἰ δ' ἔστ' ἀνάγκη τήνδε τεκνοῦσθαι βρέφος,
'Άστοργον αἰεὶ καὶ πικρᾶς χολῆς γέμον,
'Ρυτίδας ἀώρους εγχαραττέτω ταχὺ
Μητρὸς μετώπῳ, πανταχοῦ λύπην φέρον·
Δάκρυα δὲ θερμ' ἀπ' ὀμμάτων στάζοντ' ἀεὶ
Λιπαραῖς παρειαῖς ἄλοκας ἐντάμοι βαθεῖς·
Κήδων δ' ἀπάντων, τῶν τε μητρῴων πόνων
Καταφρονείτω καὶ καταγελάτω τέκος·
'Όπως ἐπαυρῇ τῆσδε τῆς ἁμαρτίας
Παθοῦσα τ' ὀψέ περ, σαφῶς ποτ' εκμάθη
'Όσῳ πάθημ' ὀξύτερόν ἐστι δήγματος
Φονίου δράκοντος, ἡ τέκνων ἀχαριστία.

A second specimen, of which a fac-simile of his own vellum copy in his own handwriting is given on the opposite page, is a translation of Wolsey's Soliloquy, beginning

" Farewell, a long farewell, to all my greatness !
This is the state of man ;—to-day he puts forth
The tender leaves of hope—to-morrow, blossoms,
And bears his blushing honours thick upon him :
The third day comes a frost—a killing frost ;
And when he thinks, good easy man, full surely
His greatness is a ripening, nips his roots ;
And then he falls, as I do. I have ventured,
Like little wanton boys that swim on bladders,
These many summers in a sea of glory,
But far beyond my depth : my high-blown pride
At length broke under me, and now has left me,
Weary and old with service, to the mercy

ΟΥΛΣΙΟΥ ΜΟΝΟΛΟΓΙΑ.

χαίροις ἂν ἤδη μακρὰ πᾶσ᾽ ἐνδοξία·
χαίροιτε δυνάμεις, αἳ πισωρεύεσθέ μοι.
οὕτως ἔχει ῾τε τἀνθρώπεια· σήμερον
ἀνὴρ τὰ χλωρὰ φύλλα τ᾽ἀλπίδος φύει·
αὔριον ἀκμάζει, πορφυρέοις τ᾽ ἐπ᾽ ἄνθεσι
τιμῶν ὅσων περ εἶυχε, πολλ᾽ ἀβρύνεται·
τρίταῖον αὖτε ῥῖγος ἐμπίπτει βαρυ,
κἀπεὶ πεποιθὼς κάρτα ῾δ᾽ ἐλπίζει τάλας
καρπὸν μεγίστων ἐκπεπαίνεσθαι καλῶν,
ῥίζῃ πρὸς αὐτῇ δύσμορος ξηραίνεται,
κἄπειτα πίπτει δειλός, ὡς ἐγὼ τὰ νῦν.
ὁποῖα παῖδες νήπιοι παράφρονες,
ἐπὶ κύστεσιν νεῖν ἐν θέρει πειρώμενοι,
ὅπως τὰ πολλὰ ῾δ᾽ ἐ῾δ᾽κεκινδύνευκ᾽ ἐγὼ
δόξης θαλάσσῃ, πρὸς βάθος μηδὲν σκοπῶν·
κόμπος δ᾽ ἀραιὸς ὃν ἐπεφυσήκειν ἅδαν
ἐσχισμένος λέλοιπέ μ᾽ ἐν κλυδωνίῳ,
῾γ᾽έροντα, μόχθῳ καὶ χρόνῳ κεκμηκότα,
κἀνταῦθα λάβροις κύμασι βυθισθήσομαι.
ὦ λαμπρότητος καὶ τρυφῆς κένη σκιά!
ἀπεχθὲς ὄνομα! νῦν δὲ καρδίαν ἐμὴν
αὐταρχίας τυχοῦσαν εὖ ῾δ᾽ ἐπίσταμαι.
φεῦ δυστάλαιναν τοῦ τρισαθλίου τύχην
χάριτος τυράννων ὅστις ἐκκρεμάννυται!

Of a rude stream that must for ever hide me.
Vain pomp and glory of this world, I hate ye!
I feel my heart new open'd.   Oh! how wretched
Is that poor man that hangs on princes' favours!"

This exercise, which was undertaken on the recommendation of Dr. Charles Burney, is not always successful in expressing fully the sense of the original, and is chargeable with some metrical and other improprieties, which a practised imitator of the Greek tragic writers would have avoided. Some of these faults are corrected in the alterations suggested in the Note below.[a] The two last months of the year 1791 he passed with his uncle Dr. Brocklesby in London, by whom he was introduced to the most distinguished literary society of his day. He has recorded, in his Journal, several conversations on subjects of Greek criticism, with Porson, Baker, Burney, and Lawrence, which show that he was already prepared to enter the lists with those distinguished scholars, and to contend with them on not very unequal terms.[b]

[a] The following alterations and corrections were inserted in the margin of the manuscript: those marked with an asterisk (*) were made upon the recommendation of Sir George Baker, and those marked with † upon that of Dr. Charles Burney.
Line 1. Or χαίροι το λοιπὸν πᾶς ἔρως εὐδοξίας.†
   „   2. Substitute χαίροι τε πλοῦτος, ὅσπερ ἦν ἐμοὶ μέγας.
   „   3. For τ' ανθρώπεια read τᾶν βροτοῖσι. †
   „   4. Or τὰ χλωρὰ φύλλ' ἄνθρωπος ἐλπίδος φύει. *
   „   5. For πορφυρέοις τ' ἐπ' ἄνθεσι read πορφυροῖσιν ἄνθεσι.†
   „   14. Or οὕτως ἐγὼ πόλλ' ἐγκεκινδύνευκ' ἔτη.†
   „   16. For κόμπος δ' ἀραιὸς ὄν read ἀλαζονεία δ' ἦν.*
   „   17. For ἐσχισμένος read ἐσχισμένη, to agree with the correction made in the preceding line.
   „   19. Or κ' ανταῦθα κῦμα μ' ἐς ἀεὶ καταβροχθίσει.†
   „   22. Or αὐτῆς κρατεῖν ἤδη καταισθάνομαι σαφῶς.
[b] 12th December, 1791.—Dr. Lawrence, Sir George Baker, Porson, and Murphy supped with my uncle ; Murphy read Johnson's Latin poem on the completion of his Dictionary.   Young.

After quitting his uncle's house, he resumed his residence at Youngsbury, and continued there until the

Young. "Will turba scholarum do?"

Porson. "No; the five or six examples that may be brought are not sufficient to justify the making à sch short."

Young. "What are we to make of immensaque stagna?"

Porson. "Most of the MSS. have immensa stagna."

Speaking of Brunck, Porson said—"He gives us τὸν τράγον ἐκ δίσσαιν ἤγετο θηροσύναιν—what can we make of this?"

Young. "It must mean that he hunted him twice."

Porson. "ἤγετο might mean that he dragged him for himself, but never brought him to another: we could not say ἤγετό σοι."

Young. "That's certain."

Lawrence. "Perhaps ἄνθετο."

Porson. "The MS. has τὸν τράγον ὠδίσσαιν ἄγετ' ἀθηροσύναιν."

Lawrence. "Philodemus was a fine fellow :—ἡ μὲν μάτρωνας τε τρόπους καὶ ἤθεα στέργειν. I read τηρειν."

Porson. "I cannot believe that any writer of the Augustan age would lengthen καί ἤθεα. I read στέργειν ἠθὴ τε τρόπους τε. Nothing is more common than to find τε and καὶ confused ; if some copyist had written ἠθὴ τε καὶ τρόπους, the change would then be natural into the vulgar reading."

On another occasion, when supping with Dr. Lawrence, and speaking of the measures of the ancients, Porson said—"We do not know exactly what their cubit or ὀργυιά was."

Young. "I believe ὀργυιά is generally translated a fathom from stretching out the arms thus."

Porson. "To confirm that, you have ὀρογυίαι in Aristophanes. Photius in his MS. Lexicon ὀρογυιὰι τετρασυλλάβως ὄντως Αριστοφάνὴς."

Young. "Then we must read Θυρωρῷ πόδες ἑπτορογύιοι?"

Porson. "Undoubtedly; and there is a line in Aristophanes beginning with ἑκατοντόργυιον which is impossible, though Toup would tell you that a vowel might be made short before ργ."

Young. "Is it known at what time the Arabic numerals were introduced? I cannot help thinking they were immediately derived from the Greek." (Young then exemplifies his views of the derivation of these figures, but adds in a marginal note that Vossius and others had made the same suggestion : it is known to be unfounded.)

Porson. "But the Arabic figures were very different at first from their present form, and the Greek characters have varied as much. How would you suppose the Latin & to have been formed?"

Young. "I think this ℥ is very clearly ετ."

Porson. "That is not the immediate derivation ; the ετ was at one time written α, and this only wants the eye to make it &."

Many similar conversations with Dr. Burney are also mentioned. Thus, speaking of Morell, Young said—"Morell has made a curious blunder :

summer of 1792, devoting himself with his accustomed regularity and diligence to his classical, botanical, entomological and other studies. In the autumn of the same year he finally quitted his residence in a family which had become endeared to him by a truly parental kindness.

It was at this point that Young's general education, as far as it may be considered as the basis of his subsequent studies, may be said to terminate, and his professional, and perhaps I may add, his ornamental education to begin; and I have been thus minute in describing its whole course and progress, as I conceive it presents many instructive lessons with respect to the proper conduct of education generally—though, on the other hand, it may be viewed as giving the history of the training of a very remarkable mind and therefore in a great measure inapplicable to ordinary students.

What then were the primary causes of the extraordinary success of an education conducted for so many years with so little communication with other minds, with so little assistance from extrinsic sources? The principal of these must be referred to the peculiar constitution of his own mind; to his great industry; to the conviction, which he always felt, that what one man had accomplished, another might accomplish also;[a]

he cites ὡς ἥδομαι καὶ τέρπομαι καὶ χαίρομαι, as good Greek, when Aristophanes calls it τὸ Δάτιδος μέλος, as completely barbarous."

Burney. "He gives you in another passage στίχοισι long too; when the true reading is τοίχοισι."

Young. "That is excellent."

Burney. "It is Richard Porson's."

[a] This was a favourite theme with Young both in early and later life. In a letter to his uncle, written in 1792, he quotes some homely lines from some stanzas addressed by Dr. Barnard to Sir Joshua Reynolds, as expressive of his opinion with respect to his own art :—

> " Thou say'st not only skill is gained,
> But genius too may be obtained,
> By studious imitation."

" This

to the determination of mastering every branch of knowledge, whose acquisition he thought necessary or desirable.

He had little faith in any peculiar gifts of genius, believing the original difference between human intellects to be much less considerable than it was generally supposed to be. His temper, also, in early youth was singularly unruffled and tranquil; he had no boyish tastes or amusements; he was seduced by no dreams of the imagination from the assiduous cultivation of the understanding.

There were many other causes to which his success was attributable. Amongst them may be mentioned his clear and beautiful penmanship, and that nice and almost artistic appreciation of form which is connected with it, whether as a result of practice or a gift of nature, which enabled him, even when a boy, to write his Greek and other exercises, not merely with the most minute attention to accentual and other diacritical marks, but which extended likewise to the most complicated contractions of the early Greek printers. I know of no practice which is more calculated to form those habits of accurate observation which are so essential to give the last finish to the edge of critical scholarship; and when we come to the examination of his researches in later life into the Hieroglyphics of Egypt, we shall trace the influence of the same habit in the exquisite copies which he made of the Rosetta and a multitude of other inscriptions, and which contributed not a little to his great discoveries in that department of research.

"This goes further," says he, "than Dr. Johnson; and I now may be allowed to hope that I have not been totally mistaken, nor too decided, in an opinion which was formed as early as I can recollect to have thought upon the subject."

Another important practice, to which the accuracy of his scholarship was not a little indebted, was the rigorous attention which he paid to the grammar and syntax of the languages, whether ancient or modern, which he studied, and the patient perseverance with which he practised composition in them. It is rarely that a student who is not compelled to do so by the rigid system of a school, will restrain his impatience of becoming acquainted with the contents of ancient authors, for the purpose of reducing his knowledge of the language in which they are written to the test of composition : a task which—in its earlier stages at least, when words are imperfectly remembered, when phrases and their construction are imperfectly understood, when it is difficult, if not impracticable, to distinguish between what is correct and what is incorrect, between what is easy and classical and what is harsh and barbarous—is always more or less laborious and distasteful to a student who rarely appreciates the importance of the end to be attained. It is probably for this reason that great facility and nicety in the practice of composition in the classical languages is seldom attained, unless under the severe discipline of a public school, where such exercises are not only greatly encouraged but rigorously enforced. Dr. Young may be considered as almost an unique example of an unassisted student, in whom this difficulty was overcome by a rare union of foresight and of perseverance in the use of the means which were necessary for that purpose with a steady view to the end to be attained.

The extent to which the practice of composition in the classical languages, as an essential part of a sound classical education, should be encouraged or required, is a question upon which public opinion has long been and is likely to continue to be, much divided. Are such compositions to be considered as auxiliary to the attainment of a critical knowledge of the syntax and construction of a language merely, or as a means of cultivating the taste by the imitation of those models of pure and refined expression and sentiment to which the whole civilized world has been so long accustomed to do homage? If the first of these views be taken, there can be little doubt but that translations from our own into the classical languages would most certainly accomplish the object proposed, as they allow of less licence in the use of words and phrases than mere imitations or original compositions. But even upon the range of such translations some limitations must be imposed : for the forms of many languages, more especially that of the Greek, are as various as those of our own from the time of Chaucer downwards, and even if it were desirable, it would not be practicable, to attain to an equal mastery of them all ; and the same observation is still more applicable to translations into verse, where the forms of versification are so multiplied. It is therefore to prose translations into the language of the best and purest authors of the best ages, whether of Greek or Roman literature, that we must look for that vigorous and well-disciplined training in their grammar and syntax, and of those other niceties in the use of words and phrases which is essential to the acquisition of accurate scholarship—and beyond these it would seem hardly necessary to proceed ; and though it may be quite true that there are many proprieties and even beauties which a student who neglected similar exercises in imitation of the great tragic, heroic, or elegiac poets of Greece or Rome, would fail to notice or appreciate, and some delicacies of construction which he might altogether overlook, yet it should always be kept in mind that the business of education is one of selection, where much must be postponed and much must be sacrificed, in order to lay a secure basis for the more important parts of the vast fabric of human knowledge.[a]

This self-education, however, eminent as was its success, was not without very serious disadvantages.[b] He had no sufficient opportunity of freely reciprocating his thoughts with other minds than his own, at that period of life when such interchanges are most cordial and spontaneous : when every impulse of feeling, every creation of the fancy, every dream of the imagination, every hope that we cherish, every apprehension that we entertain, is thrown open to our equals in age and in fortune; when the experience of life, its trials and its disappointments have not chilled the ardour of our affections, or clouded the brightness of those visions of happiness or distinction in which youth so much delights to indulge. If he had to regret no loss of time or opportunities in the pursuit of knowledge, to deplore no sacrifices to the seductive influences of boyish sports or idle com-

---

[a] See Observations on the Statutes of the University of Cambridge, p. 157.

[b] In a letter to one of his brothers, Robert, the course of whose studies he had undertaken to direct, he says :—"Although I have readily fallen in with the idea of assisting you in your learning, yet it is in reality very little that a person who is seriously and industriously disposed to improve may not obtain from books with more advantage than from a living instructor : something is wanting for the direction of application in the right path, but it must be the strength of the traveller and not of the guide that must conquer the difficulties of the journey. Masters and mistresses are very necessary to compensate for want of inclination and exertion ; but whoever would arrive at excellence must be self-taught, as I lately heard maintained by one of the first scholars in Europe." Little reliance can be safely placed upon Young's opinion in a case where he judged of other minds and dispositions by his own.

panions, he had, on the other hand, no means of observing the difficulties which they experience in the progress of their studies or of fixing upon those points, in the communication of knowledge, which, though clear and obvious to himself, were likely to be obscure or unintelligible to others : he was throughout life destitute of that intellectual fellow-feeling—if the phrase may be used—which is so essential to form a successful teacher or lecturer, or a luminous and interesting writer.

His mathematical was, if possible, still more unassisted than his classical education, and we can only form an estimate of the correctness and soundness of his knowledge, by his philosophical writings in afterlife, which, though always obscure and generally deficient in elegance and concinnity of form, yet touch upon many of the most abstruse applications of mathematics to natural philosophy, and are often remarkable for the simple means by which the most difficult problems are solved. There is, in fact, no department of his very various researches and labours, in which the resources of his genius—for a less forcible term would be inappropriate—are more remarkable than in this. We fear, however, that it would be difficult, if not impossible, to point out the causes of his success. A desultory mathematical education rarely leads to sound or accurate knowledge. One or more fundamental principles imperfectly understood or altogether misconceived, are generally found to affect the stability of the whole structure which is raised upon them. The very basis of demonstration is unsound, and there is an end of all certain distinction between truth and error. If, therefore, in the remarkable instance before us it produced a different result, it is rather referable to the peculiar character of his mind than to the discipline to which it was subjected.

We find from his journals that he studied mathematical, much in the same manner as other, books. The six books of Euclid were begun on such a day, and were finished on another; and we hear no more of them. Algebra, trigonometry, fluxions, were treated in a similar manner. The Principia of Newton must have presented to a student thus prepared greater difficulties than to the contemporaries of its author, to nearly all of whom it was a sealed book: however, he not only read it deliberately through, but we find in his journals remarks, on some of the leading propositions contained in it, which show that he had very sufficiently understood, not merely their general purport, but also the full force of the demonstrations. A retentive memory and great clearness and precision of thought would appear to have superseded in his case the necessity of a more progressive training. In other respects the effects of this irregular intrusion into the inmost recesses of philosophy were such as might have been anticipated: he never felt the necessity nor appreciated the value of those formal processes of proof which other minds require.

CHAPTER II.

MEDICAL EDUCATION : LONDON.

IN the autumn of 1792, Young took lodgings in Westminster for the purpose of prosecuting his medical and anatomical studies, and became an attendant at the lectures of Dr. Baillie, Mr. Cruikshanks, and subsequently of John Hunter, in the Hunterian School of Anatomy. The choice of his profession was greatly influenced by the wishes of his uncle Dr. Brocklesby, who had already undertaken the charge of his education, and had given him reason to expect the reversion of such a portion of his fortune as would secure him a moderate independence. He had access, also, through the same kind relative, to the most distinguished literary circles in the metropolis, including Mr. Burke, Mr. Windham, Mr. Frederick North (afterwards Lord Guildford), Sir Joshua Reynolds, Dr. Lawrence, Sir George Baker, Dr. Vincent, and others; as well as the leading members of the profession which he had chosen.

His manners, at this period of his life, are described, by one who knew him well, as very quiet and pleasing; like those of the more cultivated members of the society to which he still outwardly adhered, though he had already abandoned many of the peculiar tenets by which they are distinguished. His conversation, on classical and scientific subjects, showed a confidence and precision which were far beyond his years; whilst his ignorance of popular literature and of the habits of thinking of his equals in age and station, was in striking contrast with the range and accuracy of his other acquirements.

It was in conformity with the advice of Mr. Burke, with whom his uncle lived in habits of great intimacy, and who, on that account, had taken a more than common interest in the conduct of his studies, that he had undertaken the systematic study of the philosophical and other works of Cicero; the model on which, according to the testimony of one of his friends, that distinguished writer and statesman had laboured to form his own character, in eloquence, in policy, in ethics and in philosophy. This task he completed with his usual diligence, as the critical and other observations entered in his journals sufficiently testify. He was in the habit of copying, in his common place book, the most striking passages which he met with in his perusal both of classical and modern authors; and in the selection which he has made from the works of this great expositor of the opinions of the ancient world, it is not difficult to discover indications of the prevalent disposition of his own mind and character:—a moral tone of very unusual strictness and purity, with great firmness of purpose and reliance upon his own powers, such as we find sketched in a passage which he has quoted as peculiarly expressive of his own aims in the formation of his habits and the conduct of his studies. "For my part, judges," says Cicero, "I think the man, if any such there be, who possessed that strength of mind, that constitutional tendency to temperance and virtue, which would lead him to avoid all enervating indulgences, and to complete the whole career of life in the midst of labours of the body and efforts of the mind; whom neither tranquillity nor relaxation, nor the flattering attentions of his equals in age and station, nor public games, nor banquets would delight; who would regard nothing in life as desirable which was not united with dignity and virtue;—such a man I regard as being, in my judgment, furnished and adorned with some special gifts of the gods."[a]

In the autumn of 1793, he entered himself as a pupil at St. Bartholomew's Hospital, and devoted himself systematically to the preparatory studies of his future profession. Amongst other lectures which he attended —in addition to those which have been mentioned before—were those of Sir Alexander Crichton and also of Dr. Latham, on the Practice of Physic; on Midwifery, by Doctors Clark and Osborn; and on Botany, by Sir J. E. Smith. Mr. Wilson, the eminent anatomist, the father of Dr. Young's successor at St. George's Hospital, was the demonstrator of Anatomy. He took ample notes of the lectures which he attended. Occasionally they are written in Latin; and Greek quotations and phrases are not unfrequently introduced. It may be presumed, that before the beginning of the lecture, he sometimes amused himself with mathematical calculations and demonstrations, as many such appear among his notes. His *Prælectiones Anatomicæ* open with a notice of an introductory discourse by Dr. Baillie, which is thus characterised :—*Introductio generalis præcipuè historica et monitoria, satis elegans, laude non indigna.* Then

---

[a] Ego, si quis, judices, hoc robore animi, atque hâc indole virtutis ac continentiæ fuit, ut respueret omnes voluptates, omnemque vitæ suæ cursum in labore corporis atque in animi contentione conficeret: quem non quies, non remissio, non æqualium studia, non ludi, non convivia delectarent: nihil in vitâ expetendum putaret, nisi quod esset cum laude et cum dignitate conjunctum: hunc, meâ sententiâ, divinis quibusdam bonis instructum atque ornatum puto. Pro M. Cælio.

follows a demonstration by Mr. Wilson, on the muscles of the back, with references to numbers in Winslow's book, which mark out the course of inquiry to be pursued by the student on his return from the lecture.[a]

The medical and anatomical books which he read, in conjunction with his hospital duties and lectures, were few in number, including, amongst some others, those of Winslow, Albini, Cheselden, Monro the elder, Harvey, and Haller. He still continued to reserve, from his other studies, no small portion of his time to complete his knowledge of the philosophical and historical writers of antiquity. We also find numerous extracts in his journals from nearly all the minor Latin poets; with several sketches of monographs on various departments of entomology and natural history, some of which were communicated to the Gentleman's Magazine.[b]

In the course of his professional studies and dissections, his attention had been called to the anatomical structure of the eye, considered as an instrument of vision. It is known to be composed of a succession of curved refracting substances, of various densities and powers, which form upon the retina an inverted image of the objects of vision. If the adjustment of this machinery be imperfect or deranged, the picture thus formed, as well as the impression of sight which it produces, is defective likewise. Thus, in long-sighted persons, the focus of the rays which the eye collects, from objects at the ordinary distance of clear vision,

---

[a] Quoted from Mr. Pettigrew's very pleasing sketch of Dr. Young's Life, which he published in the Medical Portrait Gallery.

[b] His first appearance, as an author, was a Note on Gum Laudanum, with a verbal criticism on Longinus, signed with his initials, inserted in the Monthly Review for 1791. The criticism was admitted by Dr. Charles Burney (with whom he frequently corresponded on questions of Greek literature) to be perfectly correct. Works, vol. ii. p. 439.

is formed behind the retina; whilst in those who are
short-sighted it is formed before. In nearly all such
cases, this defect can be remedied by an artificial addition to the natural lenses of the eye, which tend to
shorten its focal length in one case and to lengthen it
in the other.

But there is a residual difficulty, even in well-con-
stituted eyes, which remains to be explained. By
what adjustment of its machinery does the same eye
view both near and distant objects, without being
sensible of confusion or obscurity; for it is utterly
inconceivable that the same optical apparatus should
form the images of near and distant objects at the same
distance from the iris.

Much of the confusion, which would otherwise arise,
is probably corrected by habit, and very possibly may
form an important element in those delicate laws of
aerial colouring and effect, by which the impression of
distance as well as of form is produced. It is only
when this confusion is very considerable, as in the case
of very near or of very distant objects, that we become
sensible of an effort within the eye itself, or in the
parts connected with it, by which it is partially, if not
entirely, corrected; in other words, when we look at
very distant objects, the eye assumes a state which
would make near objects appear confused, and conversely. It is inferred, therefore, that the eye possesses within itself, or in its adjuncts, the capacity of
altering its focal length.

Leeuwenhoek, in the seventeenth century, had very
accurately described and delineated the fibrous structure observable in the crystalline lens of various animals: and Dr. Henry Pemberton, of Oxford—the friend
and commentator of Newton—at a subsequent period,

had conceived those fibres to be muscles, by whose action those changes in the form of the eye are produced which are required for the adequate explanation of the phenomena of near and distant vision. Young would appear to have been aware of Dr. Pemberton's hypothesis, though he had not studied his writings; and in dissecting the eye of an ox, when very recently slaughtered, he fancied that he had discovered, in the arrangement and attachment of those fibres, very satisfactory evidences of their muscularity. The Memoir in which his views were explained was read to the Royal Society on the 30th May, 1793, and was published in the Transactions for that year. It is written in very plain and lucid language, more like the style of a practised writer and anatomist than of a youth just entering upon his professional studies. The merit of this essay was considered to be sufficient to justify his election as a Fellow of the Society in the following year.[a]

Circumstances gave to this first acknowledged publication of our author a greater degree of importance than it altogether deserved.

[a] The following is his certificate, copied from the Records of the Royal Society :—

" Mr. Thomas Young, of Little Queen Street, Westminster, a gentleman conversant with various branches of literature and science, and author of a paper on Vision, published in the Philosophical Transactions, being desirous of becoming a Fellow of the Royal Society, we recommend him from our personal knowledge, as worthy of that honour, and likely to become a useful member of the Society.

" W. Combe.	Jas. E. Smith.
G. Baker.	Everard Home.
Adair Crawford.	Richard Brocklesby.
Stephen Weston.	F. Montague.
R. Farmer.	M. Baillie.
Chas. Towneley.	John Walker.
E. W. Gray.	W. Heberden, Jun.
George Shaw.	

" March 19, 1794.

" Balloted for and elected, June 19, 1794."

It had no sooner appeared, than the great anatomist and physiologist, John Hunter, claimed the discovery, as his own, and after notifying his claim, he addressed an application to Sir Joseph Banks to be allowed to give the Croonian Lecture at the Royal Society for the following year, expressly upon the muscularity of the crystalline lens. A very small portion only of this lecture was completed at the time of his death, which took place in the following autumn,[a] and the further prosecution of the investigation was resumed by his brother-in-law, Sir Everard Home, in the Croonian Lecture of the following year, in connexion with a series of apparently very accurate and well-designed experiments made by himself and Mr. Ramsden, the eminent optician. The result of these experiments seemed very decisively to negative the existence of those changes of the form of the eye, in passing from near to distant vision—and conversely—which the hypothesis in question was designed to explain, and it was consequently very generally abandoned. Young himself, in the first instance, yielded to the force of this evidence, and in more than one publication afterwards announced that he no longer ventured to maintain his opinion in the face of such distinguished authorities.[b]

---

[a] See a short notice by Sir Everard Home, entitled 'Some facts relative to the late Mr. Hunter's preparation for the Croonian Lecture,' where the fragment which he had prepared is given.—Philosophical Transactions for 1794, p. 21. On the day of Hunter's death the following lines appear among Young's notes on the medical lecture he was attending, showing his deep sense of the loss which the science of physiology and medicine had thereby sustained :—

"Hei mihi! Quantum
Præsidium Ausonia et quantum tu perdis, Iule."

[b] In his Göttingen Dissertation, to be noticed hereafter, published in 1796, he says :—"Sententia nuper de lentis crystallinæ usu in oculo ad

The reclamation by John Hunter of the proof of the correctness of this hypothesis, and the notice, by Sir Everard Home, of his proposed memoir on it—which was read to the Royal Society in the early part of the following year—gave rise to a rumour that Sir Charles Blagden—who was generally well acquainted with all that was passing in the philosophical world, and very much given to retailing it—had spoken of the subject in some detail, at a dinner party at the house of Sir Joshua Reynolds, on the 6th of November, 1791, where Dr. Lawrence, Dr. Walker King, Boswell, Dr. Brocklesby, and Young, were also present. The circulation of such a report and the plagiarism which it implied, was so injurious to Young's character, that he felt it necessary to address letters to all these persons, requesting them to say, whether the subject of vision and any recent researches connected with it, were mentioned on the occasion referred to. A very distinct denial was given by all the parties, as far as could be authorized by the vague recollections of a conversation reported to have taken place more than two years before, and Sir Charles Blagden—who would appear to have given currency to the report—assured Young that " he was by no means so clear as to be sure that he had told him Hunter's opinion." The imputation was distinctly withdrawn by him, and was speedily forgotten ; no one, in fact, who was acquainted with the scrupulous regard for truth for which Dr. Young was always distinguished, could ever have given a moment's credit to it.

diversas rerum videndarum distantias accommodando proposita, neque nova neque vera videtur." A similar acknowledgment is also made at the end of his Memoir in the Philosophical Transactions for 1801, read in November, 1800, entitled 'Outlines of Experiments and Inquiries respecting Sound and Light.'

We shall anticipate somewhat on the current of our narrative, to refer to Dr. Young's subsequent views on this controverted subject. We have before noticed his candid abandonment of his first opinion: he resumed it, however, afterwards, and embodied his reasons for doing so in a very able and elaborate memoir, "On the Mechanism of the Eye," which was read to the Royal Society on the 27th November, 1800, and published in their Transactions for the following year.

The experiments of Sir Everard Home and Mr. Ramsden had seemed to prove, that, in the adjustment of the eye to different distances, it is the curvature of the cornea and the length of its axis—and not of the crystalline lens—which is changed ; and further that the eye of a man which had been couched, or deprived of its crystalline lens, was perfectly susceptible of this adjustment, which therefore could not be dependent upon it. It was the assertion of this startling and apparently unanswerable fact, upon such high authority, which at first induced Dr. Young to revoke his original opinion; but it was a very serious objection to its adoption, that it would require an amount of change in the cornea, and an extension of the sclerotica, which there is no adequate anatomical provision to produce, or safely to apply. Dr. Young, by means of an improved form of Dr. Porterfield's optometer, an instrument admirably adapted to measure the focal length of the eye, and by numerous experiments, both on eyes which had and which had not, been couched, was enabled to negative any sufficient change in the curvature of the cornea in all cases, and further, decisively to show that couched eyes had no power of adjustment to near and distant objects. He thus altogether reversed the conclusions of his predecessors in this inquiry, and

resumed his own.[a] Sir John Herschel, who has carefully examined the arguments and evidence adduced
in support of these opposite results, (and there is no
judge more competent and dispassionate,) pronounces
in favour of the views of Dr. Young, which are also
supported by M. Arago, with his usual precision and
vehemence of argumentation. It would not be fair,
however, to keep out of view the serious anatomical
and other arguments which may still be urged against
this conclusion ; thus the chemists will object that the
fibres of the crystalline lens do not present, when subjected to the usual tests, the character of muscles : and
the physiologists, that the palpitations which usually
accompany muscular contractions, if those fibres were
muscles, would produce unsteadiness in the picture
upon the retina.

In the spring of 1794, when proceeding from Oxford, on a visit to his friends in the West of England,
he passed through Bath, where the Duke of Richmond
was drinking the waters, under the advice of Dr.
Brocklesby, by whom he was commissioned to make
inquiries of his local medical attendant respecting the
state of his patient's health. The Duke, who had
heard of his inquiries, requested to see him. The
following letter gives a very favourable impression of
Young's manners and conversation :—

                                    "Bath, May 5th, 1794.
" My Dear Doctor,

        " I need not write much about myself, as your nephew,
who dined with us yesterday, will give you a good account of

---

[a] It is proper to observe that Sir Everard Home, in a paper in the
Philosophical Transactions for the following year, adhered to his first
opinion : he says that Mr. Henry Englefield, a very skilful observer, repeated some of the experiments made by himself and Mr. Ramsden, and
arrived at the same conclusions.

my health. I have, however, still returns of headache and my legs continue very weak. But I must tell you how much pleased we all are with Mr. Young. I really never saw a young man more pleasing and engaging. He seems to have already acquired much knowledge in most branches, and to be studious of obtaining more: it comes out without affectation on all subjects he talks upon. He is very cheerful and easy without assuming anything; and even on the peculiarity of his dress and Quakerism he talked so reasonably, that one cannot wish him to alter himself in any one particular. In short, I end as I began, by assuring you that the Duchess and I are quite charmed with him, and shall be happy to renew our acquaintance with him when we return to London.

"I am, yours most sincerely,

"RICHMOND, &c.

"*Dr. Brocklesby.*"

After a short sojourn with his parents in Somersetshire, he made a six weeks' tour in Devonshire and Cornwall, with his friend and fellow student, Hudson Gurney. He has described at great length the principal incidents of this journey; and few things, which his previous studies enabled him to observe, would appear to have escaped his observation. The heaths of Cornwall are not rich in rare plants, but he collected such as were new to him. The richest mining district in Europe, however, afforded an ample harvest of minerals. He noted the characters of such rocks as appeared to him to be remarkable, but the science of geology, at that period, had not yet furnished the clue by which such observations could be usefully interpreted. His taste for the beauties of architecture, or natural scenery, had not been cultivated, and they are rarely or very coldly noticed; but his interest was strongly excited by remarkable machinery or processes in manufactures or mining operations, which he generally very fully described. He was much struck, even in those days, either of strict conservatism or revolutionary madness, by the anomaly presented in our system of parliamentary representation by a multitude of small boroughs in Cornwall, and the enervating effects which that system appeared to produce upon their industry and material prosperity.

It can hardly be expected that letters addressed to an aged relative of somewhat formal habits, should possess a very lively character, or afford many specimens which are likely to interest a general reader ; we shall confine our extracts, therefore, to one passage relating to St. Michael's Mount, in Cornwall, as somewhat characteristic of his promptitude and skill in Greek versification.

"In the morning we went to see St. Michael's Mount, on the summit of which Sir John St. Aubin has a castle ; we of course sat in the chair—

> ' Where the great vision of the guarded mount
> Looks towards Naumanco's and Bayona's coasts.'

It is commonly said that the man who sits in this chair shall always be master of his wife. I threw this into a distich, while there, in order to inscribe it on the lead covering the tower on which it stands.

> Ὅστις ἐς ὑψηλόν τόδ' ἕδος τηλέσκοπον ἧται,
> Κεῖνον ἀεὶ κρατέειν ἧς ἀλόχου λέγεται.

The mount is a fine object from all the neighbouring coast.

"We proceeded through Penzance to the Land's End. We ought to have taken the northern road, by Chapel Carn Brae, the highest hill in the neighbourhood, affording a wide view of both channels, but not knowing its situation, we missed it by going through Buryan, straight to Sennan, where we dined at The first public-house in the kingdom. Here also I made a distich to leave behind me,

> Ἐνθάδε τηλύγετος ἐλθὼν εἰς πείρατα γαίης
> Μνῆμ' ἐς ὁδοῦ μακρῆς, γράμμ' ἐχάραξα τόδε.

This I afterwards turned into Iambics,

Ἰόγγιὸς τις ὥδε, Γορνείου μέτα,
Πόρρωθεν ἐλθὼν γῆς ἔπ' ἔσχατον πέδον
Μνῆμ' εὐπορείας τους δ' ἔγραψε τοὺς στίχους."

He visited Salisbury, on his return, on the 13th June, the day on which he attained the age of twenty-one years. Though the day was far spent when he arrived, he proposed to ride over the plain to Stonehenge, but was prevented by a storm of rain : " I had no disposition," says he in writing to his uncle, " to be wet through and benighted for the pleasure of groping over this monument, except that I had a mind for a frolic to commemorate my twenty-first birth-day." On the following day he returned to London to settle down again to his studies with renewed ardour for the remainder of the summer.

Towards the latter end of August he paid visits, amongst other friends of his uncle's, to Dr. Herschel at Slough, Mr. Burke at Beaconfield, and to the Duke of Richmond at Goodwood : the Duke, who was then and had been for several years Master-General of the Ordnance, was confirmed, upon this second visit, in the favourable opinion he had before expressed of his manners and attainments, and offered him the appointment of his private secretary, which was at that time vacant. He was himself attached to philosophical pursuits and well acquainted with the construction and use of astronomical and surveying instruments, and the great Trigonometrical Survey, which came under his department, was greatly indebted for its successful prosecution to the support which he gave to it, both privately and officially. Young was highly gratified by an offer of so flattering a nature, and which presented so favourable an opening to the most distinguished

society as well as to the honours and emoluments of
public life.   Mr. Burke, who had formed a very high
estimate of his original powers and attainments, as well
as Mr. Wyndham, who were consulted on the subject,
advised him not to accept the appointment, and recommended him rather to proceed to Cambridge, and study
the law; but he finally determined to adhere to the profession which he had first chosen, to which the position
of his uncle appeared to offer so favourable an introduction.   He was also not yet fully prepared to abandon the Society in which he had been educated, which
the acceptance of such an office would have rendered
necessary.[a]   The offer was therefore gratefully declined,
with the expression of a willingness to accept the office
for a limited period, or until such time as might be
necessary to enable the Duke to find a person who was
likely to suit him.   This proposal, however, was declined in a letter remarkable for its good sense and
considerate kindness.

In the course of this summer, he prepared for the
Linnæan Society, a scientific description of a new species of Opercularia—a plant from Australia—which
was read on the 7th of October, and published in their
Transactions for 1797.   He was soon afterwards elected
Fellow of the Society.   The interest which at one period
of his life he had taken in the study of Natural History
would appear to have afterwards given way to other

---

[a] In a letter to his mother, which was written on this occasion, he says :—
"I have very lately refused the pressing offer of a situation which would
have been the most favourable and flattering introduction to political life
that a young man in my circumstances could desire.   I might have lived
at a duke's table, with a salary of 200l. a year, as his secretary, and with
hopes of a more lucrative appointment in a short time.   I should have
been in an agreeable family, have had time enough for study, a library, a
laboratory, and philosophical apparatus at my service; and I was not
ashamed to allege my regard for our Society as a principal reason for my
not accepting the proposal."

and more pressing studies, as this was the first and the last memoir relating to it which he contributed to the Transactions of the Linnæan or any other society.

The publication of the Calligraphia Græca was designed by his friend Mr. Hodgkin, chiefly as a vehicle for examples of the correct and elegant formation of the Greek characters, in accordance with the forms given in the most carefully written manuscripts, and also as exhibited in specimens of his own penmanship. He addressed a prefatory letter to the editor, in very neat Latin, stating the objects of the work, and giving very minute details of the formation of the letters, descending even to the cutting and holding of the pen. The first part of the work, which was finished in 1794, was inscribed by the editor to Dr. Young, in very grateful and affectionate terms : the second part, entitled Pœcilographia Græca, exhibiting the various alphabets and contractions which are found in the Greek manuscripts of different ages, was not published until a much later period, in consequence of the delays of the engraver. The examples were chiefly derived from Astle's Palæographia,[a] with various important additions contributed or suggested by Professor Porson and Dr. Charles Burney.

[a] There is a letter from Mr. Astle to Young, granting permission for the use of the materials in his book, which, he says, had been collected and copied by John Caravallo, a Greek, from the ancient manuscripts of Dr. Mead and Dr. Askew.

CHAPTER III.

MEDICAL EDUCATION : EDINBURGH.

It was now determined that he should attend the medical lectures at Edinburgh during the ensuing winter session, and proceed, in the following year, to Göttingen to complete his course of professional study, and take his degree. The regulations of the College of Physicians in London confined the privileges of their fellowships to graduates of Oxford and Cambridge exclusively, granting to those of other Universities the rank of Licentiates only, and that upon the condition of a two years' residence in the same University at which they subsequently took their degree. These regulations had been recently modified, and Young's friends in the College, or those who gave him information respecting them, would appear to have somewhat mistaken their purport. The consequence was that, after the lapse of two years spent in Edinburgh and Germany, he felt it expedient or necessary to proceed to Cambridge, where he took the degree of Bachelor of Physic, and afterwards of Doctor, after the regular forms. It was not therefore until a much later period of life than usual, that he was admitted to the full honours of his profession.

Before taking up his residence in Edinburgh, he made a short tour in some of the northern counties, particularly Derbyshire and Yorkshire, examining with his accustomed activity and intelligence, the collections of art or natural history, mines, mineral springs, manufactures or other curiosities, which came in his way. A fellow traveller, the Rev. Mr. Thorp,[a] Vicar of Buxton, who had ascertained his relationship to Dr. Brocklesby, showed him many civilities, and introduced him to Mr. Bakewell, of Dishley near Ashbourn, the precursor of those useful men who have devoted themselves to the improvement of the breeds of stock, and agriculture. They were received by him in the true style of an honest farmer's hospitality.

"I viewed with pleasure," says Young, "his improvements in the various branches of his occupation; I felt his rams and sheep regularly as they were shorn, and went through all the forms of examination. What he has done is shown best by two sheep which have always lived together, one of his own improved breed, the other of his original breed from which all his stock was derived by selected mixtures without crossing with any other breed. He entirely neglects the wool, but has diminished the bone and increased the fat in a surprising degree. Some bones are cleaned as specimens, and some pieces of meat were hung up, four inches thick in fat. Another grand object which he has effected is to bring a stream of water by a cut a mile in length, so as to water nearly every part of his farm; the trenches are kept in the neatest order; he has made a comparative experiment of river and spring water, which has been somewhat in favour of the latter. The water remains twelve or twenty-four hours in summer, in winter sometimes a week, and is then properly drained off. By this management he mows it four times in the season; not for hay, for though the land would produce two crops of hay, the climate would not permit them to make more than one; but he never suffers his cows to graze on the land, finding that they spoil it and waste the grass, and therefore feeds them in stalls with mown grass." After men-

---

[a] He had bred three sons to physic, one of whom, the father of the present Archdeacon of Bristol, was for many years a very eminent physician at Leeds.

tioning some other curious particulars, he adds, "The farm is not large, about 460 acres, but probably supports about twice as many animals as most others of the same extent: the expense must be considerable, but the income is said to be 5000*l.* a-year, and very possibly may be more; for it is said that he has let three rams only for the season for more than 1000*l.*; yet at one time from the liberal entertainment of numerous visitors, and perhaps from the chance attending all schemes, he was much reduced in circumstances, but now I hope he thrives."

At Derby, Young visited Dr. Darwin, of the first volume of whose Zoonomia we find a very elaborate critique in his journals. It is a singular and not very philosophical compound of metaphysics and physiology, and has passed with his other writings—notwithstanding the magnificent versification of his poetry—into an oblivion, which is not altogether deserved and in strange contrast with their former popularity. At the conclusion of his last visit to him he says,—

"I was highly gratified with the remainder of the day which I spent almost entirely with Darwin. He gave me my choice of looking over three cabinets, of cameos, of minerals, and of plants; the two last I viewed very superficially, but spent some time with him in admiring a collection of impressions bought in Italy: he says that he borrowed much of the imagery of his poetry from the graceful expression and vigorous conception which they breathe."

On parting he gave him a letter of introduction to a friend in Edinburgh, the terms of which he quotes, with very pardonable satisfaction, in a letter to his uncle:—"He unites the scholar with the philosopher, and the cultivation of modern arts with the simplicity of ancient manners."

At Durham, he met with Mr. Hugh Salvin, a fellow student at the medical school in London, who was proceeding, like himself, to pass the approaching winter at Edinburgh.

"He has studied," writes Young, "at Cambridge, and is well read in ancient and modern languages ; he joins his knowledge with much modesty and agreeable dispositions. We called on T. Burgess,[a] whom we expected to find at home in the College here ; but he was gone into the country—I, however, left my name, with Hodgkin's plate of my Greek Translation from King Lear. The Cathedral is a noble pile of Gothic building, but far too heavy to be comparable to York ; still it affords a grand object in many rich views, with the town, the adjacent woods, bridges and banks of the river Wear; which all together form as numerous and picturesque groups as any other city in the kingdom. They are now rebuilding many parts of the abbey. Most of the land in the neighbourhood is the property of the Dean and Chapter and of the Bishop : this is considered very inimical to improvement ; a year and a quarter's rent being paid every seven years as a fine, and the incumbents being mostly old men and not disposed to grant encouragement of which they will not reap the benefit."

He arrived at Edinburgh on the 20th October, and established himself in lodgings in St. James's Square. His reputation, which had preceded him, and the various letters of introduction with which he was furnished, opened to him the best society of the place. Amongst the students were many with whom he had been previously acquainted in London, when attending the medical lectures : Bostock, afterwards a physician in London, and a physiologist of some eminence, with whom he long maintained a very animated correspondence ; Bancroft, a man of considerable attainments, with whom he lived in habits of great intimacy : he was the son of the author (amongst other works) of a treatise, entitled Experimental Researches on the Philosophy

[a] Afterwards successively Bishop of St. David's and Salisbury, and a well-known Greek scholar: he was at that time a prebendary of Durham, and rector of Winston in the same county.

of Permanent Colours, which Young made the subject
of favourable critique in the Quarterly; Turner, who
was afterwards a distinguished physician at Liverpool;
Gibbes, of Bath, and many others.

"I have found," says he, " a much more select and desirable
party of fellow students here, than I have met with before ;
there are five or six Oxford and Cambridge men, with most of
whom I associate. I dined to-day (Nov. 4) with Voght, a
German from Hamburg, who attended Higgins's lectures last
winter : he has taken a house, and is to spend the winter here ;
Schmeisser is to join him shortly. They have been travelling
together through Great Britain and Ireland, and I have been
much entertained this afternoon with Voght's very intelligent
account of the state of Ireland, of the management of the poor
in Hamburg, and other interesting conversation. I cannot yet
pretend to judge from the few introductory lectures of the different courses that I attend ; but I am inclined to suspect that
they are well worth once attending. Gregory is a very agreeable and well-informed man ; he seems to have vigorous and
rapid thought."

The Edinburgh School of Medicine enjoyed, at that
time, a very high character. Gregory, who held the
first rank in it, was one of a family singularly distinguished in the history of the sciences, which has given,
during the last two centuries, nearly twenty professors
to our universities. He was a superior classical scholar,
and his well-known treatise, entitled Conspectus Me-
dicinæ Theoreticæ, is remarkable for the purity and
ease of its Latinity. His opinions on medical questions were entitled to consideration, as much from his
great practical experience, as from the arguments with
which they were supported. Dr. Duncan, the professor
of the Institutes of Medicine, is very favourably noticed by Young. Dr. Black, one of the most illustrious of the founders of the science, was Professor of
Chemistry ; and though he had at one time been

celebrated for his skill in addressing a class and conducting his experiments, he was now old and infirm, and, before the end of the session, his duties were discharged by a deputy—Dr. Rotherham. Monro, the son of the founder of the Anatomical School in the University—the author of a celebrated work on the bones and the nerves—was Professor of Anatomy, an office which he filled for forty years, at first conjointly with his father, but latterly with his son, who still survives him, though he has for some years retired from the University. He was generally considered as the greatest of the Monros, and the last of the great physicians who united, like the late Dr. Baillie, a profound knowledge of anatomy with that of medicine. He was engaged in many controversies on anatomical subjects, frequently involving claims to priority of discovery. The chemical lectures were given by Dr. Home. The names of other occasional lecturers are mentioned by Dr. Young, particularly that of John Bell, the eminent surgeon, whose demonstrations in anatomy appeared to him to be of first-rate excellence. In writing to his uncle, he says:—

"I believe North[a] and Baker are prejudiced against Edinburgh : with respect to the study of physic, it appears to me beyond comparison preferable to Oxford or Cambridge, and in other respects little inferior. For anatomy, I am very glad that I have done with it, for I should never learn it of Monro : I think him far inferior, as a lecturer, to Baillie. I expect much

[a] The Hon. Frederick North, afterwards Lord Guildford, a man of extremely popular manners, and a patron of scholars and men of learning. Sir George Baker, an eminent physician, had been a Fellow of King's College, Cambridge : in forwarding to him a copy, in his best penmanship, of his translation of King Lear's curse, he subscribed the following distich, expressive of his opinion of his scholarship :—

Βακίρῳ Ἑλλήνων σοφίης εὖ εἰδοτι πάσης
Ἰόγγιος ᾧ καλάμῳ γράμμ᾽ ἰχάραξε τόδι.

from Gregory's practice, and something from Black and the clinical lectures: these are given by Home, who has some merit, with something ridiculous in his manner."

On another occasion, much later in the session, he says :—

"I have not time for many scientific pursuits, besides the lectures which I closely attend. Some little information on chemistry I derive from Black's copious course—hardly anything from Monro—something considerable in the medical line from Gregory and Duncan."

It is probable that Dr. Young, though generally very candid in his judgments, was somewhat prejudiced against Monro, whom he accuses of a disposition to appropriate the discoveries of other authors as his own.

"When lecturing upon the eye, he noticed," says Young, "Hunter's having claimed the discovery of its being fibrous, and said that it had been known for a century, and that he had always taught the same : this was received with applause from his pupils, who always encourage his avarice of priority : in this case, though Monro deserves nothing, I was not displeased that Hunter's pretended originality was disallowed. He is not yet come to the crystalline of the eye. I called upon him last night to show him my paper, which he said he had lately been reading, and thought it ingeniously treated, but he said he should study it more particularly, and I left him my copy with a few additional notes for his perusal. I told him of Hosack's paper, and borrowed it for him; for I have nothing to fear from Hosack's objections, and if I had I should not wish my theory to overpower a better. Monro was very polite, and asked me for my direction ; I dare say he will think the better of me for having been in any manner opposed by Hunter."

He soon afterwards received Sir Everard Home's Croonian Lecture,[a] which he lost no time in studying. It appeared to him to put an end to any question respecting the action of the crystalline lens in accom-

[a] Supra, p. 40.

modating the eye to different distances. He communicated this change of opinion to Mr. Monro, and heard
no more of it until nearly the close of the session.

"He then spoke of my paper," says Young, "with as much
respect as it deserved, and took the pains to make some objections to it, which were partly worthy of attention, and partly
groundless : not making any use of the concession which I had
made to Home's opinion, but passing over in a very slight, and,
I think, a very uncandid manner, the experiments stated in the
Croonian lecture, insinuating, as is too common with him, that
he had himself made observations of a similar nature."

Young afterwards, as we have seen, resumed his
original views.

Though his studies, during his residence in Edinburgh, were chiefly professional, they were combined
with many others of a lighter and more general
nature. He read through the whole of Don Quixote,
with the aid of a grammar and dictionary, in the
original Spanish; and the numerous extracts from,
and references to, it, which appear in his journal, show
how much he was impressed with its exquisite and in-
comparable humour. This was followed by the Orlando
Furioso of Ariosto. In a letter to his uncle, he says :—

"I have lately been studying harder than usual, and I have
deferred writing to you, as well as many other engagements,
till I had read the 'Orlando Furioso.' This I have now accomplished, with no small satisfaction ; Ariosto had one of the
most exuberant, rich, and luscious imaginations of any of the
poets ancient or modern ; as for his moralities, if I thought that
our morals depended upon those of our favourite authors, I
should think him one of the most dangerous of writers ; but this
has been said before by Cervantes, who makes the Curate determine that as long as he retains the charms of his native
language it is impossible for the severest critic to have the
heart to condemn him."

He had already begun, also, the study of German, as a preparation for his future residence at Göttingen, and availed himself of his frequent intercourse with his friend Voght to acquire a knowledge of its pronunciation and conversational phrases. He had mastered it sufficiently, before he left Edinburgh, to speak it with some degree of fluency.

We shall proceed with further extracts from his letters and journal.[a]

"November 13th, 1794.

"Last night I was highly and unexpectedly gratified by meeting Lord Monboddo and Burgess of Oxford, at Dr. Gregory's : the Dr. sent for me as a Grecian to meet them. We spent the evening in talking of ancient authors, and their editions. I introduced the mention of Aristotle to Lord Monboddo as a favourite of his ; he was warm on the subject. I do not think him a man either of the deepest learning or the finest taste ; but as a singular character, and a well-known writer, I am pleased with being acquainted with him. We sat some time, before my name was mentioned to Burgess, without literary conversation ; but he said he had a presentiment that I was that nephew of Dr. Brocklesby, whose Greek writing Porson had shown him.

---

[a] Dr. Young continued his journals during his residences in Edinburgh and Göttingen, with very full accounts of his subsequent travels in Scotland and Germany. They are contained in two small volumes, written generally with great neatness, and in some cases, as in his extracts from Spanish, Italian, and other authors, with very unusual care: he wrote German with great nicety, in the scriptive German hand, which is usually much more embarrassing to students even than the barbarous Gothic characters in which their books are printed ; a practice which long operated, in some degree at least, to produce a marked separation between their literature and that of the rest of Europe, until the barriers were broken down by the overflow of the rich treasures which it contained. Amongst the earliest entries in these journals are several pieces of music which he copied as exercises for his flute, and which are equal in neatness and finish to the finest engraving. His hand was truly that of an artist, and his memory of the minutest peculiarities of form singularly tenacious : he was thus enabled to copy inscriptions in hieroglyphics and in the Demotic characters of Egypt, not only with great rapidity, but with an accuracy and truth which are altogether marvellous.

He has subscribed to Hodgkin's work,[a] and thinks it likely to succeed. If Hodgkin should call, pray tell him that he has long promised me a letter."

On a subsequent occasion, he says :—

" I meet with very few Grecians here : many well-informed men, but hardly any deep scholars ; however, they respect learning where they believe it to exist."

Dr. Gregory and Dalzel were among the exceptions to this observation. The last-mentioned was professor of Greek and a correct and elegant scholar, who fully appreciated Young's attainments and showed him the most flattering attentions during the whole time of his residence in the University. He was at that time engaged in the preparation of the second volume of his ΑΝΑΛΕΚΤΑ ῾ΕΛΛΗΝΙΚΑ, or Collections from the Greek Poets, from Homer downwards, with annotations, partly original and partly selected : an extremely useful publication which was for many years very extensively used in our classical schools, and which has hardly yet been superseded. The task of making the selections from the Greek epigrammatists was undertaken by Young, and he added many learned notes, with the suggestion of many judicious and some happy emendations. The assistance thus rendered was very gratefully and gracefully acknowledged.[b]

---

[a] Calligraphia Græca.   Supra, p. 46.

[b] Quæ autem hic exhibentur decerpta sunt ex Brunkii analectis a *Thomâ Young*, viro planè egregio et qui juvenis adhuc dignus habitus fuit, qui in Societatem Regiam Londinensem cooptaretur. Quum is nuper in hâc Academiâ Studiis operam daret, omnibus qui consuetudine ejus utebantur, propter ingenii acumen, et variam doctrinam, mihi imprimis ob vitæ integritatem et insignem Literarum Græcarum peritiam maximi habitus ; Ego variis laboribus Academicis implicitus otioque minus abundans, eum rogavi ut ex emensâ Brunkii collectione ea seligaret epigrammata, quæ ad propositum hujus poetici nostri Delectus maxime conferrent. Neque meo desiderio (quæ fuit ejus erga me voluntas) defecit juvenis eruditus,

The epigram, which is subjoined, originated in an occurrence which the journal, which records it, assures us was not unreal; and Dalzel, who printed it at the end of the notes on the selections which Young had made for him, pronounced it to be conceived in the true spirit of the Greek epigrammatists.

ΦΙΛΗΜΑ.

Χθὲς μελὶ μοὶ προφέρεσκε Καλήδονις ἡ χαρίεσσα,
  Τοῦ δὲ μελισσογενοῦς οὐδὲν ἔφην ἐθέλω.
'Αλλ' ἀπὸ σοῦ στόματος δὸς μοὶ μελὶ, κᾆτ' ἔφιλησα,
  Κῆν γλυκίον τὸ φιλῆμ' εἰκοσάκις μέλιτος.

Young made very few contributions to the Muses, though generally very prompt, especially in later life, to answer by trifles in verse the sudden calls which the importunities of female society make upon men of celebrity, whether they be poets or not. His ear was not attuned to the easy flow of good versification : the song which we subjoin is of very slight texture, and is given in his journal, with the music adapted to it.

"SONG.

" AIR.—' Were I obliged to beg my Bread.'

" Were I of fortune's ample stores
    And bounteous nature's gifts possessed,
  I'd ask the maid my heart adores,
    And care should leave my soul at rest :—
      In one dear gentle maid
      I'd think past pain o'erpaid.

" Or if, of lowly lineage born,
    Chill want forbad her worth to shine,
  For her the gay, the great I'd scorn,
    And fondly hope to make her mine :—
      In one kind gentle maid
      I'd deem all pain o'erpaid.

---

et in poetis Græcis apprimè versatus. Quæ hic recepimus, eorum pleraque ille humanissime indicavit, quin et propriâ manu nitidissime descripsit, mihique tradidit *Corollam* variis flosculis pulcherrimè a se contextam.

"But wealth, nor I can hope to share
　　Nor she to lose can ever dread,
　　And nought is left but blank despair,—
　　For hope and fear alike are fled.
　　　I'll seek thee, peaceful tomb!
　　　And hail thy silent gloom.

"Nor distant scenes, nor length of days
　　Shall cruel mem'ry's power destroy;
　　Nor beauty's charms, nor glory's blaze,
　　Shall rouse my heart to transient joy.
　　　I'll seek thee, peaceful tomb!
　　　And hail thy silent gloom."

He had resolved, before quitting London for Edinburgh, to give up some of the external characteristics of the Quakers, though, in corresponding with his family and members of the Society, he continued the usual form of addressing them. He feared the tears of his mother, to whom he was tenderly attached, and who clung—as is very commonly the case with females of her sect—to the outward marks of membership as possessing all the sanction of religion. It rarely happens, in fact, that the garb and phraseology of Quakers can long survive extensive intercourse with literary and refined society; but in passing the conventional boundaries which separate them from other sects, they sometimes abandon the peculiar religious doctrines in which they have been brought up, without adopting those of the Established Church, or of the sect with which they afterwards appear to communicate. Such changes, therefore, are apt to give rise to charges of hypocrisy when they are not fully carried out, or of infidelity and relaxation of morals when they are so, and which are unhappily not always without foundation. From the first of these charges Young did not altogether escape when he joined in the innocent pleasures of society; though he still retained his predilection for the other great and distinctive prin-

ciples of the Quakers ;—their steady humanity and love
of peace and order, and the general purity of their moral
conduct. Such principles continued to make them, in
his judgment—in spite of much that was absurd and
unreasonable—the most respectable of all sects and the
best suited for a man of truly dignified and philosophical turn of mind; but he speedily found that the
total change of habits and associations which followed
the abandonment of external communion with them,
leads almost inevitably to a total and permanent
separation from them. So necessary in fact, as all
experience shows, are forms and discipline to protect
the integrity of special religious and other communities
from the disturbing effects of the fashions and opinions
of the world.

This result would appear to have followed in Young's
case even more rapidly and to a greater extent than he
probably had ever ventured to anticipate. He mixed
largely in society, not merely amongst his fellow students, but amongst the professors of the University
and the principal inhabitants of a city and neighbourhood proverbial for hospitality. He began the
study of music and took lessons on the flute, and
thoroughly mastered the theory of the one, and to
some extent the practice of the other, though he was
not naturally gifted with a musical organization. He
took private lessons in dancing, and what constituted
a not less serious offence against the principles of his
sect, he repeatedly attended performances at the theatre.
In writing, soon after he left Edinburgh, to his friend
and fellow student Dr. Bostock, he says :—

"I have seen Mrs. Siddons in Douglas, The Grecian Daughter, The Mourning Bride, The Provoked Husband, The Fatal
Marriage, Macbeth, and Venice Preserved. She was neither

below, nor much above, my expectation. I can form an idea of
something more perfect. My friend Cruikshanks, when I went
to take my leave of him, took me aside ; and, after much preamble, told me he heard I had been at thê play, and hoped that
I should be able to contradict it. I told him I had been several
times, and thought it right to go, &c. &c., as civilly as I could.
I know you are determined to discourage my dancing and singing, and I am determined to pay no regard whatever to what
you say. You think I shall never be able to play the flute well,
and I am pretty sure that I may if I choose ; as to dancing, the
die is cast."

Young, as might very naturally be expected, was as
much exposed to the ridicule and witticisms of his new
friends, as he was to the suspicions and reproaches of his
old : but no relaxation of morals followed, such as was
imputed or anticipated ; the purity of his conduct, according to the uniform testimony of those who knew
him best, was unimpeachable. Though passionately
fond of female society, it was in a marriage of affection
that he looked for happiness, and not in those irregular
indulgences which are only very generally overlooked
because they are so common. Whatever he thought to
be right he resolutely practised.

"What greater instance," says he, in quoting the Spectator,
"can there be of a pusillanimous temper, than to pass his whole
life in opposition to his own sentiments, or not to dare to do
what he thinks he ought to do !"

His time, during the Edinburgh session, was so
much occupied, by the medical lectures, by the study
of German, Spanish and Italian, by the acquisition of
personal accomplishments, by the claims of a very
extended society and a very large correspondence with
his friends, as to leave little opening for the reading of
many works whether of professional or general literature. The only medical book of importance which we

find noticed in his journal is Cullen's First Lines of the Practice of Physic.

"A work," to use his own words, "of great merit and sound philosophy; if others improve on him, and in the same manner as he has done on his predecessors, the science of physic will arrive at a beautiful simplicity; it may be a very positive certainty."

Even at this advanced period of his studies, when he was already recognized as an authority in· Greek criticism, and entitled to some of the honours of a master in philosophy, we are occasionally startled by some of the consequences of the severe and isolated character of his previous education. Works of an elementary nature, or of light and general literature, which have formed stock books in the early training or amusements of other students, came under his notice from time to time, with all the charms·and surprise of novelty. The following are entries from his journals.

4th Jan., 1795.—"A friend unexpectedly sent me Johnson's Rasselas to read: I began this evening, and shall soon dispatch it."

Then follow numerous extracts of some striking passages, which no intelligent reader could fail to notice.

16th Feb., 1795.—"Began Guthrie's Geographical Grammar."

12th Ap., 1795.—"I finished Guthrie: a very improving book, tolerably well written, but not free from absurdities."

14th May, 1795.—"I began, and the next day finished, Johnson's Journey. It exhibits some strength of mental powers, but with a mixture of pedantry, bigotry, and prejudice. I have not extracted from it much information of what I may find in the Highlands, but the manners of the country are well depicted."

The Scotch had not then forgiven Johnson's habitual

disparagement of their country, and Young appears to
have caught some portion of their prepossessions : the
work which he has criticized so severely will long continue to be read and admired for many just observations
and occasional tenderness of feeling, in spite of the national prejudice which it too frequently exhibits.

The lectures for the winter session terminated at
the end of April "to the mutual satisfaction," says
Young, of "professors and pupils." They were resumed
for the summer session early in May. He was accustomed to look back, with great pleasure, to the winter
he passed in Edinburgh. He had profited considerably
from the lectures. For the first time in his life, he had
enjoyed free and liberal social intercourse, altogether
unfettered by the formalities of Quakerism ; he recipro-
cated visits, and in many cases formed friendships, with
the most distinguished men in the Athens of the North,
which at that time had reached the culminating point
of its literary glory.

He now prepared for his journey to the Highlands
and other parts of the north of Scotland, examining
maps and making notes of such objects of natural or
antiquarian interest as the ordinary guide-books and
Grose's Antiquities would readily supply.

He started on his journey on the 5th of June, proceeding by Hopetown House, through Falkirk, to the
iron-works at Carron.

"My thoughts," says he, "were frequently turned back on
Edinburgh, and I believed that I could very cheerfully bear to
be compelled by the laws of the College in London to spend
another winter there ; but pleasure is not always the most
favourable to improvement. I was, as Renouard [a] observed on

[a] He had resided for some time at Edinburgh with his pupil Mr. Cust,
afterwards Earl Brownlow : he was a man of considerable learning, and
had been a contemporary of Porson at Eton and Cambridge, who often

meeting me, *in me totus teres atque rotundus*, and it may be worth while to describe my equipment. I was mounted on a stout, well-made black horse, fourteen hands high, young and spirited, which I had purchased from my friend Cathcart : I had before me my oiled linens, the spencer with a separate camlet cover ; under me a pair of saddle-bags, well filled with three or four changes of linen, a waistcoat and breeches, materials for writing and for drawing, paper, pens, ink, pencils, and colours ; packing-paper and twine for minerals ; soap, brushes, and a razor ; a small edition of Thomson's Seasons, a third flute in a bag, some music, principally Scotch, bound with some blank music paper, wafers ; a box for botanizing ; a thermometer ; two little bottles with spirits for preserving insects ; a bag for picking up stones ; two maps of Scotland—Ainsley's small one, and Sayer's ; letters of recommendation. The bags had pockets at the end, one containing a pair of shoes, the other boards with straps and paper for drying plants. I found my bags at first an incumbrance, but became afterwards more reconciled to them. They are to a saddle what pockets are to a coat, and who objects to wearing pockets? but they were wetted the first day, and stained their contents ; this will make me more careful in future."

He carried with him an ample packet of recommendations to the most distinguished houses he was likely to visit on his tour.

" I have already," says he, soon after beginning his journey, " more than forty introductory letters, and I am obliged to take more and more as I deliver them ; and as I have many acquaintances at Edinburgh who are interested in my journey, I think it necessary to keep a pretty full account of what I see, that I may amuse them with some part of it when I call there on my return."

His kind friend Professor Dalzel, in recommending him to his brother Professor, Hunter of St. Andrews, and speaking in the most flattering terms of his attain-

---

amused himself with laying traps for his almost irresistible passion for classical quotations. He was for many years Vice-Master of Trinity College, and much respected for his kind and generous disposition.

ments, proceeds to say :—" The possession of such
talents and accomplishments has not in the least
affected his manners, which are simple, unassuming and
most agreeable, and he is much esteemed by his literary
friends here." Some of his letters, to his great amusement, described him as a " Quaker of fortune and
character "—" A gentleman of fortune and a man of
letters." With such introductions in a country whose
warm and liberal hospitality had not yet been cooled
down by the crowds let loose upon it by steam-boats
and railways, it is not surprising that he should have
been almost everywhere cordially welcomed.

After admiring the works at Carron, even in those
days presenting a very striking scene of energetic
labour, he passed by Stirling and Kinross, with Loch-
Leven and its castle—the scene of Queen Mary's cap-
tivity—to Falkland, the ancient residence of the
Scottish kings, and thence to St. Andrews.

" Professor Hunter showed me the library," says Young, " a
large and elegant room, which reminded me of what I had seen
at Oxford and Cambridge. It is supported by small contributions from the students in addition to its privilege of claiming
a copy of every book which is entered at Stationers' Hall. The
students were formerly divided into three classes, primarii,
secondarii, and ternarii, something like noblemen and fellow-
commoners, pensioners, and servitors or sizars in the English
Universities ; the first of these classes is now abolished, the
sons of gentlemen commonly enter as seconders, and those of
farmers as terniers ; the seconders pay a fee of three guineas
to the lecturer, the terniers but half that sum ; their whole
board at the table furnished by the economist, costs them 10*l.*
a session ; the hire of a room in the college and of furniture
from the town, with coals and candles, will cost about 3*l.* more.
When Johnson wrote, the board was only 8*l.* The students
wear a scarlet gown, as at Glasgow and Aberdeen ; there are
apartments for about 27 in the United College ; the students
at the Philosophy College are generally from 70 to 140 ; at

the Divinity College from 30 to 40, who have passed at least three at the other, and must pass four years here before they can be taken on trial by a presbytery."

From St. Andrews he proceeded, by way of Dundee and Perth, to visit the noble domains of Scone, Taymouth and Dunkeld, with the pass of Killiecrankie, and the varied scenery of the Tay, the Tummell, the Garvie and the Bruar. At Blair he was introduced to Mr. MacLaggan, the minister of the parish, a man of considerable intelligence.

" He has made," says he, " the Gaelic, which is his native tongue, his particular study : he tells me that it much resembles the Irish and Welsh, except in pronunciation ; but that a friend of his, who has attended more to the Welsh, conjectures that this language was mixed with that of a colony from the north of Italy, which he supposes to have settled in Wales at a very early period."

He gave him much information also respecting the origin and growth of turf ; the vast primæval forests of Scotland, the remains of which are found in such abundance in removing the turf ; the remains of extinct animals which it contains—which were then rarely noticed—as well as respecting the Druidical or other monuments of the ancient religion of the country, which are observable in many places of the neighbourhood. A visit to the Falls of the Bruar, near Blair, seems to have steeled his heart against the inspection of similar objects in future :—

" He had enough," says he, like many other overtaxed travellers, " of paltry cascades. From Blair to Braemer, through Glen Tilt, a long and weary ride of extremely rugged and difficult country, my horse was obliged to creep up or to slide down steep hills, to push his way through rocks, or to step delicately over boggy ground : for once in my life, I had the pleasure of being in a bog, so that my feet touched the ground ; but we soon got out. In this glen, a village of moderate size once existed; the Duke of Athol, who is said to retain more of a highland chieftain than any other laird, whether from a wish to have the country vacant for his red deer (of which we saw many herds, which obliged the peasants to keep a constant watch over their corn), or to punish them for not entering the army as he wished, drove them all from their habitations to seek a milder master."

Hardships, such as these, which a traveller on horseback must have been daily prepared to encounter, were more than compensated by the hospitable reception which generally awaited him at the conclusion of the day.

"I have thought," says he, " that travelling through an unknown country presents not unfrequently circumstances not unlike the stories of knight-errantry; not indeed seen in so glaring colours, but making a similar impression on the mind and raising similar emotions. To lose one's way in a dark night, to have to pass through rocks and bogs, to ford deep waters, to cross steep mountains, to stand long in waiting for an asylum at a late hour in a miserable hut; to be prepared for deranged accoutrements, a lame horse, his shoes loose, his back galled, his spirits flagging; and again after a short time to be welcomed with as much hospitality, and entertained with as much splendour, as any lord of a castle could receive a knight-errant: to be at ease from every care and in the enjoyment of every amusement that men of sense and women of elegance can afford : all these vicissitudes exercise the same qualities, require the same virtues, and excite the same emotions as the obsolete chivalrous tales of fabulous ages."

At Brechin he found one of the few round towers which are to be seen in Scotland. It closely resembles the round towers of Ireland, and, as is generally the case with them, it is near the church. It is of considerable height, and the layers of stones of which it is built are spirally disposed. At Findhaven he examined one of those vitrified forts, which have so much embarrassed antiquaries.

" It is situated on a hill, called the Castle Hill, and is chiefly composed of siliceous grit, which is not everywhere firmly consolidated by vitrification. The kind of stone seems to prove that it was not burnt for strength, because they would probably have chosen the more vitrifiable whinstone, which I believe may be had here ; and I do not think the walls seem much stronger for semi-vitrification."

After examining the ruins of the monastery at Arbroath, the most considerable in Scotland, he proceeded by Montrose, Lawrence Kirk, and Stonehaven, to Aberdeen, visiting Ury with no small degree of interest as the residence of the representatives of Barclay, the Apologist of the Quakers, the grandfather of his friend, Mr. David Barclay, of Youngsbury.

" At Aberdeen," says he, " I stayed three whole days, and I thought my time not ill employed ; the town is very flourishing, some of the professors are capable of raising an university to celebrity, especially Copeland and Ogilvie ; but the division and proximity of the two Universities (King's College and Marischal College) are not favourable to the advancement of learning ; besides the lectures are all, or mostly, given at the same hour, and the same Professor continues to instruct a class for four years in the different branches. Were the Colleges united and the internal regulations of the system new modelled, the cheapness of the place, the number of small bursaries for poor or distinguished students, and the merit of the instructors, might make this university a very respectable seminary in some branches of science ; the fee to a professor for a five months' session is only 1½ guineas. I was delighted with the inspection of the rich store of mathematical and philosophical apparatus belonging to Professor Copeland of Marischal College, made in his own house and partly with his own hands, finished with no less care than elegance, and tending to illustrate every branch of physics in the course of his lectures, which must be equally entertaining and instructive. I fell in again here with Gillies of Brechin, and dined with him and a party of lairds to whom he introduced me. I remained occu-

pied in my own defence and in studying the various appearances of human nature until three o'clock in the morning."

It is hardly necessary to add that Young was
habitually temperate; a virtue not sufficiently appreciated in those days, either in Scotland or elsewhere.

We shall not attempt to follow his course through
Peterhead, Banff to Elgin, and thence by Fort George,
Cromarty, Skibo and Wick to John o' Groat's house;
and back again through Thurso, Skibo, Dingwall,
Beauly, Inverness, Calder, Forres, to Elgin again.
During his first visit at this latter place, he went to
Gordon Castle, but the Duke and Duchess were from
home. Upon his return he was more fortunate, and
the extracts from his journal which follow, present an
interesting picture of a family distinguished, not merely
as occupying the highest rank in society, but for the
good sense, frankness and cordiality of manners, personal beauty and accomplishments of its members. He
had been specially recommended to them by Lady
Caroline Lennox, the mother of the present Duke of
Richmond and the eldest daughter of the House.

"In the morning, without stopping at Elgin, I rode to
Fochabers, and was in time for dinner at Gordon Castle. The
Duke, the Duchess, Lady Madeline (Sinclair) and her son,
Lady Louisa,[a] Lady Georgiana,[b] Lord Alexander, and Mr.
Hay, his tutor, compose the family there at present. They
had a large party to day. When a moderate time had been
spent over the bottle, we found the ladies dancing. They
were dancing reels when we came in; after one or two had
been gone through I found myself standing up with Lady
Madeline, and the Duke with Miss Gordon; the Duchess
afterwards danced, and Lady Georgiana danced some high
dances with great elegance. Most of the party stayed over

[a] Afterwards Marchioness of Cornwallis.
[b] Afterwards Duchess of Bedford.

night, which seems to be the custom in this country. In the morning I went down to the inn at Fochabers to look after my horse and luggage. In returning I met the Duke; he showed me the site of the old town of Fochabers, much nearer to the house than the present, which he has built within a few years. After breakfast the Duke showed me his lathes, and a variety of objects which he has turned; the apparatus is most splendid, made at Aberdeen under Copeland's directions, and the Duke is an expert workman. I went to the library and had begun a letter to my uncle, when his Grace came in to ask me to go with him and see a stag shot: the groom was sent with four or five couple of fox-hounds to draw the woods, while the Duke was stationed at a proper place to intercept the deer, and two servants at different places to watch if they took another course. We waited here an hour or two in vain, and the Duke blew his bugle-horn to call off the huntsmen to another cover. Here we had better fortune; we soon heard the dogs in full cry and a fine buck made his appearance; he stood still at some distance; the Duke fired with his rifle, and heard the bullet strike him; the animal moved and then stood gazing; he shot again and missed; the stag did not move at first, but the dogs coming up drove him off. The German servant then fired and missed him, but, seeing blood from the Duke's shot, he let loose a bloodhound. When they are wounded, the bloodhound commonly overtakes them and kills them, but to-day all the dogs, after a long pursuit, returned without their game. We spent much time in endeavours to recover it by trailing the slopes, but in vain. We returned about four. Col. Duff and Col. Hay from Banff were at the Castle. We joined the ladies early. I brought down my notes as far as I had written them, for their amusement, and they took the trouble of looking at several parts of them. I read them some of my extracts in verse, and I thought the better of my selection when I found that Lady Louisa had some of them by heart as well as many other poems of various descriptions, of which she repeated enough to show a fine taste and an excellent memory. I had not yet seen the beauties of Gordon Castle. I met the ladies before breakfast to take a walk along the Holly-bank: there are the finest trees of the kind I have ever seen.

" The Duchess, looking over my memorandums, entertained

me with an account of a romantic tour she had made with her sister, through many of the finest parts of Scotland; of the manner in which she spent her time in solitude, and her studies during the infancy of her children : she took me into her library and presented me, for my amusement on the road, with a copy of Petrarch, on which I shall always set a high value.

"It was Lady Georgiana's birthday, the flag was hoisted, Lord Alexander's regiment of little boys was paraded, and employed in racing and dancing on the green; and in the evening a ball was given to the servants ; all the family went down stairs, and amused themselves with observing the agility of the lads and lasses. Every person employed about the house, except one man, is married, and most of them are descended from those who have served the family before them. The Duchess proposed, in honour of the day, that Sir George Abercrombie and I should dance a reel with the two younger ladies; for they danced nothing but reels : afterwards the Duke danced with one of the upper servants; some time after our party joined again in the amusement at the same time with two others; when it was late and Sir George was tired, we took a girl in his place and resumed the sport ; Lady Madeline sat by and made the music play till the other sets quitted the field, and left us victorious to reel through the whole room. I have now written as much of dancing in my Tour as Johnson has in his; and as much more as a young man may be expected to write of it than an old one.

"The next day was not the first that I had fixed for setting off, the time allotted for my whole journey was already more than elapsed ; I had for a long time heard nothing from my uncle, and I had many reasons for hastening. I could almost have wished to break or dislocate a limb by chance, that I might be detained against my will ; I do not recollect that I have ever passed my time more agreeably, or with a party whom I thought more congenial to my own dispositions : and what would hardly be credited by many grave reasoners on life and manners, that a person who had spent the whole of his earlier years a recluse from the gay world, and a total stranger to all that was passing in the higher ranks of society, should feel himself more at home and more at ease in the most magnificent palace in the country, than in the humblest dwelling with those whose birth was most similar to his own. Without enlarging on the Duke's good sense and sincerity, the Duchess's spirit and powers of conversation, Lady Madeline's liveliness and affability, Louisa's beauty and sweetness, Georgiana's naïveté and quickness of parts, young Sandy's good-nature, I may say that I was truly sorry to part with every one of them."

Quitting these scenes of enchantment, our traveller returned to Inverness, and proceeded by Fort Augustus under the foot of Ben Nevis to Fort William and Ballachulish, through the picturesque valley now so well known as that of the Caledonian Canal : after visiting (from the latter place) the valley of Glencoe, he proceeded to Oban : a six-hours' sail took him to Aros in Mull, whence he crossed the island to Torloish, the seat of Mr. M'Lean, where he found a numerous party, and all the luxuries of refined society.

"The next day I procured a boat which took me to Staffa ; I climbed up to the furthermost part of the cave, and was delighted with the grandeur and beauty of the scene ; the regularity of the columns forming the walls, the waves dashing below, and the island of Iona, with its venerable ruin, terminating the view at a distance, forming a most striking combination which I faintly attempted to sketch ; the whole island is composed of basaltes ; the pillars are mostly irregular hexagons of different sizes, some straight, some curved, some erect, some inclined, some horizontal ; the vertical ones forming a kind of stratum which stands on the bed of amorphous basaltes and is covered by another which forms (where the pillars have been washed away) the roof of the cave."

He speaks highly of the accuracy of Pennant's plates and descriptions, in his Tour in Scotland, but the island itself, its cave and other wonders, were little known and very rarely visited before Sir Joseph Banks described them. The taste of the public had not yet been formed for the search and admiration of beautiful scenery.

We next find him lodged at Inverary Castle, the
magnificent residence of the Duke of Argyle, to whom
he had been introduced by the Duchess of Gordon.

"The Duke is about 73; his two daughters, Lady Augusta
Clavering and Lady Charlotte Campbell,[a] and Lord John with
his tutor, were with him, as well as some other visitors. I was
surprised to find my old acquaintance, Mr. Crawford Campbell
of Ashnish, with him, and also Dr. Longlands, his domestic
physician : after breakfast the party were to ride, and the doctor
gravely submitted to my determination whether I would go at
a slow pace with him and the Duke, to view the country
leisurely on the way, or ride with the ladies, and be galloped
over. I told him that of all things I liked to be galloped
over, and therefore should be of the youthful party : accordingly Ashnish and myself attended the two ladies. We first
rode down by the side of the loch : Lady C. showed me one of
the barns, which are singularly spacious, with frames for drying
corn of a peculiar construction ; my horse approached nearer
to the ground than he had ever done before ; it may be guessed
what made his rider careless. After dinner the Duke rode
again, and the younger men of the party took a walk ; I left
them about nine, and joined the ladies at tea. I was showing
Lady C. some of my sketches ; she begged to see my notes,
and I showed the greatest part of them. All the family are
musical ; the ladies sing admirably ; cards and the fine piano
occupied the evening. After supper, besides other songs, I heard
a most beautiful canzonet by Jackson, beginning ' Love in
thine Eyes.' It was twelve o'clock when we retired. After
breakfast I took my leave ; not without regretting that I had
so little time to observe the beauties of Inverary. Lady Charlotte is handsomer than Lady Augusta, she sings better, but
she has less good sense, and less sweetness ; an innocent
giddiness sometimes gives her the appearance of a little affectation : she is to Lady Augusta what Venus is to Minerva ; I
suppose she wishes for no more. Both are goddesses."

He arrived in Edinburgh by way of Dumbarton,
Glasgow, Hamilton, and Lanark, on the 6th August,

[a] Afterwards Lady Charlotte Bury.

but remained there no longer than was necessary to see
his more intimate friends in the city and neighbourhood,
and to arrange his affairs preparatory to his final departure. He then proceeded southwards, through Selkirk,
Hawick, Langholme and Longtown to Carlisle, from
whence he diverged for the purpose of seeing the principal English lakes. Though extremely minute in the
record of all that he saw and did, we find few passages
which enable us to judge of the impressions which
beautiful scenery produced upon him : but it is sufficiently manifest that the phases of life and society,
collections of natural history and philosophical instruments, and works of art, such as his previous studies
enabled him to appreciate, attracted much the greatest
share of his attention.

His tour of the lakes ended at Kendal, where he found
Mr. John Gough, a man of very remarkable attainments,
though he had been blind from his infancy ; he was at
once a mathematician, a naturalist, and a scholar :

" I knew," says Young, " his sisters in London ; they supply,
with some other assistance, his want of sight ; and the accuracy
of his sense of touch, together with the inventive powers of his
mind, have rendered him so much a master of what he pursues,
that he would rather be supposed to have a supernumerary
sense than to want one."

He afterwards controverted, with considerable acuteness and ability, some of Young's speculations on the
propagation of sound.

He made a short visit to his friend Bostock at
Liverpool, and was introduced to the most distinguished
people there. Its docks were then objects of admiration, though insignificant compared with what they
are now, when adapted to the wants of the greatest
commercial emporium in the world.

" We visited also," says Young, " the Asylum for the Blind, erected in imitation of that at Paris, before any other in England ; they are taught to spin, to make mats, baskets, and various other articles, and some of them play upon the harpsichord ; one poor boy had acquired considerable execution ; it is a most interesting and useful institution.—We dined with Mr. Roscoe ; the company consisted of Mr. Yates, Bostock, Arthur Aikin, Dr. Shepherd,[a] Dr. Garnett, late of Harrowgate, and myself. Roscoe is a friend of Fuseli, and has several of his paintings ; his song on the French Revolution is well known ;[b] he is now moderate in his political sentiments ; he is about to publish the Life of Lorenzo de Medici."

From Liverpool he proceeded across the Mersey to Chester, on his way to North Wales ; he left Manchester behind him, with some regret, not merely as a great dépôt of manufactures and machinery but also as the only considerable town in the United Kingdom which he had not visited or did not propose to visit. The journal of his Welsh tour, which was very short, offers nothing which is worth extracting. He returned by way of Shrewsbury, to the Coalbrook Dale, on a visit to the magnificent iron-works established there.

" This valley runs north of the Severn between steep hills, and with its houses, woods, and iron-works, makes both by day and night a remarkable scene. Mr. R. Reynolds, at whose house I was most hospitably received, took me to the top of a neighbouring hill, from whence we had a good view of the Severn, and the Iron Bridge, the first ever erected, of a light and elegant structure, though said to be much heavier than was necessary. My chamber at night presented an appearance

---

[a] He was afterwards called Poggio Shepherd ; in consequence of having written the Life of Poggio Bracciolini : he was a man of very lively conversational powers, and somewhat allied, both in his opinions and studies, with Mr. Roscoe.

[b] " O'er the vine-covered hills and gay regions of France
       See the bright star of Liberty rise," &c.

It was written to celebrate the anniversary of the 14th August, and attacked Mr. Burke with great severity.

similar to what I observed at Carron, but greater and more picturesque. The next day, my friend, Mr. Nehemiah Lloyd, walked with me to Ketley, and we viewed the various processes going on there; the forges, the puddling, the engines, the inclined planes for raising boats instead of locks, part of an iron aqueduct which they are constructing, and various other operations and experiments on a magnificent scale. If the grand system of these iron-masters requires any improvement, it may perhaps be made by attending a little more to neatness and elegance, but the useful and convenient must be allowed to outweigh. Mr. W. Reynolds, in the afternoon, showed us his laboratory, his library, and his minerals, and told me that before the war he had agreed with a man to make a flute one hundred and fifty feet long, and two and a half in diameter, to be blown by a steam-engine and played on by barrels, and that he is determined at a future time to prosecute experiments of this nature.''

It is interesting to discover in these observations the early recognition of the importance of combining higher views of art with our manufactures, which unhappily continue to be too much neglected.

He accompanied Mr. Lloyd to Birmingham, where he sold his horse, and proceeded by coach to London ; passing one day at Beaconsfield with Mr. Burke, where he found a French emigrant nobleman, the Duke de Coigny; he reached London on the 4th September, and found a large party at the house of his uncle, who was anxiously expecting his return. After passing one week at Worthing, he went with the same kind relative on his annual visit to Goodwood, where he met the Duke and Duchess of Devonshire, Lady E. Foster, Mr. Grenville, and Mr. Spencer, besides the members of the family : they returned to London on the 23rd. The next fortnight was spent in preparations for his Continental tour.

CHAPTER IV.

MEDICAL EDUCATION: GÖTTINGEN.

" I LEFT London," says Young, " on the afternoon of the 7th of October, 1795, and arrived at Norwich the next morning. Gurney soon met me, and we spent the greater part of the day at Keswick, in a circle, part of which was gay and part grave. At the time when I first became acquainted with these families, I came very decidedly under the latter designation, and then little imagined that I should live to play a minuet on the flute, while the young —— were dancing it ; but stranger things than this happen every day. I walked over to Earlham[a] and back again with Gurney, and we returned there at night ; the next day we set off with Joseph Gurney to Yarmouth, and we had time enough to stroll and see the place, which exhibits nothing that is remarkable ; on the next morning I embarked in the packet for Hamburg, quitting for the first time my native land, expecting to be more than two years from it, and hoping to see Germany, Italy, Switzerland, and France, and to return by a shorter passage than the present deplorable war would permit me."

After six days, and not more than the usual sufferings of a first voyage, he reached Hamburg, where he was most cordially welcomed by his friends and fellow-students, Voght and Schmeisser, who were natives of the place, and connected with some of its opulent fami-

---

[a] The residence of the junior branch of the Gurney family, so justly distinguished for the public and private virtues of its members. Of those who are no more, it may be sufficient to mention the names of Mrs. Fry, Mrs. Samuel Hoare of Hampstead, and John Joseph Gurney : of the living it would be unbecoming to speak.

lies.   It was under their auspices that he formed his first acquaintance with German society; the impression was decidedly favourable.

On the 21st he took the boat to Harburg, to join the Stuhlwagen to Hanover :

" It is a waggon with a leather covering, the back part like a coach, holding six, with curtains instead of glasses, and without doors ; the front seat holds three, with a curtain also to keep out the rain. I did not much dislike the conveyance, as the motion suited me better than that of a coach ; but to be two nights and part of two days travelling less than ninety English miles would make any carriage disgusting. The country consists entirely of sand, and, being almost entirely without water, is incapable of any great improvement ; the accommodations on the road are uniformly wretched, but you get good coffee, and you are not in need of much more.—At length, about noon on the 23rd I arrived at Hanover. I went immediately upon my arrival with a letter from Mr. Burke to Mr. Brandes, the Secretary of the Regency ; he was not then at home, but I saw enough of him afterwards to make me rejoice in his acquaintance, both for the various information I gained from him, and the civility he showed me."

Mr. Burke described Mr. Brandes as one of the best-informed men in Germany, and particularly well acquainted with the complicated system of the various governments of the empire. From Hanover he proceeded to Göttingen, which he reached on the 27th of October.

After delivering his letters of introduction to some of the principal professors from Mr. Brandes, Professor Dalzel, Dr. Vincent, and others, he established himself, for the six months' session, in a house belonging to Professor Arnemann, adjoining that in which he himself resided.   On the 29th of October he matriculated, and, on the 3rd of November, entered upon his academical studies and occupations. The labours of the day were distributed as follows :—

" At 8, I attend Spittler's course on the History of the Principal States of Europe, exclusive of Germany.

" At 9, Arnemann on Materia Medica.

" At 10, Richter on Acute Diseases.

" At 11, Twice a week, private lessons from Blessman, the academical dancing-master.

" At 12, I dine at Ruhlander's table d'hôte.

" At 1, Twice a week, lessons on the Clavichord from Forkel ; and twice a week at home, from Fiorillo on Drawing.

" At 2, Lichtenberg on Physics.

" At 3, I ride in the academical manège, under the instructions of Ayrer, four times a week.

" At 4, Stromeyer on Diseases.

" At 5, Blumenbach on Natural History.

" At 6, Twice Blessman with other pupils, and twice Forkel.

" Spittler, Arnemann, and Blumenbach follow, in lecturing, their own compendiums, and Lichtenberg makes use of Erxleben's. I mean to study regularly beforehand."

For some time he was unable to seize the full import of the lectures from want of familiarity with the German language; but this difficulty was speedily conquered by confining himself strictly to the use of it in society, even when conversing with his fellow-countrymen—not more than four or five in number—who were students at the University.

The following letter describes his academical and other occupations :—

" DEAR BOSTOCK,   "Göttingen, 14th December, 1795.

" THEY say that to begin a letter is more difficult than to write all the rest of it ; I will therefore omit that form and proceed to the more essential parts. Tayleur sends you his very best compliments. I do not see him very frequently, except at the lectures, for we are both of us a little recluse, and his real or imagined indispositions frequently confine him still more ; besides we have now entered into an engagement not to speak English in each other's company, which has already been expensive to me ; for we were four Englishmen, not reckoning

Dr. Ash, whom no creature sees; Colhoun, the son of a Norfolk squire, had been here nearly a year, Tayleur and Kinglake about four months, and myself more than one, so that we could all contrive to be understood in German, and solemnly executed an obligation to speak no English in each other's hearing on pain of forfeiting twopence every half hour, when all of a sudden two Scotchmen came in upon us, and one of them speaking not a syllable but English, and obliging me and Colhoun out of civility to incur frequent penalties; the other two, who are more solitary beings, have escaped. We are not riotous nor absurd, as Englishmen in foreign countries generally are said to be, but it will require some influence to restrain young H——'s propensity to drinking. You will be pleased, as a lover of the fine arts, to hear that I am taking lessons in drawing; you will not be surprised that I receive in this study, as well as in music and dancing, full approbation from my masters, for application and accuracy, at the same time they honestly tell me that ease is wanting; and you will also readily believe that I have the assurance not to be discouraged with this character while they all assert that I may confidently expect sufficient advancement in due time. I will not enter much into particulars, because no person is a competent judge in his own case; but I draw only figures, and, with the assistance of my master's touches, they do not look amiss. I am learning the Klavier or Clavichord. I have four lessons a week for this instrument, and two for the flute. There are much better musicians here than might be expected from the size of the place; many of the students play very well, and generally exhibit their talents at the concerts. We have every Saturday a public concert to which the ladies are admitted gratis, and the students make a tea-party with a private concert on the Wednesdays. I have not yet exhibited myself at a public dance, my master, who is a very sensible fellow, advising me against it, as he observed that a person seldom loses the character which he obtains from the first impressions; but we have agreed that I may venture at the next pique-nique. I have sent Gurney an account of the public amusements here; I wish you could see it to save me the trouble of repeating it, for we have very few private parties, but Sunday is the time appropriated for all sorts of company; in the morning the professors are at leisure to receive the visits of the students, and in the afternoon we have sometimes a public assembly at the house of a professor, where the professors' wives and daughters and a few other families who reside here, generally with a majority of students, meet to play at cards and to talk, and on the alternate Sunday a dance; either a tea-dance or a supper-dance, one from four to eight, the other from five to one: this is called a pique-nique, and in its constitution resembles a Scotch oyster-dance. The professors seldom invite the students to dine or sup with them; indeed they could not well afford, out of a fee of a louis or two, to give large entertainments; but the absence of the hospitality which prevails rather more in Britain is compensated by the light in which the students are regarded; they are not the less, but perhaps the more, respected for being students, and indeed they behave in general like gentlemen, much more so than in some other German universities. There are some of the abundant German nobility among them, who in appearance are less distinguished than in England, but in family pride and connexions much more, although rank here does not confer what in England we call precedency. I have not yet formed any very intimate acquaintances, but I now begin to speak enough of the language to talk familiarly, and I shall probably visit with as much freedom in some houses, as the nature of the circumstances will permit; for the few mothers here who have handsome daughters have reason, in such a place, to fear a traitor in every young man.

" This apprehension has given rise to a club of a rather singular nature; the young ladies of the place meet in the ball-room every Thursday, to drink tea and see their acquaintances; in this compendious mode of visiting, the rules are two, that none of the male sex be admitted, and that no scandal be talked; the latter I conjecture may be rather difficult to observe; for instance it was reported to the assembly that I had talked with a young lady in a private company, although the whole conversation did not last two minutes; but this was no scandal—however I conjecture it must be necessary to be very careful. I like the place very well, everything is calculated for laborious application, and I want a little time for this. And with five or six lessons in dancing, and four in the manège every week, I have almost exercise enough, although there is no temptation to take any out of doors; the place is the very reverse of Edin-

burgh in many respects.   *   *   *   *.   *   *
I am not very punctual in some of the medical courses, yet I am reading Sydenham, and I must shortly prepare for graduating.

" Your truly affectionate

" T. Y."

He has indicated, in the preceding letter, the feeling, or rather principle, which led to this somewhat excessive pursuit of personal accomplishments. He had been precluded from their cultivation in early life, when men of refined education usually learn them, and he had already begun to feel, as we have seen before, that his want of them operated as a bar to his full participation in the pleasures of society. It was in vain that his fellow-students, whether in banter or in earnest, told him that his musical ear was not good, and that he would fail to acquire ease and grace as a dancer. A difficulty thus presented to him as insuperable was a sufficient motive to attempt to conquer it; and though different opinions have been expressed with respect to the entire success of the experiment, there is no doubt that the mastery of those arts, which he really attained, was another triumph of his unconquerable perseverance.

Young had several introductions to Heyne, and felt naturally very anxious to become acquainted with one of the most eminent scholars of the age; he was received by him with very great civility, but not invited to visit him.

" I believe he thinks himself exempted," says he, in writing to his uncle, " by his literary fame and occupations, and his various offices in the University, from the necessity of showing much attention to strangers, as is usual in most cases, for he very seldom, if ever, has any parties at his house. He is however very civil to me, and I had last week the honour of meet-

ing him with his whole family at his brother-in-law Blumenbach's.   I have not entered very deep into literary conversation
with him, and have not had any opportunity of bringing forward
any of my attempts in composition, except that he has seen a
little compliment which I paid my drawing-master Fiorillo, in
imitation of an ancient epigram, and expressed his approbation
of it; perhaps you would like to see it, though it is not worth
showing anybody.   It refers to the story of Niobe, and the first
line and part of the second are from the Anthologia.   The
head of Niobe is one of the finest antiques that we have, and
expresses calm grief in a most exquisite manner.

> Ἐκ ζωῆς με θεοὶ τεῦξαν λίθον, ἐκ δὲ λίθοιο,
> Χειρὶ Φιωρίλλου ζῶσα πάλιν γενόμην.
> Ἥρξατο μὲν Νέος, Ἄγγλος· ὃ δ' ἄπνοον, οἷα μαθητοῦ
> Ἔργον ἔην, πνεῖ νῦν, ἀλλὰ θανεῖν ἐθέλει.
> or κέυχεται ὦκυ θανεῖν.

"Blumenbach has shown me many civilities, but I am most
at home at Arnemann's, under whose roof I live, and who has
been long in Britain, and brought an English wife home with
him.   You need not be afraid of my following his example, and
marrying a German lady; I am not likely to lose my heart
here, though there are some tolerably agreeable girls, with
whom I wish to be more acquainted for the sake of exercise in
the language; for conversation with women gives both a fluency
of expression and a delicacy of manners which are never to be
learnt from men."

On other occasions he is disposed—though speaking
with great respect of the professors generally—to complain of their want of hospitality.   In one of his letters
to his uncle he says :—

"Your idea of the German manners, as far as relates to Göttingen, is perfectly correct: partly from the nature of a University, crowded with young men, not always the most prudent
nor the most temperate, and partly from the want of other inhabitants of respectability, the professors are the only established
persons who form the society of the place ; and having no superiors, being in the habit of a dogmatical delivery from the chair
of instruction, and not being so absolutely dependent on their

hearers for emolument as in some other seminaries, they are led to a formality and a distance which destroys the social pleasures. There are scarcely two families here who are sincerely cordial; either their pursuits are different, and they have no manner of connection, or they interfere and become rivals. There are, indeed, particular exceptions, and most of the professors receive visits with politeness, but scarcely in any case think of returning them ; Arnemann, in whose house I live, and Lichtenberg, the lecturer on Natural Philosophy, are the most sociable. But, on the whole, one must be content to be in Göttingen a mere student; as such one has many advantages, but the pleasure and improvement of free social communication must be sought elsewhere."

Young had been somewhat spoiled by the open-hearted hospitality of Edinburgh, and hardly made sufficient allowances, not merely for differences of national manners, but still more for the great sacrifice of time which the systematic reciprocation of the visits of students and professors would occasion. Those resident members of our English Universities who have attained to some degree of eminence, or who from any circumstances have become very generally known, can bear a feeling testimony to the severe and almost intolerable burden imposed on them by a compliance with those duties which the habits of society in other places recognize as indispensable.

The only lectures, which he attended, that were not of a professional character, were those of Spittler on the History and Constitution of the European States : of Heyne on the History of the Ancient Arts, and of Lichtenberg on Physics. The first were described by Young as—

" Possessing very great merit, as well in a moral and psy chological sense as in an historical view ; and though the mere historical facts may escape the memory of his hearers, yet they cannot fail to profit, if they have paid sufficient attention, by the conclusions-which they are taught to draw."

The second, which were given at a late period of his residence at Göttingen, were particularly interesting to him. In the course of them the professor described the characters and adventures of every work of art of importance which has come down to us, and exhibited to his class representations of them from the superb collection of prints in the University Library, where the lectures were given. These were accompanied by copious references to classical authors. It were well if such an example were followed in our Universities in connection with their collections of art, as we are rather too apt to neglect both the historical and artistic applications of classical learning.

His uncle, in one of his letters to him, had referred to some .opinions which this great critic was said to have expressed in disparagement of English public schools. Young in his reply to him says :—

" I do not know when or where Heyne can have attacked the English public schools ; soon after I wrote to you last, I copied out a passage from a review of his writing, which I will translate to you ; he acknowledged it to me as his own, and declared it expressed his true sentiments. ' The instruction . at Eton is perhaps, in comparison with ours (in Germany), in many respects very limited ; it is however shown by experience, that a firm foundation in the ancient languages, much exercise in construing the classics, and a readiness in thought and expression in the manner of their originals, formed and derived from that exercise, accompanied also by mathematical studies, will always carry the mind to a higher degree of perfection than a premature general knowledge, built upon a sandy bottom, and unfit for the foundation of a complete and regular academical education : we find in this collection (the Musæ Etonenses for 1795) several poems in which the plan, manner, and turn are perfectly classical, and which show a readiness in poetical expression which we cannot but admire.' "

Of the lecturers of the Medical School, Blumenbach was the most considerable. His text-book was his own Compendium of Natural History, which Young considered to embrace a very judicious selection of subjects, though he objects to his frequent departure from the system, and still more from the precision, of Linnæus, whose works he had himself so diligently studied, and whose authority in almost every department of this science was still very generally recognized as supreme. Young speaks of his lectures as not being very deep, but containing much general information : their interest was not a little increased by the genial manner of the lecturer, and the amusing anecdotes with which they were occasionally interspersed.

" He showed us yesterday," says Young, " a laborious treatise, with elegant plates, published in the beginning of this century at Wurzburg, which is a most singular specimen of credulity in affairs of Natural History.   Dr. Behringen used to torment the young men of a large school by obliging them to go out with him collecting petrifactions : and the young rogues, in revenge, spent a whole winter in counterfeiting specimens, which they buried in a hill which the good man meant to explore, and imposed them upon him for most wonderful *lusus naturæ*. It is interesting in a metaphysical point of view to observe how the mind attempts to accommodate itself ; in one case where the boys had made the figure of a plant thick and clumsy, the Dr. remarks the difference, and says that nature seems to have restored to the plant in thickness, that which she had taken away from its other dimensions."

It is not added that the unhappy victim of this roguery died of mortification when the imposition was made known to him.

Two other lecturers—Arnemann and Richter,—whose

courses he attended throughout, as he tells us, with very exemplary regularity, were also men of very great eminence and very voluminous medical writers. He takes no notice of the anatomical and surgical lectures, though the staff of professors, who gave them, was not less complete than that of medicine. In fact, there was no department of learning which was not well represented in this University, which was then and continued for many years, to be the most illustrious in Germany.[a]

The relative merits of English and German medical writers and medical practice were made the frequent subjects of discussion in the correspondence which passed between Young and his uncle. The latter, who was a good authority on the practice and well acquainted with the literature of his profession, was not free from the prejudices respecting German physicians and their writings, which were very generally prevalent in those days,[b] when Germany had not yet fully vindi-

---

[a] The Baron Meerman, an intelligent Dutch traveller, who visited Göttingen in 1791, and who regards it not only as the first University in Germany but in Europe, says that there were at that time forty-nine professors, of whom thirty-seven were ordinary and twelve extraordinary, besides private teachers: of the former four belonged to the faculty of theology, ten to that of law, seven to that of medicine, and sixteen to that of philosophy. In speaking of the many distinguished men whom this staff included, he says, " What student of the Bible does not honour the name of Eichhorn ; of jurisprudence, those of Böhmer, Pütter, or Runde ? What admirer of ancient and modern literature, elevated by all that judgment, style, and taste can contribute to their refinement, does not recognize a Heyne; or of philosophy, a Feder and Meiners ? What student of mathematics, natural history, chemistry, or anatomy, a Kästner, a Lichtenberg, a Blumenbach, a Gmelin, or a Wrisberg; or of geography and history, a Gatterer, a Plank, a Spittler, and a Schözer ? " Though the salary of no one of these professors, in addition to their fees, exceeded 1000 dollars, they were at that time better paid than those of any other University in Germany. The number of students was about 800.

[b] He had resided in Germany, as physician to the English army, during part of the Seven Years' War.

cated that high position in the world of science and
literature which she is now acknowledged to hold:
Young however ventures to combat the truth of these
views with his usual sobriety and good sense.

" I will venture to repeat," says he, "that your opinion of
the state of physic in this country is formed from viewing it on
the worst side ; your acquaintance with their authors is probably
almost confined to those who wrote forty years ago ; and since
that time, although something old-womanish may perhaps still
remain, yet the main bulk of the art has undergone a great
revolution.   They translate and read, but do not believe all
the new theories that start up.   Brown, Beddoes, Darwin's
works, are all well known, and Hunter's book will probably soon
be turned into German ; all the practical works are also immediately attended to ; they have also among the crowd of their
own authors many who observe and think for themselves.   The
kindred sciences of anatomy, botany, and chymistry, are upon
the whole, further advanced than in Britain ; and the lectures
here on physic and the materia medica are unquestionably
better than those which I heard on the same subjects at Saint
Bartholomew's Hospital.   From all this I do not conclude that
their practice, generally speaking, is equal to the English, but
that it is not greatly inferior, and that one who is disposed may
learn in German books, and from German lectures, something
which is not contemptible."

On another occasion he says :—

"The English physicians are quoted as familiarly here as
they are at home ; the Germans know what London contains
better than many of our own countrymen ; but the reverse does
not hold good ; the German authors are very imperfectly or not
at all known in Britain.   The English may say that the German
medical practice is theoretical and feeble ; the Germans allege
that the treatment in London is merely empirical, and that,
while one half of the faculty is led away by extravagant hypotheses, the other acts only on the narrowest experience : the
truth perhaps is in the medium ; and at any rate the science
here has one advantage—that the doctrines of both countries are
well known here, while the English attend little to any opinions
but those of their own country."

The outline of the plans for study and travel, which
he had formed soon after he came to Göttingen, and
which he submitted to his uncle for his approbation,
was as follows :—

" To take a diploma here in the spring ; to leave this place
late in May ; to travel in Germany during the summer,
reaching Vienna early in the autumn, and having spent the
winter there, in the further prosecution of my medical studies,
to proceed through Switzerland, to the North of Italy,
Rome, and Naples, and then make the best of my way to
England."

The second and larger portion of this scheme was
put an end to by the rapid progress and extension of
the war ; the rest of it was modified by a better knowledge of the difficulties which would prevent his speedy
admission as a licentiate, by the College of Physicians
in London.   Sir George Baker had told him that two
years spent in different Universities in the study of
physic, with a medical degree, would answer the purpose ; and such would really appear to have been the
intention of the framers of the regulation which had
been recently adopted.   The lawyers, however, who had
been employed to put the regulation into a legal form,
had given it a different construction, requiring that the
two years of academical study preceding the application
for a degree should have been spent at the same University.   The obvious effect of this unexpected reading of
the statute was to nullify any claim which he might
have founded upon the year which he had passed at
Edinburgh, and thus to recall to his uncle's mind the
expediency of his proceeding to Cambridge, and, by
graduating there, to secure the full honours of his profession : to this scheme he had long been favourable,
and was now enabled openly to urge it upon his

nephew, when his religious principles no longer presented an insuperable obstacle to its adoption. In the mean time Young had obtained his uncle's consent to his graduating at Göttingen, without adopting any immediate resolution with respect to his future proceedings. On the 21st of March he addressed the usual letter of application to the Medical Faculty, requesting to be examined, preparatory to his degree. On the 30th of April, he passed the examination in company with three other students, Niemeyer, Treviranus, and Grabenstein.

"I made," says he, "no preparatory study, as is usual here, and also at Edinburgh not uncommon under the name of grinding. The examination lasted between four and five hours ; the four examiners were seated round a table, well furnished with cakes, sweetmeats, and wine, which helped to pass the time agreeably ; the questions were well calculated to sound the depth of a student's knowledge in practical physic, surgery, anatomy, chymistry, materia medica, and physiology ; but the professors were not very severe in exacting accurate answers. Most of them were pleased to express their approbation of my replies. We were all previously obliged to give a summary account of the manner in which our lives had been spent."

Young had already made some progress with his Thesis, or the Dissertation which was to precede his public disputation, and which, as it is always printed and circulated, becomes an exercise of importance, which no student of high character could allow to appear without very careful study and preparation. The subject which, after much deliberation, he chose for this Dissertation, was " De Corporis Humani viribus conservatricibus." It is of considerable length, extending to eighty pages, and is written, as might be expected, in very correct Latinity. He had read, as a special preparation for fluency and propriety of expression in medical Latin, the works of Celsus, and was both pleased and instructed by this elegant writer, who, amidst much that is erroneous, exhibits no small portion of sound observation, and judicious practice, more especially in what relates to chirurgery. The Aphorisms of Hippocrates, upon a careful study, fell short of his expectation. The great library of the University, probably the richest, and certainly the best and most liberally administered establishment of the kind in Europe, supplied him with all the books bearing upon his subject, which he felt it necessary to consult; and amongst them he particularly mentions Brande Ueber die Lebenskraft and Hufeland's Ideen über Pathogenie. The Dissertation was finished and printed early in June, and received the ready approbation of the *censor* (the Dean of the Faculty), who spoke in very high terms of its merits.

On the 16th July, he proceeded with his *præses* (Wrisburg) and his two opponents (Weber and Nöden) to the summer auditorium, where he read a short thesis, called a *lectio cursoria*, the subject of which was the human voice ; disputed according to the forms ; was complimented on his performance ; and, after reading something like a prayer, was married to Hygeia, and created doctor of Physic, Surgery, and Midwifery.

The only fragment of this *lectio* which has been preserved is printed at the end of his Dissertation, professedly with a view of filling up some pages of the last sheet, which would otherwise have remained unoccupied. We there find an alphabet of forty-seven letters, designed to express, by their combination, every sound which the organs of the human voice are capable of forming, and thus adaptable as an alphabet for all languages. It is distributed into sixteen pure and five nasal vowels; ten pure, three nasal, and one mixed, semi-vowels; three explosives, six susurrants, and three mutes. Whatever were the bases upon which this scheme was formed, it is evident from reference to it in his correspondence, that it was much in his thoughts; and he assures us that it was in connection with inquiries upon the powers of vocalization of the organs of the human voice, and in order to form a perfect conception of what a sound was, that he was conducted through a series of experiments and observations on the theory of the formation of sound and the laws of its propagation, to the consideration of analogous propositions respecting the theory of light, which became the foundation of his greatest discovery.[a]

Sir John Herschel, in his valuable Treatise on Sound, which is given in the Encyclopædia Metropolitana, has called attention to the extreme imperfection of our existing alphabet to represent all the sounds required in our language :—

" We have six letters," says he, " which we call vowels, each of which, however, represents a series of sounds quite distinct from each other ; and while each encroaches on the functions of the rest, a great many very good simple vowels are represented by binary, and even ternary combinations. On the other hand, some single vowel letters represent diphthongs (as the long sound of i in *alike* and of u in *rebuke*), consisting of two distinct single vowels pronounced in rapid succession ; while again, most of what we call diphthongs are simple vowels, as *ea* in *bleak*, *ie* in *thief*, &c."

He then proceeds to an enumeration of our English elementary vowel sounds, as they really exist in our language, making fourteen vowels and six diphthongs. The consonants, which offer nearly equal confusion, are distributed into four classes, including seven con-

See Works, vol. i. p. 199.

sonants denominated by him as *sharp*, seven as *flat*, and seven as *neutral*. We thus get thirteen vowels and twenty-one consonants, which are competent, either singly or by reduplication and combination, to express all the sounds of the English language. With some additions he seems disposed to think that every known language might be reduced to writing, so as to preserve an exact correspondence between the writing and pronunciation.

The varieties of pronunciation, however, in all languages, even if a recognised standard of pronouncing them in every case could be agreed upon, are sometimes so delicate and so difficult to distinguish, as not merely to surpass the powers of the most careful analysis, but are such as would be found to extend such an universal alphabet to a length which would render it practically useless. The subject, however, assumes a high degree of importance when alphabets are proposed for languages previously unwritten, as in the translations of the Scriptures for the different tribes of Africa, America, and the islands of the Pacific and Indian Ocean, which are accessible to Missionary enterprise, as a means of materially facilitating the study of such languages, and thereby clearing the way for the instruction of those who speak them in religion and the arts of civilized life.

In the month of May—during a short suspension of lectures—he made a tour to the Harz, which has been denominated the Derbyshire of Germany, but far surpassing it in the boldness of its mountain scenery, and the richness of its mines. He was accompanied by two of his fellow-students, and also by Mr. Wedgwood and Mr. Leslie, who were making a short sojourn at the University on their way to Switzerland. Mr. Wedgwood was a man of very agreeable manners and considerable philosophical attainments, the author of a paper of some merit in the Philosophical Transactions for 1794, on the emission of light from heated bodies. Mr. Leslie, subsequently so well known, was at that time engaged in a series of observations on the temperature of springs, with a view of ascertaining whether they represented, or not, the mean temperature of the latitude, at different elevations above the level of the sea. His observations in the Harz were found to be generally accordant with this theory. The travellers were delighted with their excursion through this beautiful region. They ascended the Brocken, so celebrated in the legendary history of Germany, and in the creations of the greatest of its poets. They descended two of the deepest mines, and as usual, were very poorly rewarded for their labour.

Amongst so many objects of natural interest, they were not less pleased with the aspect of Goslar, one of the many free imperial cities, once so numerous in Germany, though now abolished, which tended so much, by their privileges, to preserve the arts and national character of the people, amidst the barbarism and military violence which prevailed around them. Its Gothic houses, its cathedral, its towers, and its ramparts, recalled forcibly to their minds an image of the middle ages.

Amongst other objects also which they visited was a cave at Swartzfeld, extending some hundred yards into the earth. It was known by the name of the Unicorn's Cave, from the bones of an unknown animal which is found there.

"We dug up," says Young, "some of them for specimens. I found the upper part of a tibia, and Wedgwood the lower part of a humerus, of what animal I cannot say, but about the size of a bear."

Cuvier and Buckland had not then shown the deep import of such remains in illustrating the past history of the world.

Young's miscellaneous studies at Göttingen, amidst so many engagements and attendance upon so many lectures, were very limited. The works of Fielding, read, for the first time, after the age of manhood, came upon him by surprise, and he was fascinated by the truth and vigour of their pictures of human nature, notwithstanding their repulsive coarseness.

The Vicar of Wakefield, a work so much and so justly admired in Germany, was found to be almost equally attractive. His previous studies of Ariosto had prepared him to appreciate the wit and vivacity of the Oberon of Wieland, notwithstanding the puerility of many of its adventures and its daring violations of probability. His opinion of the works of Kant, which he had begun to study, but afterwards abandoned, is expressed in the following extract from a letter to his uncle.

" I had begun, but now, on account of graduating, I must for the present intermit, a very deep study of the philosophy of the celebrated Kant, in his Critique of Pure Reason. Kant, in point of popularity, is more than the Aristotle of Germany. In his lifetime he makes already the text of numberless commentators; and it is as much of a compliment to say of a man that he is a good Kantian as that he is a good Grecian. I therefore thought it necessary to have at least an acquaintance with his principles, more from a knowledge of their currency than from an opinion of their worth; and I have not yet been able to see them in a better light. From what I have read of his works, Kant seems to possess great penetration, yet not without confusion of ideas. His language is unpardonably obscure; it is also one of the spurious arts of becoming popular to affect innovations in language. His system may, perhaps, be shortly described by saying that it is diametrically opposed to Hume's."

The constitution of Young's mind was essentially English, and altogether alien to those refinements of thought and niceties of expression which the developments of the philosophical systems of Kant and his followers absolutely require. The German language is as flexible as that of the ancient Greeks, and whilst it is equally capable of adapting itself to the expression of the most profound and transcendental speculations, it exercises in return no inconsiderable influence in modifying and forming the intellectual habits of those who use it. It is probably owing to these influences that the English mind has generally failed sufficiently to appreciate or understand, or the English language sufficiently to express, those philosophical views which have found such general acceptance in Germany; and that all attempts to incorporate or assimilate them with our own, have led to no small amount of confusion and obscurity both of thought and language.

On the 23rd of July, he started on foot, with a man to carry his knapsack, on a short excursion, first to Pyrmont, and thence to Brunswick and Helmstadt; returning by the skirts of the Harz Forest to Göttingen on the 25th of the following month. The rapid progress of the French armies having already involved some provinces of Germany in a war, which threatened before long to extend to the remainder, made it somewhat hazardous for an Englishman to enter upon any very extended tour; and Young had already abandoned his scheme of a winter residence at Vienna and a subsequent visit to Switzerland and Italy.

Göthe has described, in one of the most touching of his poems, the kind sympathy of his countrymen for the emigrants, who first fled from France on the breaking out of the Revolution. The great addition to their numbers, however, including many bad characters and desperadoes, upon the defeat at Valmy and the withdrawal of the royalist army from France, rapidly changed this feeling of general welcome into one of dislike and alarm. Our traveller had not completed his first day's excursion, before he was alarmed by the report that many emigrants were leading a wandering life in the country through which he was passing, who earned their subsistence by contributions forced from the travellers whom they met; and he found that whenever he presented himself in his pedestrian costume at a country inn, the first question addressed to him, before he was received, was, "Are you an emigrant?"

He arrived at Pyrmont, the most northerly of the popular German spas, on the second day from Göttingen, and remained there a week to study the habits of the place, presenting much the same succession of employments as are characteristic of such places in our own times.

At Brunswick he made his appearance at court, dressed in proper costume.

"I was presented," says he, "to the duchess (our King's sister), to the hereditary princess, the Stadtholder's daughter, and the duchess dowager, sister of the late King of Prussia. The duchess and princess each talked about two minutes with me, the mother asked me two questions, and from this time till nine I was left at my own disposal. . . . . I was glad when supper was announced: about twenty ladies sat on one side of the table, and as many gentlemen on the other; I was placed in the middle, opposite the princess: the duchess was not there. I attempted to converse with one of my neighbours, but he was either stupid or sulky, and the others were engaged among themselves. At last the duchess dowager, who looks like a spectre—has lost her teeth—and whom I fancied totally unfit for all company, began a long and amusing conversation. She asked me what I had studied at Göttingen? I told her I was a doctor of physic.—If I could feel a pulse:—how frequent the most rapid pulse that I had felt was :—whether the English or the Germans had the best pulses. I said that I had felt but one pulse in Germany, which was that of a young lady, and a very good pulse. She asked me if there was a good theatre of anatomy at Göttingen. I told her pretty good, but that I did not attend it ; I had only gone to a single lecture, and had seen the professor dance a caricature dance ; that I had been a more frequent attendant of the manège than of the school of anatomy. Our discourse awoke the attention of those who were within hearing, and now I had enough to talk with ; but supper was soon over, and the company dispersed.

"On the following morning I went to see the ducal manège ; the horses are good, but the riding must not be compared with Göttingen."

Young speaks elsewhere of Göttingen as at that time the first school of horsemanship in Europe, the still more celebrated school at Turin having been suppressed by the war. He was passionately fond of this exercise, and an assiduous attendant at the school, and there were no feats of horsemanship, however daring or difficult, which he did not attempt or accomplish. His muscular power was always remarkable, and the companion of his early studies has assured me that he was in the habit of leaping over the loftiest gates with a single spring. In writing to his uncle, towards the close of his residence at Göttingen, he says—

" I have this morning been upon the back of the Springer. To mount this terrestrial Pegasus is considered here something like *summi in re equestri honores*, and is seldom attained without long practice. I finish my lessons this week, and look back with satisfaction on the health and amusement which have repaid my time and money. It might, perhaps, be more useful to me to take some instructions how to sit in a doctor's chariot ; but it is impossible to possess any qualification which one may not want,

and capabilities are but light burdens. We have another
fashionable exercise, which I think adequately corresponds to
the athletic schools of the ancients—vaulting on a wooden horse
in various positions; and I am much more known among the
students for excelling in this, than for writing Greek, of which
they have little knowledge, and not much more respect."

He had a favourable opportunity of exhibiting his
personal activity at a court masquerade which was
given the next day, where he made his appearance with
great success in the character of Harlequin.

At Helmstadt, to which he proceeded upon quitting
Brunswick, he was introduced to Professor Bereiss, a
most singular combination of learning and talents with
the most impudent charlatanerie.

" I scarcely ever met with a more interesting man than Professor Bereiss. I should not have repented going ten times as
far to see him. Everybody allows him to be in one respect an
unique ; that he has more vanity than any other mortal creature.
As to his merit, opinions are different : those who know him
well maintain that he has great parts and industry ; but no
single dissertation of extraordinary merit, nor any one grand
original idea has been produced by him ; it is no wonder therefore that some deny him any claim to superiority, and depre-
ciate all that he possesses. But it cannot be denied, that he
has bought articles of immense value without apparent income
sufficient to purchase a tenth of them ; and he must be allowed
to be an extraordinary man, and though not one of three, as he
maintains, yet at least one of three hundred. The two whom
he is said to place by himself in the temple of Fame, are Zoro-
aster and the late King of Prussia. He formerly read fourteen
lectures, or hours, out of the twenty-four ; now he reads but ten,
on medical, chymical, and philosophical subjects, on the fine
arts, on law, and various other branches of learning. He says
that he sleeps but two hours—others say that he sleeps seven ;
he is sixty-six years old. He says that he has eleven collections,
all equally perfect—one of natural history, one of coins, one of
gems, one of diplomatic manuscripts, one of anatomical preparations, one of pictures of great masters, one of secondary

masters, one of chirurgical instruments, one of philosophical and
mathematical instruments, and some others which I do not recollect; he says that he plays on all instruments, others say
that he plays on none.   His greatest treasure is Lieberkuhn's
collection of anatomical injections and other preparations, about
one hundred and thirty-one, each placed before a microscope, and
arranged in a little box, which he reckons his greatest treasure,
and, together with a picture, keeps always within his reach, that
in case of fire he may in these rescue food for his mind throughout
the rest of his life.   The picture is about a foot square, a Jesus
and John, by Raphael; and it must be allowed to be exquisite.
He says seriously, that all the galleries in the world would be
inadequate for it.   He says that the man who pretends to be a
chymist, and has not as much money as he wants, is an infa-
mous impostor : that he can obtain, from nature, one hundred
thousand thalers whenever he pleases, but I think he does not
seem to affect that he can make gold.   He says he has a dia-
mond which all the kings in Europe together could not buy—
to which the great one in Portugal is a grain of sand—that he
seals it up in chest upon chest, and pays several thousand dollars yearly for having it kept; but it must be brought to him
once a-year that he may be assured it is safe : others who have
seen it, say it is a crystal : he says he will leave it to nobody, for
he knows none worthy of it; and he has already made a furnace
to evaporate it.   The way in which he gets his money he will not
tell, lest a bad use should be made of it.   He says he does not
write because he would lose time in answering the fools who
would oppose him; that he teaches only orally.   The whole number of students in Helmstadt does not amount to one hundred.
What I saw was, in the first place, a few minerals, good, but not
unique ; the collection of the first and the last works of the
greatest painters, whom he thus reckons : Raphael, Michael
Angelo, Correggio, Guido Reni, Trevisano, and Francisca, of
the Italian school; Albert Dürer, Lucas Cranach, Holbein, and
three more Germans; Rubens, Rembrandt, and four more
Flemish ; and four French, which he did not show.   Those
which I most admired were Jesus at Emmaus, M. Angelo ; a
holy family, Correggio ; the little Raphael ; two infants, Trevisano ; and a head of A. Dürer, by himself; there were many
more that were good, and others which he raised to that dignity.

He had a reckoning machine, which he said none but a German had diligence enough to be capable of making. Three automata, made by Vauguyon—a flute player, a pipe and tabor player, and a duck; the musicians could not play much because his servant was not there; but the duck performed many motions just as a living one, and eat and swallowed a moderate quantity of oats, which require an hour to be digested and excreted. I had a great desire to see his medals, which are said to be the best thing that he has; but I had already spent five hours with him, and could not well prolong my stay. Ramdohr, a relation of the author, was most of the time present, and was to see the coins the next day, and I had half promised to be of the party. When I told him I must go, he said, not 'I am sorry for it;' but, 'I am sorry for you.' One cannot but admire Bereiss's industry and enviable acquisitions, at the same time that one must either pity or despise his unpardonable arrogance and exaggeration. Some more particulars of him are to be found in Meerman's Travels."

On the 28th of August he took his final leave of Göttingen " with as little regret as a man can leave any place where he has resided nine months." He had been repelled by the general want of hospitality on the part of the Professors, and the few opportunities for the enjoyment of refined society which the place presented.

He proceeded, as before, generally on foot, first to Cassel and thence by Gotha, Erfurt, Weimar, and Jena to Leipsic. Germany is full of capital cities, the residences of its past or present numerous petty sovereigns, and presenting as common features, palaces, museums of science or art, and other public buildings and establishments, whose splendour is very often in striking contrast to the poverty or small extent of the territories which are attached to them. What is found in one of them may generally be expected to be found in another, and the repeated descriptions therefore of them become tedious and uninteresting. As the principal part of Young's journal is occupied with such details, we shall confine our extracts from it, or other notices of his travels, within very narrow limits.

At Gotha he inspected the fine observatory built in a noble situation on the Seeberg, and made the acquaintance of the observer, the Baron de Zach, afterwards so well known for his various and interesting contributions to astronomy and astronomical literature.

Of the great poets who for so many years made the little city and court at Weimar the most distinguished in Germany, all were absent but Herder, to whom he brought letters from his son, who had been Young's fellow student at Göttingen.

" Herder expressed a curiosity to see more of my attempt to illustrate the human voice. I wrote out for him a little specimen of the manner in which I would describe the pronunciation of the most current European languages, and this afforded conversation with him and Mr. Böteker in the evening, which passed away very pleasantly at his house. Mr. Gore, an English gentleman, who has long resided at Weimar, was there also, with his two daughters; as well as the little Princess with her governess and one or two other ladies. Herder is very well versed in the English poets, but does not speak the language. We had a little debate on the subject of rhyme, which he would reject altogether."

At Jena the University was not in session, and nearly all the Professors were absent. Young, however, found Bütmer the eminent philologist there, by whom he was most kindly received.

" He has applied himself particularly," says Young, " to the study of languages, and, at the age of eighty-three, is going to enter on the publication of a general dictionary of all existing languages, which is already written but not copied for the press. He was formerly Professor at Göttingen, and taught natural history, but has long retired to pursue his grand object. He has already published comparative tables of Alphabets, and now he is publishing a scheme of the pronunciation of all European languages. He asked me to drink coffee with him in the afternoon. I carried him my Dissertation, and wrote out some additional examples of orthography; and he showed me his manuscripts, particularly on the elements of the Chinese language. His library consists of 60,000 volumes, and is particularly complete in natural history. At his death, the Duke of Weimar purchases it for the University."

"Jena is said to have about 1000 students, and those who distinguish themselves find sufficient access to familiarity with the few families resident here. It is considerably less expensive than Göttingen, and money is said to attract less attention here than there."

"The country from Jena to Nuremberg is highly romantic. It follows nearly the course of a fine river, which in the course of ages has worked itself a deep valley, in a country which is otherwise nearly flat, of which the sides are now clothed with vineyards and cottages, the bottom with trees and pasture—here crowned with a city and a castle, and there hanging over a little town. About Leipsic, the country is perfectly flat and void of all natural beauties. I stayed a week there, and met with many civilities from the relatives of an intimate acquaintance in Göttingen; but in general I found little to interest a stranger. I was in one large company of the gay, and in another of the learned world, but I found both too much occupied with old friends to be anxious to become intimate with a new. I saw little of the University; it is lost among the other inhabitants, who are 40,000 in number. There are said to be 1200 students, about as many as in Edinburgh. I met with a Silesian count, who gave me a seat in his chaise upon condition of my being at the cost of an additional horse, and brought me to Dresden in a moderately short time. We travelled in the finest moonshine, and in the morning reached the Elbe at Meissen, one of the finest river views which I have ever seen."

At Dresden, our traveller engaged lodgings for a month, and was much interested with the study of the vast collections, in almost every department of the fine arts, for which that city is so celebrated. He found here also many acquaintances, both English and foreign, and passed his time both profitably and agreeably. He paid visits to Kœnigstein and the Saxon Switzerland, and also to Freyberg, where he was introduced to the celebrated Werner.

" We looked curiously," says he, " at the academic collections, and saw the collection of models of machines and mines. Among the minerals there is a separate division for the illustration of Werner's terms, and subservient to his introductory lectures. The Amalgamir Werk is in every respect the pride of Freyberg. The building is a quadrangle ; in the centre of the court stands a building for throwing water over every part of the works, to prevent such a conflagration as took place a few years ago.

" At first sight, the neatness and order observable throughout the whole are striking to a stranger. It belongs to the Elector, and all the ore of the proper kind found in the neighbourhood is brought here.   It contains, on an average, 3¾ ounces of silver in 1 cwt. After being roasted, it is sifted, and twice ground ; then 11 cwt. of ore and 3 or 4 cwt. of water are put into a barrel, 5 cwt. of quicksilver is added, and the barrel turned round its axis, by means of a water-wheel, for eighteen or twenty hours ; the mercury is then suffered to subside, and the greatest part separated by straining through linen bags ; the rest is distilled off *per descensum*, and leaves the silver with something more than a sixteenth part of other metals ; it is afterwards assayed. The ore remaining is washed in a peculiar machine, separating the remaining mercury ; and if on trial with the test more than a drachm of silver remains in a cwt. of ore, it is again heated with mercury. They lose about three-quarters of an ounce of mercury for every cwt of ore. None of this seems to be evaporated, nor are any prejudicial consequences found on the health of the workmen. The ore, previous to roasting, is mixed with about a tenth part of its weight of salt. There are twenty barrels, all in continual motion. The silver produced should at this rate be worth 70,000*l.* per annum ; but I think they reckon it at about one-third of that value. The mines belong partly to private companies, and partly to the Elector. The miners receive five groschen (8½d.) a-day, for eight hours work ; they sometimes work more than one spell (schichte) in twenty-four hours. They seldom contract. This is about as much here as 9s. a week in England, and in Cornwall the miners earn from 12s. to 18s.

" My friends had never been in a mine ; we therefore went to the bottom of the Churprinz, something more than one hundred and thirty fathoms in depth. It is a convenient mine for descending, and affords a very good specimen of mines in general, but has nothing very singular to distinguish it. Everything is very similar to the method commonly used in England. The external appearance of the buildings, and their situation in the valley, are very agreeable. The ore is carried down a little court to the Amalgamation Work. The smelting-houses and blowing-furnaces adjoining this work have nothing very peculiar."

We have given this extract at length from his Journal as a good specimen of the minute accuracy of his observations and descriptions.

On the 19th of November he started for Berlin in company with Mr. Grey, the Secretary of the Embassy at Dresden, and reached it after three weary days' travelling over the sandy and featureless district which characterizes, for the most part, the approaches to that capital. The extension and probable continuance of the war had put an end to all reasonable expectation of his being able to carry into execution the scheme which he formerly entertained of passing the winter in Vienna and the following summer in Italy, and he finally acceded to the wish which his uncle had frequently expressed, that he should return to England at an early period, and then proceed to Cambridge to take his degree ; for it had now been distinctly ascertained that there were no means of obtaining his licence to practise in London, without a continued residence in the same

University for two years previous to graduation. In a letter addressed to his uncle, written on the 12th of December, after a three weeks' residence in Berlin, announcing his determination, he proceeds to say :—

"I have not formed many connections in this place, neither have I seen any great curiosities; indeed I am glad to have a little respite from the perpetual pursuit of novelties, which seldom equal expectation. I have been to-day in the Royal Library, which is tolerably good and extensive, and in a day or two I am to make an excursion to Potsdam to see the palace, with its paintings and statues. I have dined twice with the English ambassador, Lord Elgin, and once with Dr. Brown, a Welch physician and in great favour with the king.

"There are some other Englishmen here, but most of them about to leave Berlin; amongst them is a Mr. G——, who was turned out of the Guards for democratical principles : I believe you know his father. I am acquainted with one or two Jew families, who are very respectable; the women are generally more accomplished and better informed than those of other denominations, and associate as little as they can with men of their own nation. I have not yet seen any of the professors, but I mean to call upon Walther, Klaproth, and one or two others. You say my Thesis is caviare to the general; but do not you think people have a greater respect for anything out of the common way? Perhaps indeed few people will give it attention enough either to like or dislike it, yet I do not know that I have any reason to avoid distributing it among my friends. It seems a fatality that almost everything I do or produce should be termed stiff: in this case it may arise from my having been obliged to treat the subject in a short compass."

He left Berlin for Hamburg on the 14th of January, 1797.

"On the whole road there was nothing to amuse or even to call off the attention; the country is a flat sand, now covered with half-thawed snow; the inns poor and dirty, the weather cold, perpetually threatening rain or snow; the carriages are the coarsest and simplest open waggons, without any other seat than straw. I was very happy the greatest part of the night in such beds as I could get, and in four days and a half I reached my destination."

After passing a week with his hospitable friends at Hamburg, he hastened to Cuxhaven, in order to join the packet for England, the sailing of which was delayed by adverse winds until the 7th of February. He was invited, on the day of his arrival, to dine with Mr. Heise, the Governor and Amptmann of the town, to whom he had letters of recommendation from his friends in Hamburg. He met at his table, besides his four daughters, several of the French emigrant nobles, and some English naval officers :—

" The evening," says he, " was concluded with dancing a cotillon, to the simple music of the flute. I felt no impatience for change of wind : I could read and write almost as well here as in England. The inn was not very good, but the people agreeable and civil, and there was a spirit of hospitality and a sufficient portion of good company among the inhabitants.

" It seems the most natural employment for leisure hours, when we are on the point of leaving a country which we have endeavoured to view with the eye of a philosophic traveller, to take a retrospective view of some of its most remarkable characteristics.

" The country of which I am qualified to speak is only the northern part of Germany : in natural advantages perhaps inferior to the southern, but in activity and cultivation much superior. From the Northern Sea, all the way to the neighbourhood of Hanover, to that of the Harz Forest, to Leipsic, and almost to Dresden, the country, except the banks of the Elbe and a few other rivers, is a flat barren sand, covered here and there with heath, fir-woods, and now and then other trees. But the Weser, and the country near it, from below Hameln to Cassel and further up, then the whole tract between this and Gotha, many parts of the Harz Forest, the Elbe in Saxony, the banks of the Saal, and perhaps some other parts, are equal in beauty and apparent fertility to almost any portion of England of equal size.   Much is said of Bohemia, of the banks of the Danube and Rhine, and of Tyrol.   These I have no expectation of visiting at present; whether I may hereafter seek an opportunity of doing it I cannot determine, but I should not be disposed to attempt it without a combination of the most favourable circumstances.   ' Ist nicht Deutschland von einem Ende zum andren durchreist, durchkreutzt, durchzogen, durchkrochen und durchflogen?' says Göthe, as he is relating the manufactory of a journal by a person who had not made the journey.—' Give me thy route, before you come to me.   I will promise you sources of information and materials for assisting your work : there shall be no want of square miles which have never been measured, and of population which has never been reckoned.   The revenues of the countries we will take from almanacks and tables, which, as is well known, are the best documents.   When we do not happen to travel through the residence of any celebrated men, we will take care to meet them in some inn, and make them talk nonsense to us in confidence, and especially we will be careful to interweave with spirit a love adventure with some lively beauty ; and this will give you such an interest to the whole as to ensure the attention of every reader.'

" I have often been inclined to doubt whether a general character of a people can with any certainty be laid down ; it is probable that a few distinguishing characteristics may in some cases be described, but there is scarcely any one common cause which can produce a similar effect over the whole of Germany. If we analyse the idea of countrymen, and look for the bond of mutual attachment, there is scarcely anything but the use of the same mother-tongue that can give any rational determination of the idea.   The facility and promptness of a mutual communication of ideas, and the habit of having absorbed from the earliest infancy similar principles from the same or similar writers, are perhaps the only marks of belonging to the same country that can be found throughout Germany ; and indeed even the language can scarcely be said to be universally the same, except among those of the first ranks.   Where the different parts of the same country are united by a community of government, of laws, and of opinion, the attachment is still closer and the resemblance greater. But the liberal mind must rise above the little prejudices of local attachment; the love of our country sounds well in the mouth of an orator or in the lines of a poet, but it is one of the most dangerous tools in the hands of ambition, and has often been converted to the worst of purposes. It is not to be expected, nor perhaps to be wished, that the vulgar should desert every principle but those which are founded in cool reason and philosophy; yet too little attention is paid by popular writers and speakers to the important maxim conveyed in the short answer of Socrates to the men who inquired of what state he was a citizen. A man who has formed intimacies and friendships with inhabitants of different parts of the globe will find enough to love and to disapprove among every people; and perhaps one who has acquired the faculty of communicating his thoughts with equal ease and pleasure to the individuals of several nations, will find himself as much at home in the one as in the other. Certainly one who is totally destitute of this attainment can never be admitted to judge with impartiality of the character of any country. Many men of enlarged minds see clearly the want of common spirit in Germany, but it may be doubted whether they do not act unphilosophically in lamenting so much the absence of national attachment, with respect to its moral effects, however pernicious the political influence of so many jarring interests may be.

" The complicated system of so many hundred independent governments, with all possible variation of constitutions, is productive of numerous inconveniences in almost all public works. The States monopolize many undertakings, and attempt to derive as much revenue as possible from them, and not unfrequently, from the pride of being independent, interfere with the beneficial projects of their neighbours. Thus the roads lie unimproved; the provision for travelling, for want of sufficient emulation, is seldom in any tolerable degree of perfection : it is true none are prohibited from establishing conveyances of different kinds at their private expense, but there is not yet sufficient encouragement to tempt any adventurers. The number of petty courts serve to spread over the country some degree of the forms of refinement : but a ready communication with a single animated centre would have more effect than a greater number of less perfect ones.

"In the learned world the great majority are mere mechanical labourers;—the names of a Schiller, a Wieland, and a Göthe are but rare luminaries among an infinite number of twinkling stars and obscure nebulæ. The established custom of the booksellers, who pay every ordinary writer exactly in proportion to the number of sheets, and at their periodical fairs exchange bulk for bulk of every kind of publication, is the grand impediment,—among those who are necessitated to subsist in part by writing,—to the laconic efforts of a brilliant genius, and the cause that the innumerable and ever increasing heap of volumes envelops from day to day more and more the sciences which it is designed to illustrate.

" The pride of independence in the petty states is the cause of the great existing number of universities, all furnished with numerous professors, who are generally ill paid by the institutions, and to increase their fame and fill their purses are tempted to undertake an unreasonable diversity of lectures, which their diligence raises to the merit of minute prolixity, but which their genius seldom elevates above the rank of mediocrity. The students, from diligence or vanity as well as from universal custom, are prompted to attend to a superficial course of study in every imaginable subject of literary information, which they take implicitly from the tribunal of the school, retain in some shape by a mechanical memory, until time and other pursuits—unless fortunate circumstances have favoured them —wash out those slight impressions, which, if infixed, would have been both ornamental and useful.   Hence one advantage of the usual education in England, however grossly deficient it may be in some particulars; the ancient languages are generally so impressed as never to be entirely forgotten, and having attained a considerable degree of perfection in any one branch, the influence of this positive acquirement may extend into the remotest pursuits."

*   *   *   *   *   *

" Here I was interrupted by an invitation from the governor to spend the evening at the Castle, with a large party assembled to celebrate his birthday; it was the last that I passed in Germany, and one of the pleasantest: after supper we had a little dance, in which I was so fortunate as to have the two prettiest of his daughters and a prettier cousin for

partners.   The wind was already changing, and I took a final
leave : the next morning we received the welcome summons.
I went immediately to bed, and by this means avoided any
material sickness till the third day, when the wind was a little
high.   I was imprisoned in the same disgusting hole the
remaining five days, for, if I attempted to sit up or go on deck,
I became giddy.   On the eighth day we saw land, and made
Yarmouth Roads about noon.   We were several times alarmed
lest we should meet with privateers ; once I was in full expectation of an engagement, which was perhaps as bad as the thing
itself.   I could eat almost nothing, but slept soundly and
dreamt of feasting.   The trouble and vexation at the custom-
house was almost as bad as being at sea for the time ; but I
settled everything, and slept at Yarmouth that night, which
was the conclusion of all dangers and difficulties.   I must now
resume my observations.

" There are many points in which Germany differs from
England that almost baffle all description.   Whether the human
mind is on the average in a more cultivated state in this
or that country, it is very difficult to say : there are more
learned men in Germany than in England, but we have, and
ever have had, some individuals in many branches who are
almost unequalled.   Latin is much better understood in Germany, Greek but little ; commercial men speak French and
often English.   In the mathematics and in chymistry the
Germans are making rapid advances ; as painters they copy
better than the English, but have perhaps less invention ; in
engraving the English confessedly excel them ; and the Germans still more decidedly bear away the palm in music, in
which they rival the Italians.

" The spectators in a German theatre applaud with more
taste than the English ; the actors follow more closely the delicate touches of nature, but have less force in expressing violent
passions ; their plays too are seldom raised above common life.
A poor strolling actress in a barn has sometimes excited as
much emotion in me as Mrs. Siddons has done.   They never
act Shakspeare's pieces well.

" Generally speaking the Germans are less handsome than
the English ; the greatest difference that struck me on my
return was in the elegant forms of the women ; half of the

girls that one meets in the streets would be pointed at in Germany as remarkably well made. The German women are, on the other hand, in general more accomplished than the English ; they almost always speak French well, often English and Italian, and mostly play on some instrument, but they have very little scientific knowledge. The Jewesses, especially at Berlin, are among the most cultivated and agreeable of the inhabitants, and mix more with the world than in London.

" The great number of independent states reduces the courts more nearly to the resemblance of private companies than elsewhere ; it is usual for all those to be introduced who have a title to that privilege, and this keeps up a marked distinction between the numerous and poor nobility, and the richest or most accomplished of the commonalty ; and even a nobleman of late creation is not admitted into the first circles at Vienna, nor permitted to dine with the Elector of Saxony. The idea conveyed by the English word gentleman cannot be expressed in German ; they translate it nobleman, and sometimes make the distinction of lesser nobility. The professions are of little esteem, and a degree is thought a degradation rather than an honour to one who wishes to be in good company. I found it an impediment to me, and never made use of the title. ' I do not know,' says Göthe's Wilhelm Meister, ' how it may be in foreign countries, but in Germany a nobleman alone has the power of attaining a certain universal, or, if I may so call it, a personal, cultivation and refinement. A commoner may have merit and may form his mind with the utmost labour, and bring it to the highest state of perfection ; yet his personality is lost, let him place himself as he will. A nobleman may everywhere push forwards, a commoner can do nothing better than feel in silence the boundary that is prescribed to him. He must not ask himself, What are you? but What have you ? This difference originates, not from the encroachments of the nobility and the concessions of the commonalty, but from the constitution of society ; whether, and how, this will ever be altered concerns me but little ; as things now are, I must do my best to attain that which I feel as an absolute and undeniable want.' Much more to the same purpose is to be found in this interesting work. Whoever becomes rich can easily purchase nobility, and then all their descendants for ever are equally noble, and

enjoy in some cases certain privileges : hence it is easily understood how there is so great a difference from the state of
society in England.

" The ornamental exercises, especially among the nobility,
are more attended to than in England,—riding, fencing, vaulting, and dancing; the prevalence of a military life is also in
part a cause of this, as well as of some other differences. The
union of literature and fashionable elegance is very rare ; the
learned never aspire to make a figure in the gay or in the
political world ; and those in power look upon a man of
letters at best merely as an ornament to their court, like a
musician or a dancer. On a certain gala day at Dresden, the
actors are allowed to pay their court to the Elector ; but professional men, I believe, never.

" The laws in most parts are guided by the Roman civil law ;
the depositions taken in writing, and the sentences given in
private. Their physic is composed of that of all other nations ;
for they read all books in all languages, but they select too little,
and do not seem to know the beauty of simplicity. Scarcely a
work of any consequence can appear in any country, but that
one or more translations of it are immediately promised. The
Germans have sometimes been accused of too great an attachment to the imitation of foreigners ; their Anglomania in physic
has of late been rather too rashly censured. In their dress
and furniture they follow the English at present much more
than the French ; and in general everything that is English
is reckoned the best of its kind. An Englishman, known no
otherwise than as an Englishman, is universally treated with
respect, and thought admissible into all companies ; he feels
himself nearly of the same rank with a count—though a German count is less than an English baronet ; but the English are
generally more feared than beloved : one man very innocently
told me in conversation in a mixed company, that he never had
met with an Englishman that he could like.

" A stranger finds the table d'hôte very convenient ; at a
good one the best company is to be found ; each is independent
and pays moderately. They seldom drink to excess, except
occasionally a few students and officers ; but not more than the
English ; they are generally near two hours at dinner, and rise
before the cloth is removed. Smoking is carried to such an

excess that it must have a pernicious effect both on the health and character of individuals. The marriage state is a medium between what it is in England and was in France ; divorces are easily and not unfrequently obtained ; the couple interferes less with each other's pursuits than in England ; they sleep often in separate rooms, and almost always in separate beds ; a bed large enough for two is a rarity in Germany.

" The German language is easily so far learnt by an Englishman, that he can read a common author ; but the connection of sentences and order of words is so intricate that it is difficult to speak and write it with perfect delicacy. It is capable, by the facility with which it admits of all manner of combinations, of expressing readily many compound ideas which can less easily be rendered into any other language : some of its guttural sounds, and some combinations of consonants, are rather unpleasant to the ear, but the general tenor of the language is sufficiently soft, and the accent and cadence diversified, and, at least to an English ear, agreeable. It has more dignity than the French, and more force than the Italian ; I think it has a vigour of expression hardly equalled by any other language ; but such a comparison is very difficult to make. A foreigner is puzzled with the variety of pronunciation in different parts ; after many times changing my practice, and making repeated inquiry, I find that Adelung's rules are almost universally the best ; in Dresden and Berlin they speak ill and acknowledge it ; in Hamburg and Brunswick they have some peculiarities ; Austria is confessedly *solœcous ;* Hanover and Göttingen seem to be the nearest to correctness.

" Schiller, Wieland, and Göthe, are the three reigning authors of the present day, both for poetry and prose. Göthe has a strong party, especially among the ladies, many of whom extol him far above all other mortals ;—Werther, Iphigeneia, Egmont, and Tasso, are said to be his best pieces. Wilhelm Meister is by no means unworthy of Göthe's genius ; but it vanishes in comparison of some of our English novels.—Schiller is grand ; Wieland elegant, fanciful, and pleasing ; Klopstock, Voss, and Herder, are also among the first of the living authors.

" The low German is half way between German and Dutch, and deserves well the notice of one who wishes to study the

English etymology: Mr. Croft is now very laudably employing himself with it at Hamburg.

"What impressions a stranger would receive from France and Italy I cannot exactly judge : but I should think Germany at present the most interesting country to a traveller of any in Europe; not so much from its original merit, but from its being a kind of compendium of everything that is excellent, and everything that is remarkable in every country existing; nor do I in the least repent the time and labour employed in seeing and learning as much of it as circumstances would allow me.

*   *   *   *   *   *

" From Yarmouth it was natural that I should visit Norwich in my way to London. Mrs. Rich took me up after sleeping at Keswick; the next night we arrived at Wade's Mill; not that the fatigue of travelling in England could be said, in comparison of Germany, to make rest necessary; but it was more convenient to sleep there : in the morning I took a walk up to the house at Youngsbury where I resided so many years, and we arrived about noon in London."

The reader who might be disposed to criticise the preceding views of the national character and literature of Germany should keep in mind the great changes which both of them have undergone since the time that they were written. The common calamities which nearly all the members of that vast empire suffered from the French occupation and the common exertions which were called forth in its defence, during the war of liberation, have created a common feeling for their fatherland, which no subsequent dismemberment, and we may likewise add, no subsequent misgovernment, has been able to destroy : whilst the rapid developments of every department of their national literature have tended to inspire, with a just pride, all those who have the privilege of using the language in which it is embodied.

CHAPTER V.

MEDICAL EDUCATION : CAMBRIDGE.

Almost immediately after his return to England, he was admitted a Fellow Commoner of Emmanuel College, Cambridge. The Master, Dr. Farmer, the well-known author of the Treatise on the Learning of Shakspeare, was a friend of his uncle, a circumstance which probably determined the selection of this college, which was at that time the resort of many students in the higher classes of life. The tutors under whom he was admitted were the Rev. R. Towerson Cory, who shortly afterwards succeeded to the mastership, and the Rev. R. Hardy, afterwards Rector of Loughborough in Leicestershire.

We have received from a gentleman who succeeded Dr. Cory as Tutor of the College, some particulars respecting his academical habits and occupations and the general estimate which was formed of his character and attainments by his fellow students and contemporaries. The writer of them was a man of great energy of character and of very acute observation, but possessed of no great learning ; he was evidently not very partial to Dr. Young, and by no means disposed to recognize, even after the death of their author, the importance of those discoveries which the most eminent scholars and men of science of the age had long since acknowledged.

" When the Master," says the writer, "introduced Young to his tutors, he jocularly said : 'I have brought you a pupil qualified to read lectures to his tutors.' This, however, as might be concluded, he did not attempt, and the forbearance was mutual ; he was never required to attend the common duties of the college.

" He had a high character for classical learning before he came to Cambridge ; but I believe he did not pursue his classical studies in the latter part of his life—he seldom spoke of them ; but I remember his meeting Dr. Parr in the college Combination room, and when the Doctor had made, as was not unusual with him, some dogmatical observation on a point of scholarship, Young said firmly : ' Bentley, sir, was of a different opinion ;' immediately quoting his authority, and showing his intimate knowledge of the subject. Parr said nothing ; but, when Dr. Young retired, asked who he was, and though he did not seem to have heard his name before, he said, ' A smart young man that.'

" He had a great talent for Greek verse ; and, on one occasion, I remember a young lady had written on the walls of the summer-house in the garden the following lines :—

' Where are those hours on airy pinions borne
    That brought to every guiltless wish success ?
When pleasure gladdened each succeeding morn,
    And every ev'ning closed with dreams of peace ? '

" On the next morning appeared a translation in Greek Elegiacs, written under them, in Young's beautiful characters. It may be here mentioned, that when his mode of writing Greek was laid before Porson, he said, that if he had seen it before he would have adopted it."

" The views, objects, character, and acquirements of our mathematicians were very different then to what they are now, and Young, who was certainly beforehand with the world, perceived their defects. Certain it is, that he looked down upon the science and would not cultivate the acquaintance, of any of our philosophers. Wood's books I have heard him speak of with approbation, but Vince he treated with contempt, and he afterwards returned the compliment. I recollect once asking Vince his opinion of Young : he said he knew nothing correctly.

'What can you think,' says he, 'of a man writing upon mechanics, who does not know the principle of a coach wheel.' This alludes to a mistake of Dr. Young's on this subject in his Natural Philosophy.[a]

"He did not seem even to have heard the names of most of our poets, or literary characters in the last century, and hardly ever spoke of English literature. I remember having invited him to meet at dinner Mr. Whiter, of Clare Hall, who, though an admirable scholar, was a wit and a bon-vivant, while Young took no delight in the pleasures of the table, and never could either make a joke or understand one. Whiter quoted something from the *Oxford Sausage*, and when our philosopher betrayed his ignorance of the existence of such a work, with his total inability to taste or relish the allusion, it was almost painful to witness the ridicule which he was obliged to sustain; but to do him justice, he did sustain it with perfect good humour."

An observation of his own has been sometimes quoted, with reference to this peculiar result of his early education and course of study, which we have elsewhere had occasion to notice. "When I was a boy, I thought myself a man; now that I am a man, I find myself a boy." Nothing is more humiliating to a young man, who is conscious of great powers and of the possession of superior attainments, than to find himself the object of the banter or the patronizing airs of those who are in advance of him in their knowledge of the habits of good society and of the popular topics of conversation, though in other respects immeasurably his inferiors.

"He never obtruded his various learning in conversation; but if appealed to on the most difficult subject, he answered in a quick, flippant, decisive way, as if he was speaking of the most easy; and in this mode of talking he differed from all the clever men that I ever saw. His reply never seemed to cost him an

---

[a] See note, Works, vol. i. p. 361. Dr. Young formed a just estimate of the great merits of Dr. Wood's elementary books, but was generally very unjust to Vince.

effort, and he did not appear to think there was any credit in being able to make it. He did not assert any superiority, or seem to suppose that he possessed it; but spoke as if he took it for granted that we all understood the matter as well as he did. He never spoke in praise of any of the writers of the day, even in his own peculiar department, and could not be persuaded to discuss their merits. He was never personal; he would speak of knowledge in itself, of what was known or what might be known, but never of himself or any other, as having discovered anything, or as likely to do so.

"His language was correct, his utterance rapid, and his sentences, though without any affectation, never left unfinished. But his words were not those in familiar use, and the arrangement of his ideas seldom the same as those he conversed with. He was, therefore, worse calculated than any man I ever knew for the communication of knowledge. I remember our once asking him to answer an objection to Huygens's theory of light, which he preferred to Newton's, and, though there were many very competent persons present, he attempted in vain. But this perhaps was no wonder; the objection was that, on this supposition, there would be no shadow, and it has not yet been removed.[a] I remember also his taking me with him to the Royal Institution, to hear him lecture to a number of silly women and dilettanti philosophers. But nothing could show less judgment than the method he adopted; for he presumed, like many other lecturers and preachers, on the knowledge and not on the ignorance of his hearers.

"In his manners he had something of the stiffness of the Quaker remaining; and though he never said or did a rude thing, he never made use of any of the forms of politeness. Not that he avoided them through affectation; his behaviour was natural without timidity, and easy without boldness. He rarely associated with the young men of the college, who called him, with a mixture of derision and respect, ' Phænomenon Young;' but he lived on familiar terms with the Fellows in the Common-room. He had few friends of his own age or pursuits in the university;

---

[a] See Works, vol. i. p. 151. It was a mistake in a proposition of Newton that was the foundation of this objection, for the removal of which the weight of his own authority was the chief difficulty to be overcome. See *infra*, p. 140 and 170.

and not having been introduced to many of those who were distinguished either by their situation or talent, he did not seek
their society, nor did they seek him : they did not like to admit
the superiority of any one *in statu pupillari*, and he would not
converse with any one but as an equal.

"It was difficult to say how he employed himself; he read
little, and though he had access to the college and university
libraries, he was seldom seen in them.   There were no books
piled on his floor, no papers scattered on his table, and his room
had all the appearance of belonging to an idle man.   I once
found him blowing smoke through long tubes, and I afterwards
saw a representation of the effect in the Transactions of the
Royal Society to illustrate one of his papers upon sound ;[a] but
he was not in the habit of making experiments.   He walked
little, and rode less, but having learnt to ride the great horse
abroad, he used to *pace* round Parker's Piece on a hackney : he
once made an attempt to follow the hounds, but a severe fall
prevented any future exhibition.

"He seldom gave an opinion, and never volunteered one.
He never laid down the law like other learned Doctors, or uttered apothegms, or sayings to be remembered.   Indeed, like
most mathematicians, (though we hear of abstract mathematics,)
he never seemed to think abstractedly.   A philosophical fact, a
difficult calculation, an ingenious instrument, or a new invention,
would engage his attention ; but he never spoke of morals, of
metaphysics, or of religion.   Of the last I never heard him say
a word, nothing in favour of any sect, or in opposition to any
doctrine ; at the same time, no sceptical doubt, no loose assertion, no idle scoff ever escaped him."

The preceding spirited and clever sketch expresses
with some, but not very great, exaggeration, the views
entertained of Young's character, attainments, and
discoveries, especially in early life, by the great majority of his contemporaries, to whom they were but
superficially known.

Young's first impressions of Cambridge, (if we may

[a] See Works, vol. i. p. 68, Outlines of Experiments and Inquiries
respecting Sound and Light.

judge from a letter to his uncle,) were decidedly favourable.

" I have been invited," says he, " in the course of the week to several agreeable and rational parties both of scholars and fellows; the manner of life and behaviour here is much more civilized and refined than in the foreign universities, and I begin to see many advantages in our institutions, however abused, for the promotion of learning. The retaining a body of men who have time and opportunity of associating with the students, must tend to fill up the void places in their intelligence, and to repress the ferocity, roughness, and levity of manners which are too apt to be carried to excess, where very young men are left entirely to themselves. "

His subsequent letters indicate no change in this opinion, though he occasionally complains of the barriers which custom opposes to a free interchange of society with the senior and more distinguished members of the University, with whom the claims of a letter of introduction were considered to be generally discharged by a single dinner, to be succeeded afterwards by a formal and somewhat distant recognition.

There was at that period no proper system of medical instruction at Cambridge, no anatomical or other collections, and only one course of lectures on human and comparative anatomy, given by Sir Busick Harwood, a man of vigorous intellect and considerable attainments, who addressed them rather to a general audience than to the medical students, who were not even required to attend them. A proposal which he made to compel them to do so was not encouraged by the authorities of the University, and was thrown out by the Senate.

The superintendence of the medical faculty was entirely entrusted to the Regius Professor of Physic,

who presided at the medical disputations in the schools
and whose certificate of competency and a compliance
with the statutable forms, were the only conditions required by the senate for admission to a medical degree.
The requirements of the statutes, which were framed in
the early part of the reign of Elizabeth, were adapted
to a much younger class of students than those of the
present day, and were rigorous and unalterable in all
that regards the time and form of graduation. Thus
six entire years were required to elapse between the
admission of a student and the degree of M.B., and
five more before he was allowed to attain the mature
honour of the Doctorate ; and the University possessed
no power, unless in virtue of a special mandate of the
Crown, to reduce the length of these intervals, even in
extraordinary cases, where a combination of age and
merit might appear to require it. We thus find that
Young was not admitted to the degree of M.B. until
the year 1803, when he was thirty years of age, nor to
that of M.D. until five years afterwards : he had begun
the practice of his profession in virtue of his former
degree, before the expiration of the first of these periods,
but did not attain the honour of the fellowship of the
College of Physicians before the conclusion of the
second.

Notwithstanding the repressive influence of mediæval
statutes, and the want of any organized system of
medical instruction, the medical students of the English Universities very generally attained the highest
rank amongst the physicians of the metropolis and
elsewhere. They entered the profession generally late

---

[a] A grace of the Senate, founded upon a somewhat violent stretching of
the words of the statute, has reduced this period to five years : it is now proposed to reduce the first of these periods to four years and the second to two.

in life, but with all the advantages of a classical as
well as medical education, and were thus associated
more intimately in rank and estimation with the higher
classes of society, than those whose early studies had
been of a less refined and general character; and there
are many reasons which should induce us to conclude
that the high social position which physicians have
hitherto been enabled to maintain in this country—so
different from that which they occupy on the Continent
of Europe—is not a little owing to this admixture of
well educated gentlemen, so many of whom have been
supplied by the English Universities. The privileges
also which were accorded to the College of Physicians,
though long stigmatized as unjust and illiberal, and
the cause of frequent litigation, especially about the
period of which we are now speaking, had a similar
tendency; and it may be reasonably doubted, now that
those privileges are to a great extent abandoned,
whether the medical profession will long be able to
maintain, as hitherto, the same estimation in society
with the members of the professions of the Church
and the Law. If it should succeed in doing so, it can
only be effected, as of late years, by a liberal distribution of honours by the Crown.

It is often contended that Oxford and Cambridge—
considered in their double capacity as Universities and
towns—do not furnish adequate materials for the formation of good medical schools. But is such an opinion
well founded? Some of the teachers whom they now
possess are men of eminent ability, and the services of
others might be easily obtained if they were adequately
paid. Their anatomical collections are very considerable, and there exists a more liberal access to many
extensive libraries for the purposes of private study

than is afforded by the metropolis or any other cities in the kingdom. Their hospitals are admirably administered, and better suited for the clinical instruction of a limited number of pupils than those much larger establishments, where, as is generally the case, a vast mob of students encumbers the progress of the lecturer, and makes deliberate observation difficult or impossible. Neither is the objection, so commonly urged, of the very limited range of medical practice, arising from the small population of Oxford or Cambridge much better founded than the others; for those hospitals are not confined to the towns alone, but extend to the counties in which they are situated, the most difficult and interesting medical or surgical cases being generally forwarded to them; whilst the experience of other medical schools has shown that a large population is not necessary to their success.

The inhabitants of Montpelier, Göttingen and Heidelberg are less in number than half those of Oxford and Cambridge, whilst those of Pavia, the first of Italian schools, do not exceed them.[a]

On the 13th of December, 1797, upon his return from Cambridge, he met, for the last time, his uncle Dr. Brocklesby, who had just returned to town from a visit to the widow of Mr. Burke at Beaconfield, to receive his other nephew Mr. Beeby and himself. At dinner he appeared to be in his usual good health and spirits, but he expired suddenly a few minutes after retiring to bed. He had attained a considerable rank in his profession, and lived on terms of intimacy and friendship with the most distinguished men of his day, to whom he was equally

[a] See Report of the Cambridge University Commission on the evidence of Professor Fisher, M.D., of Downing College, Cambridge.

recommended by his medical skill, his benevolence and his literary attainments.

His generous offer to Dr. Johnson of an annuity to enable him to resort to a warmer climate, and also of apartments in his own house when his confined dwelling in Bolt Court, Fleet Street, was considered injurious to his health, is well known; and having bequeathed in his will a legacy of one thousand pounds to Mr. Burke, he gave it to him in his life time, before the grant of an ample pension had made such a gift no longer necessary for his comfort.

He bequeathed his Irish estates, which were considerable, to Mr. Beeby; to Young, he left his house and furniture in Norfolk Street, Park Lane, his library, his prints, a choice collection of pictures, chiefly selected by his friend Sir Joshua Reynolds, and about 10,000*l.* in money: other legacies were made to his servants and other members of his family. Young had just reason for regarding with affection the memory of this kind and liberal relative who had fostered his rising talents, provided so judiciously for the completion of his general and professional education, and left him a fortune amply sufficient for his establishment in life, though not so large as to impair those motives for exertion which are generally found necessary for eminent success. It is quite true that even the kindest actions of this excellent relative were not altogether unmixed with some root of bitterness, such as dependence of every kind, except that of a child upon a parent, is apt to bring along with it: he was somewhat querulous in his temper, and somewhat exacting in his claims to respect and deference; though liberal in great things, he was somewhat parsimonious in small; and though generally judicious in the course which he recommended Young to pursue, he was sometimes rather unreasonably suspicious when his wishes (though often very obscurely intimated) were not fully carried out.

Dr. Young was now entirely at liberty to form his own scheme of life. He retained apartments in his uncle's house for his own occupation when in London, but continued to reside in Cambridge, as before, during such portions of every term as the statutes of the university required, and sometimes likewise during part of the summer vacation. We find him occasionally residing for a few weeks in Bath, with professional views, and at another time in Southampton and its neighbourhood. He paid yearly visits, as he was accustomed to do with his uncle during his lifetime, to the Duke of Richmond's, at Goodwood; but his longest sojourns during the summer months were at Worthing, in the house of Mr. John Ellis, a very rich West Indian proprietor, the brother of the late Lord Seaford, and the cousin of George Ellis, of Sunninghill, the well-known editor of the Specimens of Early English Poetry and Metrical Romances. Mr. Ellis had always been a most welcome guest at the choice dinners which his uncle Dr Brocklesby—who was fond of the pleasures of the table—was in the habit of giving, and had received from him the *sobriquet* of Squire Allworthy, in compliment to the kindness and generosity of his character. With the other members of this family and more especially with the last of those mentioned above, —whom Walter Scott denominated the most accomplished man of his age—Young continued through life to live on terms of the greatest intimacy.

During his residence at Cambridge he availed himself of every opportunity of entering into general

society, so much so as sometimes to interfere ma=
terially with the prosecution of his studies. Amongst
others with whom he was accustomed to associate, and
whose friendship he continued to retain, may be mentioned, the late Lord Brownlow, then a student of
Trinity College, whom he had known in Edinburgh;
Mr., afterwards Sir William Gell, a member of the
same college with himself, an accomplished artist,
archæologist and scholar, who in later life maintained
with him a most lively and agreeable correspondence
on hieroglyphics and other subjects; Mr. Dodwell, of
Trinity College, who afterwards published a magnificent work on Greece; Mr. Caldwèll, afterwards Tutor
of Jesus College, a man of cultivated manners and an
excellent classical scholar; Dr. Pearce, Master of Jesus
College and Dean of Ely, a man of considerable acuteness and some learning; Sir Busick Harwood, who
fully appreciated his attainments; Dr. Raine, the well-
known Master of the Charter House, to whom he was
made known by Dr. Charles Burney; Sir Isaac Pen-
nington, the Regius Professor of Medicine, and at
that time in possession of the first medical practice
in the University; Mr. Kempthorne, a Fellow of
St. John's; Mr. Holden, Fellow of Sydney College,
at whose musical parties he was accustomed to take
a part; Mr. Tavel, likewise a musical amateur and
a well-known Tutor of Trinity College, and many
others. The records however of his college life are
very scanty, and the few incidents which we have
been able to collect concerning it have not been
derived, either from his correspondence and journals,
as heretofore, but from extraneous sources. The
academical life of the editor was too far separated

ᵃ See Works, vol. iii. *passim.*

from that of Dr. Young to enable him to supply the deficiency.

In writing to his friend Dr. Bostock, in the month of June of this year, 1798, he refers to an occurrence, which, by keeping him at home, had recalled him to his usual habits of application.

" I met with an accident," says he, " about five weeks ago in London, which has prevented my walking ever since, and I think I broke one of the metatarsal bones ; this has been a favourable circumstance, for it has increased my literary application in a considerable degree ; I have been studying, not the theory of the winds, but of the air, and I have made observations on harmonics which I believe are new. Several circumstances unknown to the English mathematicians which I thought I had first discovered, I since find to have been discovered and demonstrated by the foreign mathematicians ; in fact, Britain is very much behind its neighbours in many branches of the mathematics ; were I to apply deeply to them, I would become a disciple of the French and German school ; but the field is too wide and too barren for me."

It would indeed have been fortunate for his scientific character, and would have greatly aided the ready reception of his subsequent discoveries, if he had been tempted, at this early period of his career, to study systematically in this school of mathematics, and had adopted the elegance of form and completeness of development for which the works of Euler, La Grange and La Place are so justly distinguished.

The experimental researches which are referred to above, were embodied in a Memoir which was prepared at Cambridge in the summer of 1799, and read to the Royal Society on the 16th of January of the following year—it is entitled Outlines and Experiments respecting Sound and Light. Some of the conclusions and speculations to which these investigations lead, are of great theoretical importance, not merely as tending to correct many prevalent errors and misconceptions respecting the propagation of sound, but especially as establishing the great principle of the interference of sounds, and the explanation of the phenomena of beats and of the grave harmonics which is founded upon it: a principle which speedily conducted him to the discovery of the kindred principle of optical interferences,—

"Which has proved," says Sir John Herschel, "the key to all the more abstruse and puzzling properties of light, and which would alone have sufficed to place its author in the highest rank of scientific immortality, even were his other almost innumerable claims to such a distinction disregarded."

In the course of this Memoir, he noticed an erroneous statement respecting the crossing of the vibrations or rather undulations of air which constitute musical sounds, without affecting the same individual particles by their joint forces, which appears in the well known Harmonics of Dr. Robert Smith. In proposing, at the close of it, a system for the temperament of musical intervals, and in noticing—amongst many others which had been recommended or made use of for the same purpose—the system put forward by the same author, he spoke of the work in which it was given as "a large and obscure volume," and of the system itself as "leaving the subject, except for the use of an impracticable instrument, exactly where it found it." The first of these observations, though undoubtedly well founded, called forth the indignant remonstrance of Mr. John Gough, of Kendal, who had been accustomed, like many others, to regard this work of Dr. Smith with great admiration; the second, of more questionable validity, subjected its author to a rebuke—not unmixed with commendation—of the celebrated Dr. Robison of Edinburgh, which appeared shortly after the publication of the Memoir, in an admirable article on music in the supplement to the first edition of the Encyclopædia Britannica. It should be observed that Dr. Robison regarded the very method which Young disparages, as practically superior to every other which had been proposed.

"We are surprised to see this work of Dr. Smith greatly undervalued by a most ingenious young gentleman in the Philosophical Transactions for 1800, and called a large and obscure volume, which leaves the matter just where it was, and its results useless and impracticable. We are sorry to see this, because we have great expectations from the labours of this gentleman in the field of harmonics, and his late work is rich in refined and valuable matter. We presume humbly to recommend to him attention to his own admonitions to a very young and ingenious gentleman, who, he thinks, proceeded too far in animadverting on the writings of Newton, Barrow, and other eminent mathematicians."

The admonitory criticism to which Dr. Robison refers, and partially quotes, appeared in the third of a series of nine essays, published in the British Magazine for 1800, under the title of The Leptologist, upon the subjects, and in the order, indicated in the following motto :—

> " Grammaticus, rhetor, geometres, pictor, aliptes,
> Augur, schœnobates, medicus, magus, omnia novit
> Græculus esuriens."

It is a Treatise on Cycloidal Curves, displaying geometrical resources of no mean order, preceded by some prefatory remarks on the superior precision and clearness of geometrical above algebraical investigations, as well as upon the danger, without adequate examination, of putting forward as new, "propositions and discoveries which have long since been known and forgotten." He exemplifies the necessity of such caution by referring to a young gentleman of Edinburgh, "a man who certainly promises, in the course of time, to add considerably to our knowledge of the works of nature," who, in a memoir printed in the Philosophical Transactions for 1798, had proposed one problem as new, which was familiar to the mathematicians of the seventeenth century; and had put forward a solution of another problem as superior to that which was given by Newton, but which only differed from it by being less simple, and by erroneously giving the name of cycloid to a curve, which was, though closely allied to it, in reality the companion of the trochoid.

The author of this paper, which contains several porismatic propositions which are curious and original, was Mr. Brougham, then a very young man, whose enterprising genius seemed to have prepared him to grapple with every branch of human knowledge; and though the particular criticism referred to was just, it was somewhat flippant and ungracious, and was probably not without its influence in provoking the severe retaliatory treatment which Young's own Memoirs shortly afterwards experienced at the hands of one who, though not himself invulnerable, was armed at all points and always prepared to come to close quarters with his enemies.

Dr. Robison was well entitled, by the high position which he held in the scientific world, as well as by his profound practical and theoretical knowledge of the science of music, to assume the office of a critic; and the great and just respect with which Young was accustomed to regard his writings was not likely to lessen his anxiety to rebut the force of his censure. He addressed therefore a letter to Nicholson's Philosophical

Journal for 1801, in which he attempts to justify the opinion which he had expressed respecting Dr. Smith's theory of imperfect consonances, by showing that it was not altogether original, and also that the method of temperament founded upon it was practically inapplicable ; at the same time he fully recognised the great merits of his optical writings.

What is most worthy of notice, however, in this reply, is the first public announcement which it gives, of the extension of the principle of interferences from sound to light, and the consequent establishment of its propagation by undulations.

"I am of opinion," says he, "that light is probably the undulation of an elastic medium, because

"1st. Its velocity in the same medium is always equal.

"2nd. All refractions are attended with a partial reflection.

"3rd. There is no reason to expect that such a vibration should diverge equally in all directions, and it is probable that it does diverge in a small degree in every direction.

"4th. The dispersion of differently coloured rays is no more incompatible with this system than with the common opinion, which only assigns for it the nominal cause of different elective attractions.

"5th. Reflection and refraction are equally explicable on both suppositions.

"6th. Inflection is as well, and, it may be added, even much better explained by this theory.

"7th. All the phenomena of the colours of thin plates, which are in reality unintelligible on the common hypothesis, admit of very complete and simple explanation by this supposition. The analogy which is here superficially indicated will probably soon be made public more in detail; and will also be extended to the colours of thick plates, and to the fringes produced by inflection, affording from Newton's own elaborate experiments a most convincing argument in favour of this system."

It was in the month of May, 1801, as he himself

elsewhere informs us, that he first recognised this principle.[a]

The first memoir, On the Theory of Light and Colours, in which this discovery was developed, was read to the Royal Society on the 12th of the following November. It was succeeded by a second, entitled An Account of some Cases of the Production of Colours, which was read on the 1st July, 1802; and by a third, entitled Experiments and Calculations relative to Physical Optics, read on the 24th November, 1803. The first and last of these memoirs, now so justly celebrated, received from the Council of the Royal Society the compliment of being selected as Bakerian Lectures, which entitled their author to receive the produce of a small pecuniary bequest. The publication of these three memoirs constitutes the first great epoch in the history of his optical discoveries, which will be made the subject of special discussion in the following Chapter.

After the completion of this memoir, which had employed so much of his time, and which gave rise to so many important speculations, Young established himself, for the remainder of the summer, in London, attending the hospital very closely, in order to refresh his memory and to add to his stock of observations; he availed himself also of the ample medical library which had been bequeathed to him by his uncle, to increase his knowledge of medical literature, which had hitherto been somewhat limited.

In the autumn of 1799 he returned to Cambridge for his last term of residence; and in the early part of the following year he made a commencement of medical practice in the metropolis, establishing himself

[a] See Works, vol. i. p. 202.

in a house in Welbeck-street (No. 48), which he continued to occupy for five-and-twenty years.

A physician in London, however fortunate in his outset, must be prepared to pass many years of involuntary leisure before he can hope to secure a sufficient footing in his profession to afford him constant occupation. It was a happy circumstance for the fame of Dr. Young that this period never arrived, and though some of the best years of his life were diverted to professional studies and occupations, he was enabled to devote many more of them to those literary and scientific pursuits in which so few could compete with him.

The first subjects which would appear to have occupied him were the Essays under the signature of The Leptologist, and the Memoir on the Mechanisn of the Eye, to which we have before alluded. Upon this last production he put forth all his powers. The optical and anatomical investigations which it contains are of no ordinary difficulty and importance, more especially the happy adaptation of an instrument called the Optometer, originally invented by Dr. Porterfield, for accurately measuring the focal distance of the eye both in a vertical and horizontal plane, which in many eyes are unequal to each other; the determination of the refractive power of a variable medium, and its application to the constitution of the crystalline lens; the pointing out the nice and accurate adjustment of every part of the eye for viewing at the same time the greatest possible range of objects without confusion; the measurement of the collective dispersion of coloured rays in the eye; and the ingenious and multiplied experiments for ascertaining, in some cases beyond the reach of controversy, what parts of the eye are changed, and what are not, when passing from the view of near to distant objects, and conversely.

Like most of his other memoirs, it is very obscure, partly from the great condensation of the subjects which it embraces, and partly from the intrinsic difficulty of the subject and the constant references which it requires to an instrument and apparatus which cannot easily be understood, unless it be seen and used. It has probably arisen from this cause that, though this Memoir has often been referred to, it has been very rarely read.

In the year 1801, Young accepted the office of Professor of Natural Philosophy at the Royal Institution, which had been established in the year preceding, chiefly by the exertions of the well known Sir Benjamin Thompson, Count Rumford. It was designed as a great metropolitan school of science, where lectures should be given, models of useful instruments exhibited, and collections of books on science and of chemical and philosophical apparatus, formed, on the most magnificent scale. Its founder, if such he may be termed, had further views also of making it subsidiary to the promotion of many useful projects and inquiries which he had recently proposed in his Essays, which enjoyed an extraordinary popularity. After managing the affairs of the Institution for a few months, and commencing the editing of its Journal, he quarrelled with some of the directors and abandoned the scheme altogether. The conducting of the Journal was thenceforward entrusted to the joint care of Dr. Young and his colleague, Mr. Davy, at that time Professor of Chemistry, in whose hands and in those of his not less distinguished successor, Mr. Faraday, the chemical laboratory of the Institution has become the most celebrated in Europe.

Dr. Young's first lecture was delivered on the 20th of January, 1802, and the last on the 17th of May. The whole number of lectures given during this Session was thirty-one, which was increased, by the introduction of new subjects in the following year, to sixty, assuming that they correspond, in arrangement and number, with those which appear in his great work, entitled " A Course of Lectures on Natural Philosophy and the Mechanical Arts," which was published four years afterwards. They are divided into three parts, containing twenty lectures each. The 1st, including Mechanics, theoretical and practical ; the 2d, Hydrostatics, Hydrodynamics, Acoustics, and Optics ; the 3rd, Astronomy, the Theory of the Tides, the Properties of Matter, Cohesion, Electricity and Magnetism, the Theory of Heat and Climatology. They form altogether the most comprehensive system of Natural Philosophy, and of what the French call Physics, that has ever been published in this country ; equally remarkable for precision and accuracy in the enunciation of the vast multitude of propositions and facts which they contain, for the boldness with which they enter upon the discussion of the most abstruse and difficult subjects, and for the addition or suggestion of new matter or new views in almost every department of philosophy.

We propose to reserve the more particular consideration of these Lectures to a subsequent Chapter.[a]

Dr. Young, by his own confession, and for reasons which we have before alluded to, was not adapted for a popular lecturer. His style was too compressed and laconic, and he had not sufficient knowledge of the intellectual habits of other men, to address himself

[a] Infra, p. 188.

prominently to those points of a subject where their difficulties were likely to occur. If, indeed, these lectures were delivered nearly in the form in which they are printed, they must have been generally unintelligible even to well-prepared persons, notwithstanding all the assistance which models, drawings, and diagrams could afford.

We have heard it remarked, that no writer, on any branch of science which these lectures treat of, can safely neglect to consult them, so rich is the mine of knowledge which they contain; and it is a well known fact, that many important propositions and discoveries have been more or less clearly indicated in them, which have only been recognised or pointed out when other philosophers discovered them independently, or announced them as their own.

One very striking example of such an anticipation Dr. Young has himself noticed in a review [a] of Dr. Wells's well-known Essay on Dew. In a passage of his fifty-sixth Lecture, he says—

" There are frequently some local causes of heat and cold, which are independent of the sun's immediate action. Thus, it has been observed, that when the weather has been clear, and a cloud passes over the plane of observation, the thermometer frequently rises a degree or two almost instantaneously. This has been partly explained by considering the cloud as a vesture, preventing the escape of the heat which is always radiating from the earth, and reflecting it back to the surface."

This observation, combined with others which connect the theory which it indicates with the discoveries of Leslie and Prevost respecting the radiation of heat and the deposition of dew, sufficiently show that Young was, in the year 1807, when this work was published,

[a] See Works, vol. ii. p. 424.

in full possession of the principle which Dr. Wells, seven years afterwards, so happily brought to bear upon a vast mass of meteorological phenomena; but though Dr. Wells had read and studied, as he himself allows, those parts of the works of Dr. Young which relate to the subject on which he was writing, there is every reason to believe that the passage which we have quoted, and the principle which it involved, had escaped his notice.

" There are, however," says Young, in the Review referred to, "some modern philosophers, who, whether from their own fault, or from that of their hearers and readers, or from both, appear to be perpetually in the predicament of the celebrated prophetess of antiquity, who always told truth, but was seldom understood and never believed. And the author of the lectures in question has not unfrequently reminded us of the fruitless vaticinations of the ill fated Cassandra."

In the year 1802 he was appointed Foreign Secretary of the Royal Society, an office which he held for the remainder of his life, and for which he was well qualified by his knowledge of the principal European languages.

Ten years afterwards, Sir Joseph Banks, in a letter, in which he urged Young to accept the office of Secretary, which was at that time vacant, expressed in very grateful and flattering terms, the sense of the great services he had rendered to the Society, not merely by his contributions to its Transactions, but in the discharge of other duties. The offer was declined from an apprehension lest the tenure of an office conspicuously connected with the cultivation of science would operate prejudicially to him in the practice of his profession.

CHAPTER VI.

OPTICAL DISCOVERIES.—FIRST EPOCH.

THE contributions made by Dr. Young to the science of Physical Optics, and the relations which they bear to the labours, in the same field, both of his precursors and contemporaries, have been discussed by Dr. Whewell, in his History of the Inductive Sciences, with so just and philosophical an appreciation of their full value and significance, that we should do little more than obscure the lucid picture which he has drawn, if we should attempt to reproduce it in our own colours and with our own less perfect execution. In addition to the sources of information which are open to all, he had access to the interesting series of letters of Young, Arago, and Fresnel, which have been printed in the first volume of the present edition of Dr. Young's works, and which supply some very important facts in the history of the Undulatory Theory at the most critical and, in many respects, the most triumphant period of its progress; and we have found, after a very careful examination of his references to them as well as other documents, that there is nothing to correct and very little to add. In entering now, therefore, upon a short examination of the first and, hereafter, of the second of the two great epochs of Young's optical researches, we shall rarely notice the labours of other writers, unless they are essentially connected with his own.

What are our ordinary conceptions of a vibration and undulation? We usually connect the first with a reciprocating motion of the particles of the same body, without their transfer in space; with the second, a single vibration, of the same class, in the particles of a medium which is transmitted to similar portions of it in perpetual succession—the same series being renewed as long as the exciting cause of them continues to act.

But how various are the circumstances in which such movements originate, and how complicated are the results which follow from them! How difficult, also, is the accurate conception of a wave and of the mode of its propagation, even when the form which it assumes, the law of its formation, and the properties of the medium which transmits it, are cognisable by our senses! But how much is that difficulty increased, when its almost infinitesimal magnitude and the enormous rapidity of its movement altogether remove it from the sphere of immediate observation!

The pulses of air, which produce the key-note c of the natural scale of music, form an undulation whose breadth is about 212 inches, and of which 64 are propagated in a second of time. We can discover their origin; we can analyse their form and progress, and we are familiar with the medium through which they are conveyed. But if we assume light to consist in the undulations of an ethereal medium, and adopt the consequences to which such a theory leads, we shall find the length of a wave of green light, near the middle of the prismatic spectrum, to be one ten-millionth part of that of the wave producing such a sound; and that it is propagated with a velocity nine million million times as great, or at the rate of nearly 190,000 miles in a second of time. The human mind is equally embarrassed in dealing with numbers or magnitudes both so great or so small, and it is therefore only through the aid of symbolical language that the analogies which exist between the motions of sound and of light can be brought within the compass of our understanding, and that we are fully enabled to seize upon, not only the points in which they agree, but also those in which they differ.

The objection which Newton most strongly urged against the undulatory theory of light was founded upon the tendency of all undulations, in whatever medium they are excited, to diverge into the surrounding space.[a] Such is confessedly the case with the waves of water, an incompressible fluid, where the force which propagates them is that of gravity. Such he asserts to be the case with waves of sound which are transmitted through a medium of moderate elasticity. The same reasoning and the same analogy would appear to extend, therefore, to the undulations of light, requiring a medium to transmit them of an elasticity proportionate to the velocity which it communicates.

" Are not all hypotheses erroneous," says he, " in which light is supposed to consist of a pression or motion, propagated through a fluid medium ?   If it consisted in pression or motion, propagated either in an instant or in time, it would bend into the shadow.   For pression or motion cannot be propagated in a fluid in right lines beyond an obstacle which stops part of the motion, but will bend and spread every way into the quiescent medium which lies beyond the obstacle.   The waves on the surface of stagnating water, passing by the sides of a broad

_____

[a] Principia, prop. xlii., sect. viii., lib. ii. Dr. Young's Works, vol. i. p. 152.

obstacle which stops part of them, bend afterwards and dilate themselves gradually into the quiet water behind the obstacle. The waves, pulses, or vibrations of the air, wherein sounds consist, bend manifestly, though not so much as the waves of water. For a bell or a cannon may be heard beyond a hill which interrupts the sight of the sounding body; and sounds are propagated as readily through crooked pipes as straight ones. But light is never known to follow crooked passages, nor to bend into the shadow. For the fixed stars, by the interposition of any of the planets, cease to be seen, and so do the parts of the sun, by the interposition of the moon, Mercury, or Venus." [a]

Young combats these conclusions on several grounds. He doubts the validity of the demonstration of the proposition upon which they are chiefly founded, though his objections refer less to the reasoning by which it is supported than to the consequences to which it leads; asserting, also, in opposition to Newton—as the result of later and more extended observations— that sound is not equally loud when diffused in spaces which are perfectly free and when passing round corners and obstacles;[b] and that its easy propagation through bent tubes is rather due to reflexions on their surfaces than to the perfect facility of its diffusion. If, therefore, any sensible reduction of this diffusive tendency is observable in the undulations of a medium like air, how much greater must it be in the ether, whose undulations constitute light, the elasticity of which is incomparably greater!

This was the conclusion at which Huygens arrived, in a work replete with remarkable anticipations of the great truths which form the basis of the undulatory theory,[c] upon grounds which will be afterwards more

[a] Newton's Optics, query 28, quoted by Dr. Young, Works, vol. i. p. 153.
[b] Works, vol. i. p. 74.
[c] Théorie de la Lumière, written in 1678 and published in 1790.

particularly noticed, and which enabled Fresnel, when combined with the principle of the interference of light, to give a complete answer to this the most popular and the most potent of all the objections which have been made to this theory. The suggestion and establishment of this second principle was almost entirely due to Dr. Young,[a] though he failed to perceive its full bearing upon the question which we are now considering.

The following is the account which Young himself has given of the train of reasoning by which he was led to the recognition of this important principle :—

" It was in May, 1801,[b] that I discovered, by reflecting on the beautiful experiments of Newton, a law which appears to me to account for a greater variety of interesting phenomena than any other optical principle that has yet been made known. I shall endeavour to explain this law by a comparison :— Suppose a number of equal waves of water to move upon the surface of a stagnant lake, with a certain constant velocity, and to enter a narrow channel leading out of the lake ;—suppose

[a] " A doctrine " (the interference of light), says Sir John Herschel, " which we owe almost entirely to the ingenuity of Dr. Young, though some of its features may be pretty distinctly traced in the writings of Hooke (the most ingenious man perhaps of *his* age), and though Newton himself occasionally indulged in speculations bearing a certain relation to it. But the unpursued speculations of Newton, and the *aperçus* of Hooke, however distinct, must not be put in competition, and indeed ought scarcely to be mentioned, with the elegant, simple, and comprehensive theory of Young,—a theory which, if not founded in nature, is certainly one of the happiest fictions that the genius of man has yet invented to group together natural phenomena, as well as the most fortunate in the unexpected support it has received from all classes of new phenomena, which, at their first discovery, seemed in irreconcilable opposition to it : it is, in fact, with all its applications and details, a succession of *felicities*, insomuch that we may be almost induced to say, if it be not true, it deserves to be so."—Optics, Encyc. Metrop., art. 595. There is now no sufficient ground even for the fragment of doubt which is here insinuated : the evidence upon which this theory rests, though inferior in completeness, is hardly so in force to that which exists for the theory of gravitation.

[b] Supra, p. 71. Works, vol. i., p. 132.

then another similar cause to have excited another equal series of waves, which arrive at the same channel, with the same velocity, and at the same time with the first. Neither series of waves will destroy the other, but their effects will be combined: if they enter the channel in such a manner that the elevations of one series coincide with those of the other, they must together produce a series of greater joint elevations; but if the elevations of one series are so situated as to correspond to the depressions of the other, they must exactly fill up those depressions, and the surface of the water must remain smooth; at least I can discover no alternative, either from theory or from experiment.

" Now, I maintain that similar effects take place whenever two portions of light are thus mixed ; and this I call the general law of the interference of light." [a]

The law itself is enunciated in the following form, in the first of the three Memoirs which we are now considering :—

" When two undulations from different origins coincide, either perfectly or very nearly in direction, their joint effect is a combination of the motions belonging to each."[b]

All movements in the same elastic medium, of whatever nature, whether gentle or violent, small or great, are known to be propagated with the same velocity; and all vibrations whether great or small, produced by a force varying as the distance from a central point, provided it be the *same* at the *same* distance, will be completed in the same time. It will follow, therefore, that the undulations will be of the same length, when the vibrations are isochronous, but different for those vibrations, which, though following the same law, are not completed in the same time. It will be found that the first is the case with light which is homogeneous—

<hr/>

[a] Reply to the Edinburgh Reviewers, Works, vol. i. p. 202.
[b] Works, vol. i. p. 157.

but the times of vibration and therefore the lengths of the undulation of light of different colours, will be found not to be the same but to vary from red at one extremity of the prismatic spectrum to violet at the other, very nearly in the proportion of 5 to 3.

The most important consequences will be found to follow from these different lengths of the undulations of light of different colours, giving rise to phenomena of endless variety and beauty. We shall afterwards have occasion to refer to some of the remarkable observations by which those lengths admit of being measured with an accuracy which is not surpassed by any other determination in philosophy.

The *amplitude* of an undulation is measured by the greatest excursion of a vibrating particle from its initial position or place of rest, considered with reference to the vibrating particles themselves : its *phase* by the time elapsed from the beginning of the vibration, or more commonly, by the angle which would be described in that time by a radius whose extremity describes a circle uniformly in the whole time of an undulation. The movement of a vibrating particle is *positive* or progressive during the first half of an undulation, or between the *phases* 0 and 180°, and *negative* or retrograde during the second half, or between the phases 180° and 360° or 0° : its greatest positive or negative velocity is at the end of one quarter or of three quarters of an undulation, and in all other positions it is proportional to the product of the amplitude of the vibration and the sine of its phase.

The *intensity* of a vibration, or its light-producing power, must be assumed, upon dynamical considerations (the conservation of the *vis viva*), to be proportional, not to the simple power, but to the square, of its amplitude.   Light may be extinguished, but can never become negative.

With these preliminary explanations, we shall be in a condition to enter upon the consideration of some of the more simple cases of the interference of such undulations. Such are those where they are of the same length and intensity, and in complete accordance or discordance with each other, that is, in the *same* or *opposite* phases. Other cases would require for their explanation the use of analytical processes, which, though not in themselves difficult, could not easily be rendered intelligible in ordinary language.

Let there be assumed, for convenience of illustration, two sources of homogeneous light of equal intensity ; and let us consider the undulations which they transmit, in the same direction, in the line which passes through them ; and let us farther assume that the undulations which emanate from both these sources are equal in length, in intensity, and, therefore, also in amplitude, and that when they issue from them they are in the same phases of their vibrations.   If under such circumstances we suppose the sources of light to be distant from each other by an *exact* multiple of the length of one of those undulations, they will be found, when they concur, in *exact accordance* with each other ; every particle of the medium being agitated by a double force and producing a single vibration of *double* amplitude and *quadruple* intensity, performed in the same time, and therefore transmitted by an undulation of the same length as before.   In such a case the separate undulations are said to *interfere*, producing the maximum effect by their corroborative action.

Again, if we consider the undulations transmitted from two such sources of light, not upon the line

which passes through them but upon two lines issuing
from them which are very slightly inclined to each
other, and whose lengths, when they meet, differ from
each other by an exact number of undulations: in
this case, also, when they concur, they will be found in
precisely the same phase, and so nearly coincident
in direction, that their divergence will produce no
sensible effect upon their mutual action. The result
will therefore be the same as in the former case, and
the interference of the undulations will be entirely
corroborative, doubling the amplitude of the vibration,
but not altering the length of the undulation.

If in either of the preceding cases (and it is the latter
of them which we shall have most commonly occasion to
consider) the distances from the sources of light, at the
point where the vibrations transmitted along the lines
issuing from them concur, should be found to differ
from each other, not by an *exact* multiple of an *entire*
undulation, but by an *odd multiple* of *half an undulation*, they will be found, when they interfere, to be in
opposite phases, or in *complete discordance* with each
other, the same force urging each particle of the medium in opposite directions. In this case the particle
will remain at rest, the vibration will altogether cease,
and there will be no resulting impression of light:
this is an example of complete destructive interference.

If the light which thus concurs be white or common
light and not homogeneous, the effects which have been
above described will strictly apply to that portion of the
prismatic spectrum, the lengths of whose undulations
alone answer the required conditions; if the interference
of such undulations be destructive and complete, colour
will be developed by the abstraction of one portion of
the prismatic spectrum from the rest; if it be corrobo-

rative, colour will be developed by increased intensity of the corresponding portion of the interfering light. It thus happens that in nearly every case of such inter- ference, colour will be produced, and to this cause are referable many of the most varied and brilliant effects of coloration which are presented to our observation.

Whatever be the source of light which we employ (and in the practical application of this theory we are necessarily confined to that derived from one source only), it is assumed that the undulations which produce light continue to be issued, during the whole course of the observation, in the same phase of their vibrations. It will form an essential part of the investigation of every special case of interference which we have to consider, to trace the paths of the two beams, which interfere, from their common source of light, whether real or virtual, to the point of concurrence, assuming that the difference of the phases of their undulations will be entirely dependent upon the different lengths of the paths which they respectively describe.

The only case in which the principle of interference, in another science, had been applied before the time of Young, was to the phenomena presented by the tides of the port of Batsha, in the East Indies.   They had been described by Halley, in the Philosophical Trans- actions,[a] two or three years before the publication of the Principia, and the explanation of them which New- ton has given in that work has been always considered as one of the happiest efforts of his genius.   Twice in each lunar month the tides in question advance, by channels, whose lengths are so related to each other that, after they reach the port, they differ by exactly half an undulation, and the tide entirely disappears.

[a] Phil. Trans. for 1684, vol. xiv. p. 681.

For the next seven days, the tide gradually increases until it attains its maximum, and then falls off gradually during the same period until it disappears : these tides therefore present successive examples, not merely of completely destructive and corroborative interferences, but of all their intermediate gradations.

The spring and neap tides also, derived from the combination of the simple solar and lunar tides, afford, as has been observed by Dr. Young, a magnificent example of the interference of two immense waves with each other ; the spring tide being the joint result of their combination when they coincide in time and place, and the neap tide when they succeed each other at the distance of half ·an interval, and so as to leave the effect of their difference only sensible. The beating of two musical sounds, when nearly in unison, resembles a succession of spring and neap tides, considered as undulations related to each other in frequency, as twenty-nine to thirty ; and the combination of these sounds is still more analogous to that which takes place when the undulations of light interfere, in virtue of the closer analogy which exists between air and our assumed luminiferous ether than that between air and water.[a]

One of the first and most satisfactory applications which Young made of his theory was to the colours of striated surfaces ; a class of phenomena which Newton had left altogether unnoticed, and which were not explicable by any recognized theory of light which had previously been proposed. When two or more scratches, forming concave, cylindrical, or other polished surfaces, capable of reflecting light in all directions, are drawn extremely near each other, the light issuing in all directions from a luminous source may be reflected from points in

[a] Works, vol. i. p. 329.

those surfaces in directions so nearly coincident as to meet and interfere at the eye, after describing paths which differ in length by one half or by a whole of the undulation, which is appropriate to the coloured light, if homogeneous, or to some one of its constituents, if white, light be employed. The appropriate colour in one case will be destroyed by interference and corroborated in the other; and if we take into account a series of such points on each surface in lines very near to each other, the combined effect of such interferences will become sensible to the eye, and lead to the pro-duction of colour, or to a flash of darkness or light.[a]

Young employed, in his observations, Mr. Coventry's micrometric scales, the principal lines upon which were composed of two or three nearly parallel and much finer lines, not more than one ten-thousandth part of an inch from each other, and therefore capable of reflecting light under such conditions as the observation requires. Still finer examples of lines drawn on glass have been produced by Dr. Wollaston and Mr. Barton, the latter of which, when transferred to steel —as in the case of the buttons which are known by his name—produce a very brilliant effect of coloration. The effects also caused by the light reflected from the polished surface of mother of pearl have been shown, by Sir David Brewster, to be referable generally to the same class of appearances.

The most remarkable, and, in many respects, the most instructive application of the principle of interferences is found in the explanation of the rings of colours of *thin* plates, or Newton's rings. The examination of the phenomena which they exhibit, had been a labour of predilection of the great man, by whose name they are

[a] Works, vol. i. p. 158 and 298.

commonly known, and the account which he has given of them has always been considered as a model of delicate observation, of the careful exclusion of extraneous circumstances, of accurate measurement, and of the comprehensive classification of the results. These rings show themselves with great distinctness, in horizontal zones of colour, about the highest point of a soap bubble, when reduced to extreme tenuity, by carefully protecting it, when formed, from the disturbing effects of currents of air; and whenever two transparent bodies are brought very nearly into contact with each other, with air or any other transparent medium interposed, they are observed with greater or less regularity of form and succession, according as the distances between them follow or do not follow any determinate and regular law. But under no circumstances can the phenomena which they exhibit be so conveniently examined, and the diameters of the rings and the corresponding distances of the two surfaces from each other be so accurately measured or determined, as when they are formed by a double convex lens of well ascertained and considerable focal length, resting upon another surface of glass or polished metal which is accurately plane, such as the flat surface of a plano-convex lens.

In one of his observations, Newton employed a lens the surfaces of which were parts of a sphere whose diameter was 184 inches, and the measured diameter of the fifth of the dark rings was found to be 2037 inches. The corresponding distance of the surfaces—a third proportional to the diameter of the sphere and the radius of the ring—was therefore equal to ˙0000366 inches only; and as it was found that the successive distances from the point of contact, at which the suc-

cessive rings, both bright and dark, appeared, were
proportional to the square roots of the natural numbers, and that therefore the corresponding distances of
the surfaces themselves followed the order of the
natural numbers, or the squares of the former, it would
appear that the dark or obscure rings would present
themselves at distances which were successively represented by ·0000122, ·0000366, ·000061, &c., inches,
and the brighter rings at the distances of ·0000244,
·0000488, ·0000732, &c., inches, respectively.

The first remark which is naturally suggested by
such observations upon the formation of these rings,
when made by the aid of a lens of known radius, is
the wonderful power which they afford of measuring,
with great accuracy, spaces not otherwise measurable, from their extreme smallness.   A space equal
to ·2037, or little more than one-fifth of an inch,
which was, in this instance, the diameter of the fifth
ring, is measurable with considerable accuracy, by
ordinary means—even by the aid of a pair of compasses
and a common divided scale—and incomparably more so,
when observed by a telescope, as it is now usually done,
with a micrometer attached to it.   But the corresponding distance of the surfaces is only about one 7400th
part of this space ; and if we pass from the fifth to the
first of the rings, assuming the law which governs their
distances to be established, it will be found to be one
37000th part of it only, or about one 180,000th part
of an inch.

There is no refinement of art in the construction and
use of micrometers, aided by all the artifices of calculation which the discoveries of analysis have enabled us
to apply to the reduction of repeated observations, which
can give the absolute measure of a magnitude so minute

as this, though we can sometimes make an approximation to it in the estimate of the minute differences
of greater magnitudes from each other.[a]

Upon the accuracy of measures, such as those which
are now under our consideration,—though many other
means are available for the purpose,—will be chiefly
founded (as we shall afterwards see) our knowledge of
the lengths of the undulations of the different rays of
the prismatic spectrum.

It is not our intention to attempt a detailed description of the whole progress of the light concerned in
the production of these rings, and it would hardly be
practicable to do so, without the aid of figures to guide
the eye as well as the understanding of the reader.
When they are produced by white light, they present
a succession of colours very variously intermixed, and
of very various intensities, the first of the series, or
the central spot, being black, followed by rings of very
faint blue, brilliant white, and then yellow, orange and
red, and so on, forming a succession of orders between
the dark and bright rings which Newton has very
accurately defined and which, from being capable of
perpetual reproduction, possess no inconsiderable philosophical value, as an invariable scale or standard
with which any observed colours may be compared.

If, however, instead of white, we employ homogeneous light, whether red, or yellow, or blue, the
rings are increased .in number and distinctness,

[a] Frauenhofer, the justly celebrated theoretical and practical optician
of Munich, is said to have constructed a micrometric apparatus of a
delicacy so extreme as to enable him to appreciate as minute a quantity
as 1-50,000th of an inch. See Sir J. Herschel's Treatise on Light, § 741.
The arrangements made by Mr. Sheepshanks for the measurement of the
bars, which have been selected for the Parliamentary standards, have
hardly attained an accuracy equal to this.

but are mere alternations of colour and blackness
or obscurity, the colour developed being that of
the homogeneous ray only ; the series of rings also
which correspond to the more refrangible rays of the
spectrum are wider and the corresponding distances
of the surfaces of the lenses greater, than for those
which are less so. But in all cases, the dark rings
correspond to distances which follow the order of the
even numbers, and the bright or coloured rings to
those which are odd: those distances for the red being
greater than for the violet rays nearly in the proportion of 5 to 3, or, as Newton observed, more nearly
that of 14 to 9.

This recurrence of dark and bright or coloured rings,
more especially in homogeneous light, at successive
points where the distances of the surfaces are determined by multiplying the first distance, where a bright
ring appears, by the natural numbers, necessarily connects the phenomena with those distances.

Such are the appearances presented by the rings seen
by reflection. Let us now endeavour to trace the course
of the light which appears to be concerned in their production. In this examination we shall confine our attention to those cases where the direction of the light is
perpendicular to the surfaces of the lenses which bound
the interposed lamina of air ; for oblique incidences,
the explanation is by no means so simple, involving
some considerations of a much less obvious nature.

Of the light which reaches in succession the two surfaces of the lamina of air interposed between two lenses,
a portion is reflected at each of them, and it will be found
of importance to keep in mind, in the case under consideration, that the first of these reflections takes place
at the surface of a rarer, the second at that of a denser

medium: and assuming the quantity of reflected light to bear the same proportion—and a small proportion only—to that which is transmitted—the reflected beams at the two surfaces will not be very different in intensity.[a] Now it is obvious, that the light reflected at the second surface, after traversing, from one surface to the other and back again, twice the thickness of the interposed lamina, will *interfere* with the light reflected from the first; and as they are nearly equal in intensity they will destroy each other or nearly so, and produce darkness when they are in opposite phases, and will corroborate each other—producing a quadruple illumination or nearly so—when they are in the same. Such are the minimum and maximum effects. For intermediate distances the effects will be also intermediate, gradually increasing in illumination in passing from one to the other and conversely.

At the central point where the distance of the reflecting surfaces is evanescent, there is a black spot, or the two beams of reflected light destroy each other by interference: but inasmuch as they traverse the same space, this effect can only take place by supposing one of them either to lose or to gain half an undulation by the act of reflection. Other observations, which Dr. Young has pointed out, will show that this effect always takes place, when light is reflected at the surface of a rarer medium, as in the case of the upper of the two surfaces which bound the intermediate lamina of air.[b]

---

[a] The series of such reflections and transmissions will be indefinite, but as much the greatest part of the beam reflected at the second surface is transmitted at the first, the portion of it which is again reflected is very small, and does not very materially influence the circumstances of the phenomenon. In the complete solution of the problem, by analysis, all the terms of this series are taken into account.

[b] Works, vol. i. p. 175 and p. 287. c.

If we pass from the central spot, the successive dark
rings will appear at successive points where the duplicate distances of the surfaces are in arithmetical progression: if λ be the second term of this series—0 or
the evanescent distance at the central spot being the
first—the series of distances will be represented by
0, λ, 2λ, 3λ, &c., &c.; and it is manifest that if we assume
λ to be the length of an undulation, the two reflected
beams from the two bounding surfaces of the interposed
lamina—assuming half an undulation to be lost at the
first reflection—will be found to be in opposite phases
of their vibrations when they concur, and therefore in
entire discordance with each other :—under such circumstances therefore no light or very little is reflected
and reaches the eye.

If the series of bright rings be likewise observed,
they will be found to appear at successive points, whose
duplicate distances will be similarly represented by the
terms of the arithmetical series $\dfrac{\lambda}{2}, \dfrac{3\lambda}{2}, \dfrac{5\lambda}{2}, \dfrac{7\lambda}{2}$, &c.,
which are exactly intermediate to those of the former
series. When, therefore, the portion of the beam
transmitted at the first surface—without suffering
any change in the state of its vibration—returns
to it again, it will be found in an opposite phase
and therefore in entire accordance with the inverted
phase of the beam reflected from the first surface :
the undulations will therefore entirely corroborate each
other, and the light will be quadrupled or nearly so.

Again, if different coloured rays are employed in
these experiments, the rings of the same order will
be found widest, and therefore the corresponding
distances, from the central point longest, for the red or
most refrangible rays, and the corresponding rings

narrowest and the distances least for the violet, or least refrangible rays : and if, instead of homogeneous, we employ white, light, the succession of rings will form what has been termed *Newton's scale,* produced by the overlapping and irregular intermixture of the rings corresponding to the different rays of the prismatic spectrum ; these rings are consequently less numerous, and those which are more remote are much less distinct, than such as are formed by homogeneous light.   The distances of the two points of reflection at which the successive dark or obscure and bright rings appear—the first of the latter of which is a brilliant white—is such as would correspond nearly to the length of the undulation of a mean ray of the spectrum, intermediate between the yellow and the green.

The lengths of the undulations of light of different colours which are deduced from the preceding theory, will be found to enter as essential elements into the explanation and calculation of many other cases of the production of colours, and more especially of the bands of diffraction, under the very various circumstances under which they are observed ; and the determinations of those lengths founded upon these different classes of phenomena will be found to be entirely consistent with each other.

It was to one of the earlier and most remarkable of the speculations of Newton, that Young was indebted—as he has fully acknowledged[a]—for the important suggestion of the unequal lengths of the undulations of light of different colours, and for their connection with the production of the particular phenomena which we have just been considering : but there was wanting his principle of the *interference of light* to make this sug-

* Works, vol. i. p. 145.

gestion available for its application to their complete
analysis and the removal of the nearly insuperable difficulties which were otherwise presented by their theory.
    At a later period of life Newton proposed his hypo-
thesis of the fits of easy *transmission* and *reflection*,
not as a consequence of his theory of emanations—with
which it is hardly possible to connect it—but as a convenient mode of enunciating the law which is found to
determine the formation and succession of the rings.
It is not possible to do justice to this celebrated hypothesis by any brief description of it, as it requires to
be guarded by many conditions to make it generally
applicable to the phenomena : but if we assume the
intervals which separate the alternate state of the rays
of different colours, when they are *easily transmissible*
or *easily reflexible*, to be equal to half the lengths of
the corresponding undulations, the consequences to
which it leads will be immediately translateable into
those which we have just deduced from the undulatory theory.
    We have before referred to the necessity of supposing
that light reflected at the surface of a rarer medium
loses half an undulation ; a conclusion which Young felt
to be inevitable, if it was attempted, upon the principles of his theory, to account for the black spot at the
point of contact of the two lenses, or at the summit of
a soap-bubble, when, before bursting, it is reduced to
an evanescent thinness.
    In order to test the correctness of this hypothesis, he
ventured to predict, that if the substance of the interposed lamina bounded by the reflecting surfaces, was intermediate in refractive power to the two mediums which
contained it, the order of the rings would be reversed and
that a white central spot would replace the black which,

under other circumstances, was always observable : for
this purpose he interposed oil of sassafras, which answers
the required conditions, when one of the two lenses, between which it was interposed, was of flint and the
other of crown glass ; he then found as he had anticipated that the central spot seen by reflected light
was white and was succeeded by a dark ring.[a] This
was a *crucial* experiment and completely established
this interesting and very important fact.

A similar loss of half an undulation is observed to take
place when reflections are made at the surfaces of some
metals, as gold and silver ; also in some extraordinary
refractions, and very generally in very oblique reflections.

We shall not enter upon the discussion of the
dynamical or other considerations which have been
suggested both by Young and Fresnel to account
for this inversion of the phase of the undulation,
under the circumstances above enumerated : the principles involved in such suggestions are necessarily to
a great extent hypothetical, in consequence of our
ignorance of the physical constitution of the ethereal
medium, whose vibrations are assumed to constitute
light.

It was further ascertained by Newton, that if water,
oil, or other transparent media, instead of air, be interposed between the lenses, the rings continue to follow
the same law, but are contracted in diameter, and the
corresponding distances between the surfaces, and consequently the intervals between the fits of easy transmission and reflection, and therefore the *velocity of
progression* of the undulations, is diminished, and that
in the inverse proportion of the refractive powers of the

a Works, vol. i. p. 175.

media. The necessary inference to be drawn from this fact is, that the velocity of light is also less, the greater the refractive power of the medium through which it is transmitted; a fact of fundamental importance and in direct contradiction to the only conclusion, when light is considered as the emanation of material particles, which is derived from that theory.[a]

It was assumed by Huygens[b] in his proof of the constancy of the sines of incidence and refraction in passing from one medium to another, that the velocity of propagation of the undulations was in the inverse proportion of the refractive powers of the media through which they are propagated; the same conclusion therefore, as Young has most justly remarked, which is so adverse to the truth of one theory, is absolutely necessary to that of its rival.

Young again followed in the footsteps of the admirable observations of Newton in the application of his doctrine to the explanation of the colours of thick plates; and he was not less successful in its application to a class of phenomena, of what he terms *mixed* plates, not previously observed. When two pieces of plate glass, with drops of moisture intermixed with air interposed between them, were viewed against a candle or other strong light, fringes of colour were observed to be produced, which are accounted for by conceiving one, of two neighbouring rays of light, to

---

[a] Principia, lib. i., prop. 94.

[b] Théorie de la Lumière. No subsequent addition has been made to the completeness and conclusiveness of this investigation. Dr. Young refers to Barrow's demonstration of it in his Lectiones Opticæ, published in 1669; but it not only does not involve the theory of undulations, but, though edited and corrected by Newton himself, it is partly founded upon considerations of circular motion more worthy of the philosophy of the schoolmen than the opening era of the true laws of mechanical action.

pass through water and the other through air; and inasmuch as the velocity of the ray through water is about one-third less than the velocity of that through air, the first will be found in entire discordance with the other—forming a dark fringe—when the plates are distant from each other by the length of an undulation and a half. This distance is six times as great as that of two surfaces, when the same destructive interference takes place in a thin plate of air. If oil and water be employed, whose refractive powers differ much less from each other than water and air, the differences of the velocities of the rays transmitted through them will be much reduced and the same succession of phenomena will be observable, when the plates are still further separated from each other.[a]

The progress of Dr. Young in the application of his theory and of the principle of interference derived from it, to some of the most remarkable cases of the production of colour, had thus far been triumphant: he had hitherto met with difficulties, but no failures; and subsequent investigations and experiments have fully established the general correctness both of his reasoning and conclusions.

He now approached the great problem of Diffractions, in which we shall find that his success was much less complete: and though he was singularly fortunate in devising a fundamental experiment, which removed all reasonable doubt with respect to the connection of the phenomena which they exhibit with the great principle which he had discovered, and though he succeeded in founding upon it a general explanation of them which was not very different from the truth, he failed in the complete solution of the problem, chiefly,

[a] Works. vol. i. p. 173, and p. 300.

though not entirely, in consequence of its requiring analytical processes for estimating the results of the interference of any number of undulations and under any circumstances and also of integrating their effects, which Fresnel was the first to investigate and apply at a much later period.

When an object is placed in a very small beam of light or in a cone of rays diverging from an extremely small point, such as a sunbeam admitted through a small pinhole into a dark chamber, its shadow—if received upon a screen or the opposite wall—will exhibit fringes of colour, following its contour, whatever be its form, at nearly the same distance from it, " like the lines," says Sir J. Herschel, " along the sea-coast in a map." In ordinary light, three only of these fringes are to be seen ; the first being very bright and the last extremely faint : but in homogeneous light their number is much greater.   They are absolutely independent of the form of the edge or of the nature of the substance of the body which forms them, whether one be thick or thin, or the other be dense or rare.

The first of these circumstances would naturally lead us to conclude that the fringes were not dependant, for their formation, upon the reflection of rays from the edge ; the second that they were not inflected or deflected by an attractive or repulsive force, as in other cases of material action.

If a very thin slip of card, a wire or a hair, be placed within a similar beam or cone of light—so that the light passes on both sides of it—besides the external fringes on each side of the shadow, there will be observable within it bands of colour parallel to its edges, of which the central and brightest band is always white.   If the angle of a square object be similarly interposed, internal coloured bands will be observed in the form of hyperbolic curves, on each side of the diagonal which is luminous and white.

It was with reference to these internal bands that Dr. Young made the fortunate observation, that if all the light on one side of the object be intercepted, the bands will entirely disappear: thus showing decisively that the concurrence, or in other words, the *interference* of the rays of light passing on both sides of the object, is necessary to their formation.[a]

This was a *crucial* experiment, and may be considered as having constituted an important epoch in the history of the undulatory theory.

The phenomena of the external bands and the laws to which they are subject were observed and determined with his usual completeness and accuracy by Newton. He supposed the rays, on passing the object, to be deflected by a repulsive force; those nearer more so than those more remote, those more refrangible than those which were less so : in passing the edge also they were further supposed to be bent several times backwards and forwards by a motion *like that of an eel*, and the luminous molecules to be thrown off at one or other of the points of contrary flexure of the serpentine curve which they thus describe. To account for the interior bands, he supposed the repulsive forces to become attractive, and the rays to be *inflected* and not *deflected*; but it would appear that his more critical examination of their phenomena and formation was interrupted at the time he was first engaged in these researches, and was never afterwards resumed.

He was enabled by this theory to account for the

extension of the visible beyond the geometrical shadow, for the hyperbolic form of its outline and also of its conterminous fringes, as well as for the brightness of the fringes themselves, which are thus made to absorb all the light which would otherwise have occupied the space between the visible and geometrical shadow.

Though these hypotheses led to a tolerably correct representation of the form of the shadow and of its fringes, they were not reconcileable, for reasons which we have already referred to, to any recognised laws of material action. We trace their influence, however, in various subsequent speculations connected with the explanation of the phenomena of diffraction, and they would appear to have conducted a very distinguished writer to a very complex theory—which makes the rays of light to differ in inflexibility as well as refrangibility, and also in their capacity of deflection as well as inflexion, when they pass near the edge of a body which repels or attracts them—which makes colour devclopable by reflection as well as by refraction—which ascribes the colours of natural bodies generally to the different reflexibilities of the rays, and sometimes to their flexibilities—which makes the different rays of the spectrum material particles of different sizes.

The hypotheses of Newton with respect to the origin and formation of the exterior bands in diffraction were replaced, in Young's solution of the problem, by others more conformable to his own theory : he supposed the rays reflected from the edge of the body, by which the light passed, after losing half an undulation in the act of reflection, to interfere with the rays whose course was uninterrupted.

This hypothesis was found sufficient to explain the

formation of the bands of colour, the extension of the
visible beyond the geometrical shadow and the hyperbolic curves, in which they were always found; and
upon a comparison of the results of this theory with
Newton's measures and his own,[a] he found an agreement between them so close, as appeared to afford a
sufficient warrant of its truth. Differences, however,
were remarked by him, which were afterwards found,
as we shall see, to be due to an error in the hypothesis.
These bands, in fact, are not produced, or at the most
in a very slight degree, by the interference of the
reflected with the unobstructed rays.

If the accordance between the results of observation
and this theory had not been so close as it was found
to be, some very obvious objections to its correctness
could hardly have failed to receive from him much
earlier consideration than was given to them; for the
bands were found to be independant of the form and
substance of the reflecting edge, whether thin or thick,
polished or rough, polygonal or curved; all of them
circumstances which could not fail to affect both the
quantity and the direction of the reflected rays.
Neither was the quantity of such rays, which this
source could be reasonably supposed to supply, sufficient for the production of the phenomena.

The further condition which required the assumption
of the loss of half an undulation in the act of reflection
at an extreme obliquity, would appear, however, to
have been sufficiently justified by its loss in similar
reflections in other cases.

The problem of diffraction was made the special
subject of a memoir which Fresnel presented to the
Institute in 1815, and which was published, with seve-

---

[a] Works, vol. i., p. 181.

ral modifications in the *Annales de Chimie* for the
following year. The distances of the bands made by
a wire placed in a diverging beam of light, from the
axis of the beam, were determined by a method more
accurate and complete than any that had been applied
to their measurement before; and he also repeatedly
observed, as Young had done previously, the disappearance of the interior bands when the light which passed
on one side of the wire was intercepted before it
reached the screen, or rather the eye-glass of the
observer which was made use of in its place.

It was by reflecting upon this last fundamental
observation, that he was led to the conclusion that, as
the light from both sides of the wire was thus absolutely necessary to the existence of the bands within
the shadow, their formation was produced by the mixture or interference of those streams of light, under
certain conditions, with each other : from thence he
was led to the re-discovery of the principle of interference and many of its applications, which Young had
made thirteen years before, but of which he would
appear to have been ignorant at the time that his memoir was first presented to the Institute.

It was his friend Arago—who had been appointed
by the Institute, in conjunction with Prony, to
report upon this Memoir—who first made known to
Fresnel that both his theory and his most important
experiments had been long since anticipated by Dr.
Young; and it is but an act of justice to the memory of
that eminent philosopher, to acknowledge that neither
on this nor on any subsequent occasion did he claim for
himself the merit of the discoveries which others had
made before him.

The solution of the problem of diffraction, which is

given in this memoir of Fresnel, though mathematically much more complete than that of Young, involves precisely the same principles which he had assumed, and leads to few conclusions which he had not fully indicated, though he had omitted altogether, as he was too much in the habit of doing, the mathematical investigations upon which they rested, replacing them by reasonings expressed in ordinary language; Fresnel followed also the example of his predecessor in deriving his interfering rays from reflection at the edge of the interposed object, and also assumed, what the calculations required, that they lost half an undulation in the act of reflection.

The results of his subsequent investigations on this subject were embodied in a second memoir, which was crowned by the French Academy in 1819, and which has contributed more than any publication which preceded it, to bring the laws of the undulatory theory under the dominion of analysis.

We have already seen that Dr. Young had considered the interference of undulations in two extreme cases only, when they were equal in the amplitude of their vibrations, and either in the same or in opposite phases; the amplitude of the resulting vibration being doubled, and its illuminating power quadrupled in one case, and both of them reduced to zero in the other.

Fresnel viewed the problem in a much more general sense, where the amplitudes and the phases of the interfering vibrations differed in any manner whatever. If the undulations were of the same length, the resultant or equivalent undulation was of the same length likewise, and therefore produced light of the same colour, however different those undulations might be in phase

and amplitude, and therefore in illuminating power;
and whatever was the number of such interfering
undulations, the amplitude and phase of a single
undulation equivalent to them, was determinable by
processes analogous in their form and equally easy
in their application, with those which are employed
for determining the resultant of mechanical forces,
however different in magnitude and direction, when
acting upon a material point.

The undulations issuing from a luminous point are
found in successive instants of time in spherical surfaces expanding with the velocity of light, the intensity
of illumination in passing in succession from one to
another of those surfaces varying as the inverse square
of their distances from their common centre.   If we
suppose any one of these expanding spherical waves of
light to continue to be maintained in the same state,
by the perpetual issue of streams from the primitive
source, we may altogether suppress the consideration
of this primitive source of supply, and suppose all the
undulations, which reach any point of space beyond it,
to issue from every point of this spherical surface, as
forming innumerable though immeasurably feebler new
sources of light, from which it is propagated by the same
laws; thus if we suppose any portion of this diverging
sphere to be cut off by an obstacle, or even the whole
of what is not transmitted through a circular or other
aperture to be thus arrested, we may consider this
unobstructed portion of the spherical surface, whether
adjoining such object or aperture or at any point of
space beyond it, as alone concerned in the illumination
of any ulterior point of space : in other words, " *the
vibrations of a luminous wave at any one of its points
may be considered as the sum of the elementary move-*

ments conveyed to it at the same moment, from the separate action of all the portions of the unobstructed wave considered in any one of its anterior positions.[a]

This is the principle which Huygens has very distinctly announced in his *Théorie de la Lumière*. He had derived it by reasoning upon the constitution of elastic fluids, considering every point of a wave as a new centre of disturbance, from which undulations are propagated, similar in character, though less in degree, to those which originate in the primary cause which excites them. The conclusion to which this principle would apparently have led him, would have been the same as that which formed the chief obstacle, in Newton's mind, to the admission of the undulatory theory, if it had not been limited by another principle of hardly less importance, by which it was assumed that those undulations alone which *concur*, at any given point, not only with each other but with the primary wave which passes through it, so as to form a common tangent with it, are efficient in producing the impression of light; this *principle of concurrence* or *non-concurrence*, may be shown, from very simple geometrical considerations, to be equivalent to the *principle of interference*, which alone gives a demonstration of its truth, and without which it would otherwise continue to rest upon a bare assumption only.

But even subject to this limitation—important and fundamental as it was—the conception and enunciation of these principles does immortal honour to this great geometer, who applied them with singular clearness and sagacity, not merely to the explanation of the

---

[a] This is the form in which this principle is enunciated by Fresnel. By a wave is meant the great spherical wave which embraces at the same moment all the undulations issuing in every direction from the common luminous point.

reflection and refraction of light in accordance with this theory, but also, with the aid of spheroidal instead of spherical waves, to the determination of the course of the extraordinary ray in Iceland spar; a problem of the highest order of difficulty, whose solution, equally remarkable for its completeness and geometrical elegance, was unfortunately left unnoticed or unknown until the beginning of the present century. We are indebted to Dr. Young for the first suggestion and to Dr. Wollaston for the first complete demonstration of its value, as giving results which are in strict accordance with the observed laws of double refraction, which Newton had unfortunately mistaken and misstated.

By the aid of the principle of Huygens and of the interference of light—viewed in its widest sense—as applied to the estimation of the effect of the concurrence of any number of undulations with each other, however different in phase and amplitude, Fresnel was enabled to effect the complete solution of the problem of diffraction in those cases where the difficulties in the integrations which it involved, were not beyond the powers of his analysis.

Such, among several others, were those where light passed on one side of an object with a straight edge, forming the external fringes only, or by both sides of a thin card, wire or hair, so as to form the internal as well as external fringes; no account was, in either case, taken of the light reflected from the edges of the object, as in all former investigations. The results of calculation for homogeneous light were found, after the most accurate measurement, to agree· almost exactly with observation, thus enabling him to show, not only that the reflected light was not required for the production of the phenomena, but also, though in a very slight degree, inconsistent with them.

It is not easy to estimate too highly the importance of the principles developed, of the formulæ and processes investigated and of the problems solved, in this justly celebrated Memoir. Questions which had previously been treated vaguely and imperfectly by estimating general effects and tendencies only, were henceforth brought within the reach of accurate calculation, where every element contributing to the result was capable of being taken into account. The particular results also, which the application of these principles lead to, were such as were calculated to remove many prepossessions to which Newton himself had given way and which had exercised a fatal influence upon the progress of optical science. A complete answer was thus given to the great objection to the undulatory theory, that it was not reconcileable with the existence of shadows, and an end was finally put to the necessity of seeking for the explanation of the principal phenomena of diffraction by the aid of hypotheses which in most cases were not only arbitrary, but altogether opposed to all just conceptions of mechanical action.

The first feeling which was produced on Dr. Young's mind, when Arago communicated to him the results of Fresnel's investigations, was one of mortification.

" Perhaps you will suspect," says he,[a] "that I am not a little provoked to think that so immediate a consequence of the Huygenian system, as that which M. Fresnel has most ingeniously deduced, should have escaped myself when I was endeavouring to apply it to the phenomena in question; but in fact I am still at a loss to conceive the possibility of the thing ;

[a] Works, vol. i., p. 388.

for if light has at all times so great a tendency to diverge into the path of the neighbouring rays, and to interfere with them, as Huygens supposes, I do not see how it escapes being totally extinguished in a very short space, even in the most transparent medium, as I have observed in my first paper on the subject."[a]

The subsequent perusal of the Memoir, and an explanatory and very flattering letter from its author, removed every remaining doubt and hesitation from his mind.

"I return you a thousand thanks," says he, in writing to M. Fresnel,[b] "for the gift of your admirable Memoir, which deserves a very high rank amongst the writings which have most contributed to the progress of Optics. I have not the least intention of insisting upon the influence of the rays reflected from the edges of the opaque body. I was perfectly aware, that when light is admitted through two parallel slits, the interfering rays must be derived from the middle of each of them, as may be seen from figure 442 in my Lectures; but I had not conceived the happy idea of analyzing the results of the several undulations, in which you have succeeded so completely, and what prevented my doing so, was the difficulty I felt of appreciating the just effect of the obliquity, which you have not found it necessary to include in your calculations."

After noticing a slight error in a calculation contained in his letter to M. Arago, which Fresnel had very obligingly corrected, he adds:—

"You will see by the little table of tides which I have sent with this letter, that the true mode of considering a combination of undulations was sufficiently familiar to me."[c]

He then describes a construction, by which the amplitude of the resultant of two or more equal undulations of given phases is determined.

[a] Works, vol. i., p. 149.   [b] Works, vol. i., p. 393.
[c] Works, ibid.

There are some other subjects, noticed in these optical Memoirs of Dr. Young, to which we shall very briefly refer.

The repetitions of colours, which are sometimes observed within the common primary rainbow, and without the secondary, are capable of a sufficient explanation by the principle of interference, if we suppose the drops of rain or vapour, where such supernumerary rainbows appear, to be of nearly uniform size.[a] Under such circumstances the faint light, which would otherwise be diffused for a very considerable space beneath the ordinary bow, is distributed, by the effect of interference, into concentric rings, whose magnitude will be dependent upon the diameter of the drops : but if the drops, as is most commonly the case, are not equal to each other, the several sets of rings corresponding to different classes of drops of the same diameter, will be mixed up with each other, and, by their combination, produce the effect of white light.

Again when a very fine fibre is held near the eye before a very small hole in a card, so as to intercept a great part of the light of a distant luminous object, fringes of different colours are formed, whose distances are greater the less the diameter of the fibre; and if, instead of such a fibre, a great number of fibres of uniform diameters, crossed in all directions, are held before it, these fringes will form rings by their combination. Such would be the effect produced by a lock of wool of uniform texture, whose fibres cross in all directions; such also would be the effect produced by the minute particles of blood or the extremely minute seed-vessels of some plants, such as those of the *lycoperdon bovistæ*; and inasmuch as the smaller the diameter of

---

[a] Works, vol. i., p. 185 and p. 293.

the fibre or particle, the greater is that of the ring which it forms at a given distance from it, we are enabled, by measuring the distances at which a ring of given diameter is produced, to form a scale by which the diameters of such particles or fibres can be not only compared with each other but determined also, when the unit of the scale is once ascertained, by measuring the distance corresponding to some other fibre or spherule whose diameter is otherwise known : but if the fibres or particles are of different sizes, no such ring will be formed.   This was the principle of the Eriometer—an ingenious instrument devised by Dr. Young, admitting of many useful applications, and which has not received the degree of attention to which its real importance entitles it.[a]

The invisible rays, formerly known as the dark rays of Ritter, the existence of which beyond the violet end of the spectrum was ascertained by their chemical action, and which had been recently noticed by Dr. Wollaston,[b] were made to form, by an ingenious application of the solar microscope which was devised by Dr. Young, dark impressions upon paper or leather dipped in muriate of silver, of the rings reflected from a thin plate of air, as in the colours of thin plates,[c] at distances corresponding to their proper place in their spectrum.   This experiment was of great interest, not merely as establishing the close analogy which exists between the visible and invisible rays, but also as one of the first attempts to form a real photographic picture, though without any anticipation of the very important uses to which the principle involved in it was afterwards to be applied.[d]

---

[a] Works, vol. i. pp. 172, 305, and 346. [b] Philosophical Transactions, 1802.
[c] Works, vol. i. p. 190.   [d] See Philosophical Magazine for May, 1854.

We have before had occasion to refer to the attacks which were made on Dr. Young's Optical Papers, almost immediately after their publication, in the early numbers of the Edinburgh Review. They are assumed, upon sufficient internal evidence, to have been written by Lord Brougham, and exhibit all the characteristics of his vigorous style, and truly formidable sarcasm: and it would be difficult to refer to another example where the irresponsible power of anonymous criticism has been so unscrupulously exercised, or where the effects which it produced were so long and so injuriously felt.

We have given some specimens of these criticisms in a footnote at page 192 of the first volume of Dr. Young's Works. We shall subjoin a few others in connection with some observations of our own on the subjects to which they refer.

After noticing some changes of opinion and of views which the progress of his researches had induced Dr. Young to make—and which were pardonable in so novel and difficult an inquiry—the reviewer adds:—

"It is difficult to deal with an author whose mind is filled with a medium of so fickle and vibratory a nature. Were we to take the trouble of refuting him, he might tell us, ' *My opinion is changed*, and *I have abandoned that hypothesis, but here is another for you.*' We demand, if the world of science which Newton once illuminated, is to be as changeable in its modes as the world of fashion, which is directed by the nod of a silly woman or a pampered fop? Has the Royal Society degraded its publications into bulletins of new and fashionable theories for the ladies of the Royal Institution? *Proh pudor!* Let the Professor continue to amuse his audience with an endless variety of such harmless trifles, but in the name of science, let them not find admittance into that venerable repository which contains the works of Newton, and Boyle, and Cavendish, and Maskelyne, and Herschel.

" These remarks lead us to observe, that perpetual fluc-
tuation and change of ground is the common lot of theorists.
An hypothesis which is assumed from a fanciful analogy or
adopted from its apparent capacity of explaining certain appearances, must always be varied as new facts occur, and must be
kept alive by a repetition of the same process of touching and
retouching, of successive accommodation and adaptation, to which
it originally owed its puny and contemptible existence. But the
making of an hypothesis is not the discovery of a truth. It is
a mere sporting with the subject; it is a sham fight which may
amuse in the moment of idleness and relaxation, but will neither
gain victories over prejudice and error, nor extend the empire of
science. A mere theory is in truth destitute of merit of every
kind, except that of a warm and misguided imagination. It
demonstrates neither patience of investigation, nor rich resources of skill, nor vigorous habits of attention, nor powers of
abstracting and comparing, nor extensive acquaintance with
nature. It is the unmanly and unfruitful pleasure of a boyish
prurient imagination, or the gratification of a corrupted and de-
praved appetite.

" If, however, we condescend to amuse ourselves in this
manner we have a right to demand that the entertainment shall
be of the right sort, and that the hypothesis shall be so consistent with itself, and so applicable to the facts, as not to
require perpetual mending and patching; that the child that
we stoop to play with shall be tolerably healthy, and not of
the puny, sickly nature of Dr. Young's productions, which have
scarcely *stamina* to subsist until the fruitful parent has furnished
us with a new litter, to make way for which, he knocks on
the head, or more barbarously exposes the first."

Dr. Young, in his reply, has very justly defined the
proper limitation to be imposed upon the use of hypotheses in the conduct of philosophical inquiries, and
has shown that he was not guilty of the charge, either
of rashly fabricating or capriciously abandoning those
which he had proposed, which was brought against
him in this eloquent tirade.

" In order to answer the charge of inconsistency in my

opinions respecting the nature of light, I must begin by observing, that there are two general methods of communicating knowledge ; the one analytical, where we proceed from the examination of effects to the investigation of causes ; the other synthetical, where we first lay down the causes, and deduce from them the particular effects. In the synthetical manner of explaining a new theory we necessarily begin by assuming principles, which ought, in such a case, to bear the modest name of hypothesis ; and when we have compared their consequences with all the phænomena, and have shown that the agreement is perfect, we may justly change the temporary term *hypothesis* into *theory.* This mode of reasoning is sufficient to attach a value and importance to our theory, but it is not fully decisive with respect to its exclusive truth, since it has not been proved that no other hypothesis will agree with the facts.

" It is exactly in this manner that I have endeavoured to proceed in my researches. By analysing the experiments of Newton, and comparing them with my own, I had arrived at principles, to which I gave, in my paper on the Theory of Light, the unassuming title of hypotheses ; after comparing these principles with all the phænomena of light, and showing their perfect consistency, I thought myself authorised to make a conclusion, in my ninth proposition, which converts the hypothesis into a theory. I was justified in doing this, because no man had ever attempted to advance a theory which would bear to be compared mathematically with the phænomena that I enumerated. But according to the nature of the only mode of reasoning which the circumstances allowed me, it was impossible to infer, from this synthetical comparison, that no other suppositions would agree with the phænomena ; and *I expressly remarked*, with respect to one of the four hypotheses which I laid down, that it was possible to find *others which might be substituted for it.* It is in this hypothesis and its consequences only, that I have since attempted to make any improvements." [a]

After endeavouring to show that Newton had never spoken of the undulatory theory of light, even in his earlier essays, except as a vague hypothesis which

[a] Works, vol. i., p. 203.

deserved no credit, except for its applicability to a few facts, and that in later life he had entirely repudiated it, the reviewer proceeds as follows :—

" It is hardly possible to conceive a wider difference than that which subsists between the philosophy of Newton and the philosophy of Dr. Young. While the former utterly rejects hypotheses and asserts that our stock of facts is insufficient : the latter says we have enow of experiments and that we only require a stock of hypotheses. Newton proposes queries for the investigation of his successors. Dr. Young claims the inheritance and vainly imagines that he fulfils this destination by ringing changes on these hypotheses, arguing from them, as if they were experiments or demonstrations, twisting them into a partial coincidence with the clumsy imaginations of his own brain, and pompously parading what Newton left as hints, in a series of propositions, with all the affectation of system. After all, it may be said, Newton amused himself with hypotheses, and so may Dr. Young ; admitting that the Doctor's relaxations were the same with his predecessor's, it must be remembered that the queries of Newton were given to the world at the close of the most brilliant career of solid discovery, that any mortal was ever permitted to run. The sports in which such a veteran might well be allowed to relax his mind, are mere idleness in the young soldier who has never fleshed his sword ; and though the world would gaze with interest upon every such occupation of the former, they would turn with disgust from the forward and idle attempts of the latter to obtrude upon them his awkward gambols."

It will be found, however, upon an examination of his works, that at no period of his life was Newton indisposed "to amuse himself" in the framing of hypotheses. It is true, that in the Principia, they very rarely appear : but the great laws of the material world which form the subject of that work were so distinct and patent before him, that the resort to hypotheses was almost entirely unnecessary.

The case is very different, however, with his Optics,

the materials of which, though chiefly prepared in early, were put together and published, in later life—where we find hypotheses proposed, not merely with a view to give expression to the laws which appear to govern observed phenomena, but also as suggestions of the probable or possible physical causes in which such phenomena originate. The mind of this illustrious man was, in fact, naturally imaginative, and his early communications to the Royal Society—many of which are found in Dr. Birch's History only—show how much he delighted in the most adventurous speculations on the cause of gravity and of those various mysterious powers to which light, heat, magnetism, and electricity owe their origin and propagation.

The theory of light, as might be expected from the zeal and success with which he studied its laws, naturally occupied the first place in these speculations.

Was it solely caused by the vibrations of an ether, whose unequal undulations produced the impressions of different colours, like those of sound producing different tones, though all of them were propagated with the same velocity? Or were the rays corporeal, producing the vibrations of this ether, as an exciting cause? Or were they simple emanations of corporeal particles of different magnitudes, producing their impressions without the intervention of any ether whatsoever?

A quotation given by Dr. Young, in support of one of his fundamental hypotheses,[a] develops the first of these proposed theories—more especially as affecting the different refrangibility of the rays of light and the explanation of the colours of thin plates—with a

---

[a] Hypothesis III., Dr. Young's Works, vol. i., p. 144.

sagacity and clearness of conception, which is worthy of the highest admiration. It was in an answer to Hooke,—who either raised objections to every discovery or theory that Newton made or proposed, if he did not claim it as his own—that we find this remarkable exposition of what he terms, "the plain, genuine, and necessary conditions of such an hypothesis."

" But how," he further adds, " he will defend it from other difficulties I know not. For to me the fundamental supposition seems to be impossible ; namely, that the waves or vibrations of any fluid can, like the rays of light, be propagated in straight lines, without a continual and very extravagant spreading and bending every way into the quiescent medium where they are terminated by it. I mistake if there be not both experiment and demonstration to the contrary."

It was the influence of this fatal prepossession which induced him to combine, with his ether, the additional hypothesis of the corporeity of the rays, with a view of accounting with less difficulty for their rectilinear propagation ; and it was only in later life, when writing the Principia, that the naked theory of emanation was proposed, independently of any necessary combination with an ether.

After referring to the second of the theories of light which Newton suggested rather than maintained, the Reviewer proceeds to contrast it with Young's theory, which he somewhat strangely identifies with that of Euler :—

" But the clumsy hypothesis of Euler and Young is, that ether itself constitutes light ; and their object is to twist the facts into some sort of an agreement with what they conceive to be the laws of this fluid.

" From such a dull invention, nothing can be expected. It only removes all the difficulties under which the theory of light laboured, to the theory of the new medium which usurps its place. It is a mere change of name; it teaches no truth, reconciles no contradictions, arranges no anomalous facts, suggests no new experiments, and leads to no new inquiries.

" It has not even the pitiful merit of affording an agreeable play to the fancy. It is infinitely more useless and less ingenious than the Indian theory of the elephant and the tortoise. It may be ranked in the same class with that stupid invention of metaphysical theology, which, in order to account for the existence of evil, supposed the independent existence of an evil spirit; or that other notable contrivance, which to explain the power of the Deity over matter, ingeniously supposed that all matter was the Deity."

The objection, which is put in the preceding observations, refers rather to the difficulty of applying such a theory, than to the truth of the theory itself. We can subject to direct observation the properties of a fluid like water, as well as of the waves which it forms, and our knowledge of one set of properties can be made subservient to the extension of our knowledge of the other. The same course may be, and has been, pursued with respect to the elastic medium of air, its vibrations and the sounds which they produce. But the existence of the ether, whose vibrations are assumed to constitute light, is hypothetical only, and we are consequently precluded from all *a priori* knowledge of its properties as an aid to the investigation of their effects; and even the analogy with those effects in other elastic fluids is less instructive than it would otherwise be, in consequence of the enormous numbers which connect the lengths and the velocities of propagation of the real and observable, with the hypothetical, undulations which are supposed to constitute light.

But it is in the absence of those analogies—and even our assumptions respecting the general constitution of an elastic fluid must be founded on analogies with

those of such as are known—that we are left, when there
are no known physical principles to guide us, to those
hypotheses which the reviewer stigmatizes with such
unsparing severity. But such hypotheses, as the history of this and other sciences abundantly teaches us,
may be made—if the predictions which they afford us
are sufficiently verified—the secure bases of the most
certain conclusions.

The law of gravitation, when once discovered or
assumed, admitted not merely of a definite expression,
but required the aid of no supplementary principles, in
order to enable Newton to deduce from it the whole
system of the material world: although it presumed
not to reach as high as the final cause of gravity, it
caught up the chain of consequences deducible from
it, above the *nodal* point, as it were, from which its
various ramifications might be said to diverge. Our
position, however, with respect to the theory of light,
is very different. We have attained to various important truths respecting it, but much more remains
unexplained, and new facts are daily arising which may
or may not be explicable by principles already known,
or by others which are yet to be discovered. We
are still, therefore, far removed from the common
principle from which all others are derivable and which
may be hereafter destined to bind up, even the truths
which are established, into one consistent whole. It is
this want of physical principles which have a common
derivation, that renders all the resources of science and
skill inert and powerless before problems which may
hereafter be found, in another stage of our knowledge,
to admit of a complete and satisfactory solution. Such,
amongst many others that may be mentioned, are the
causes which produce the unequal dispersion and the

absorption of light of different colours in different media, or the changes in their refractive powers which some media have been recently shown to produce.

The appearance of the third and last of Dr. Young's Memoirs [a] which had been honoured, like the first, by being chosen, by the Council of the Royal Society, as the Bakerian Lecture for the year, was the signal for the renewal of these vehement outbursts of critical vituperation.

Determined, however, as the Reviewer had shown himself in his former critiques, to deny all merit, both to his experiments and his reasonings, he could hardly fail to be somewhat startled by the result of the well-known experiment which this Memoir records, of stopping the rays which passed on one side of a thin card or wire, exposed to a sunbeam admitted into a dark chamber, and which was found to obliterate the internal bands formed in its shadow whenever the light passed freely on both sides of it. After resorting to every expedient to explain away or evade the conclusion to which the experiment seemed inevitably to lead, the Reviewer, apparently dissatisfied with other solutions of the difficulty, concludes by cutting the Gordian knot, and denies altogether the accuracy of the experiment.

" The fact is," says he, " we believe the experiment was inaccurately made ; and we have not the least doubt, that if carefully repeated, it will be found either that the rays, when inflected, cross each other and thus form fringes, each portion on the side opposite to the point of its flection ; or that in stopping one portion, Dr. Young in fact stopped both portions ; a thing extremely likely, where the hand had only one-thirtieth of an inch to move in, and quite sufficient to account for all the fringes disappearing at once from the shadow."

[a] The three Memoirs were read to the Royal Society on the three successive years, 1801, 1802, and 1803.

" The Reviewer " (as Dr. Young justly observes in his reply) " has here afforded me an opportunity for a triumph as gratifying as any triumph can be where an enemy is so contemptible. Conscious of inability to explain the experiment, too ungenerous to confess that inability, and too idle to repeat the experiment, he is compelled to advance the supposition that it was incorrect, and to insinuate that my hand may easily have erred through a space so narrow as one-thirtieth of an inch. But the truth is, that my hand was not concerned, the screen was placed on a table and moved mechanically forwards with the utmost caution ; the experiment succeeded in some circumstances when the breadth of the object was doubled or tripled. Let him make the experiment and then deny the result if he can."[a]

Unjust and intemperate as these criticisms were, and utterly erroneous as were the views which they attempted to support, they were expressed generally in language so choice and felicitous as could hardly fail to charm an ignorant or indifferent reader. We find them intermixed also with passages which are remarkable for the correct and comprehensive view which they express of the proper mode of conducting philosophical inquiries, and quite worthy of those varied powers, the application of which, during a long and eventful life, will make the name of the great man to whom they have been commonly attributed, for ever memorable in the civil, the political and the literary history of this country. The effect which these powerful and repeated attacks produced upon the estimate of Dr. Young's scientific character was remarkable. The poison sank deep into the public mind, and found no antidote in reclamations of other journals of co-ordinate influence and authority. We consequently find that the subject of Dr. Young's researches remained absolutely unnoticed by men of science for many years.

The pamphlet which he wrote in reply to these

[a] Works, vol. i., p. 210.

criticisms, from which we have made several quotations, not only sufficiently vindicates his own scientific character, but retaliates upon his Reviewer with just severity.[a] If this reply had fallen into the hands of readers who were competent to appreciate the force of its statements, it could hardly have failed to secure a prompt recognition of the important discoveries which his Memoirs contained. It is stated, however, by Dr. Young, that one copy of it only was sold, and it would appear that no private means were resorted to, to make it generally known. It produced, therefore, no effect whatsoever in correcting the impressions which had been produced upon the public mind by the attacks of the Reviewer.

A letter from George Ellis shows the opinion which Dr. Young's more intimate friends entertained of this reply. "I thought it would be more satisfactory to you to hear the opinion entertained of your reply by persons more impartial than your Sunning Hill audience, and at the same time so intelligent as to make their opinions worth procuring. Canning read it with great attention, and the impression it made on him was exactly what I could have wished, namely, that the *malice and want of candour* of the Edinburgh Reviewer was fully made out, and that your explanation of your own meaning was perfectly satisfactory. He added that he thought if you had as good reasons as he supposed for feeling certain that Mr. Brougham was the author of the attack, you had treated him with rather too much lenity, and that you would have been fully justified in retorting on his Dissertation concerning 'inflection' all the ridicule which he had endeavoured to fix upon your 'interference of vibrations.' With this judgment I was

[a] Reprinted in Works, vol. i., p. 192.

well pleased, as I think that your answer, as it appeared to unprejudiced persons sufficiently full and satisfactory, is all the better for being too temperate."

It is but an act of justice, however, both to those who neglected as well as those who opposed the conclusions of these Memoirs, to admit that there is much in the form which they assumed, which made it very difficult to appreciate their value. Like all Young's early scientific writings, they were extremely obscure. The system also which he followed in this and other cases of superseding the usual forms of demonstration, whether geometrical or symbolical, by the use of ordinary language, and not unfrequently by suppressing such demonstrations altogether, imposed upon his readers a burden which few of them were able, and still fewer willing, to bear.

The correct conception also of undulations and their interferences, when not aided by the use of formulæ by which their conditions are very clearly and concisely expressible, is so difficult, that in default of such formulæ they could hardly have conveyed more than a very indistinct impression of their entire purport to the mind of the best instructed of his contemporaries. It was only by making Dr. Young's experiments the subject of special research, expanding his demonstrations when given, and replacing them when merely hinted at or omitted, that the entire correctness and coherence of his views, could be fully recognized.

It was reserved for Arago and for Fresnel to become, at a much later period, the expositors and interpreters of these Memoirs, and to rescue them from the neglect, which they had so long and so unhappily experienced from his own countrymen.

The reverence also attached in this country to whatever was sanctioned by the authority of Newton, operated not a little to retard the adoption of any methods of investigation which he had not used, or the acceptance of any conclusion or theory which he had repudiated.

At the period, of which we are now speaking, we had continued to retain, in this country, the notation of fluxions, in preference to that which was founded upon the much more expressive notation of Leibnitz, for fear of compromising the claim of his rival to the priority of its discovery; and we were thus, to a great extent, insulated, as it were, from the writings of the great mathematicians of the continent, who were greatly in advance of our own.[a]

It was the same principle which had nearly for three quarters of a century caused implicit trust to be placed in Newton's assertion that the dispersion of light, in every species of glass, was proportioned to its refractive power — notwithstanding some contemporary observations to the contrary—an assertion which effectually checked for many years the progress of inquiries for the improvement of refracting telescopes, by the correction of their chromatic aberration.

It was the same principle which also assigned to his erroneous statement of the law of double refraction in Iceland crystal, a superior authority to the correct measures and also to the correct theory of Huygens.

The influence of this hero-worship, which the history of the sciences shows to have prevailed from the age

---

[a] It was the writer of this Memoir who first introduced the notation of the differential calculus into the mathematical examinations in the Senate House at Cambridge: the effect was the production in a few years of a total revolution in the whole course of mathematical study.

of Aristotle to that of La Place,[a] is not much overstated, though carried to its utmost extent, in the following passage of a review of Dr. Young's Lectures, which refers to his theories of light.

"There is, it must be confessed, a presumption against the Huygenian theory, arising from the constant opposition which it experienced from Newton himself, and this presumption must derive weight from the known candour and modesty of his character, from his general indifference about speculative opinions, and from his exclusive anxiety to establish his facts on an irrefragable foundation. The phænomena of electricity, of heat and of light, have so many points of resemblance, that we seek to be led, by a sort of instinct, to consider them either as different affections of some highly rare and elastic fluid, which, in imitation of Newton, we call *ether*, or as separate fluids possessing, like ether, the power of traversing without resistance the pores of solid and fluid bodies, but distinguished from each other by some peculiar qualities. Since, therefore, Newton preferred to these simple hypotheses, the supposition that light is composed of seven species of particles of different dimensions, which are successively propelled in right lines from all luminous bodies with a velocity perfectly uniform, and which are accompanied and assisted in the production of certain phænomena by an attendant ether, we must conclude that he was compelled to adopt this mixed hypothesis, by the absolute impossibility of reconciling the facts, which he had ascertained, to any simpler theory. *If, therefore, he had contented himself with barely stating his dissent from every other opinion, without assigning his reasons for such dissent, we confess that our veneration for his high authority might have led us to acquiesce in his decision, and to conclude that a difficulty, which he was unable to solve, was in itself insoluble.*"

[a] See Works, vol. i., p. 220, note. So great was the influence of La Place's vehement opposition to the undulatory theory, that it was with the utmost difficulty that the powerful advocacy of Arago could secure from the Institute not favour, but justice, to the labours of Fresnel.

CHAPTER VII.

LECTURES: COHESION OF FLUIDS.

AFTER fulfilling, for two years, the duties of the Professorship of Natural Philosophy at the Royal Institution, Dr. Young resigned the appointment,—finding his longer tenure of it, in the opinion of his friends, incompatible with the pursuits, or rather with the prospects, of a practical physician. He was strongly impressed with the persuasion that the public would regard his medical skill and competence with some degree of suspicion, if a very large portion of his time and attention was known to be devoted to occupations, which were alien to his profession. Upon quitting this position however, he felt it to be equally due to his own credit and to that of the Institution with which he had been thus honourably connected, that the result of his labours, throughout the whole extent of natural philosophy and the mechanical arts, should be rendered of some permanent utility : and he immediately proceeded to revise and arrange the substance of his lectures for publication, with the addition of a most elaborate classed catalogue of works and memoirs published upon the various subjects to which they referred accompanied with copious notes, calculations and extracts;—a very laborious task, the execution of which was likely to prove of not less service to a student than the lectures to which they were appended, by enabling him to ascertain not only what had been, but what remained to be, done, in any department of research upon which he might be engaged. "When this work is finished," says he, " my pursuit of general science will terminate ; henceforwards I have resolved to confine my studies and my pen to medical subjects only."[a]

This great work consists of two quarto volumes of about seven hundred and fifty pages each. The first volume contains the lectures, with forty plates, including nearly six hundred geometrical and other figures, maps, &c., all very carefully drawn by his own hand : the second, of nearly equal extent, embraces the mathematical elements of Natural Philosophy—the systematic catalogue above referred to—a republication of his optical and some other memoirs—and a most carefully prepared index of contents. The publication was delayed until the year 1807—partly from its attaining a magnitude which had not been anticipated—and still more from the not unusual want of punctuality of the engravers. The sum of 1000*l*., which it had been stipulated to be paid to the author, was unfortunately never received by him, in consequence of the bankruptcy of the publisher.

It is not easy to speak in too high terms of the systematic catalogue in the second volume. It extends to four hundred pages, and includes references—with many valuable original observations interspersed—to the best sources of information on almost every department of mathematics and their applications, arranged in an order which is equally comprehensive and convenient. Some notion may be formed of the vast labour required

[a] Works, vol. i., p. 215.

for making this compilation, from the fact of its embracing more than twenty thousand articles which were not only to be selected and the works which contained them to be consulted—whenever they could be found in the libraries of the Royal Institution, the Royal Society, the British Museum, or of Sir Joseph Banks—but to be afterwards distributed and arranged under the various subjects to which they belonged. Few students, engaged in works of research, could then afford to dispense with the use of a classification so completely carried out in all its details; and even the lapse of half a century, which has produced so many changes in the aspect of the sciences, has not altogether deprived it of its value.[a]

The mathematical Elements of Natural Philosophy, which form another portion of this volume, were partly reprinted from the Syllabus of his lectures, which appeared in 1802. They would appear to have been regarded with no small degree of favour by their author; for we find them again introduced, with some modifications, into his Elementary Illustrations of the Celestial Mechanics of La Place, a small volume published in 1821, embracing not merely a great number of the most difficult investigations of that work, but likewise some very important propositions of his own. In these elements, we find Algebra, the Differential Calculus, Geometry, plane and solid, the Sections of a Cone and the Properties of Curves, concluded in twenty-six pages—whilst little more than double that space is devoted to Dynamics, Hydro-dynamics, Optics, Sound—embracing the most elementary as well as many of

---

[a] The republication of this catalogue, with the addition of the Works and Memoirs, which have appeared during the last half century, would confer an invaluable boon upon scientific students.

the most abstruse propositions to which they severally lead.

" They comprehend," says he, " all the propositions which are required for forming a complete series of demonstrations, leading to every case of importance that occurs in Natural Philosophy, with the exception of some of the more intricate calculations of Astronomy. The best use that a student could make of these elements, would be to read over each proposition superficially, then to endeavour to form for himself a more particular demonstration and to compare this again with that which is here given; for the exertion of a certain degree of invention is by far the surest mode of fixing any principle of science in the mind."

It is hardly necessary to add that any student who followed Dr. Young's advice—without possessing his extraordinary intuitive capacity of connecting distant points of a demonstration without the aid of the intermediate framework, whether of geometry or analysis, which ordinary minds require—would most probably have risen from his labour without retaining a single definite conception either of the propositions or their proofs.

We have elsewhere referred to the merits as well as to the defects of these lectures :ª to the causes which prevented their becoming a popular manual for students, notwithstanding the remarkable completeness of the view which they exhibited of the state of the sciences at the time they were written. He was fully aware of the charge of obscurity which had been brought against his former memoirs, and he would appear to have endeavoured to avoid it in his lectures, though not always—in consequence of the system which he followed—with entire success. In writing to Mr. Gurney he says :—

ª *Supra*, p. 135.

" I hear that your townsman, Woodhouse,[a] is now connected with the ' Critical Review,' and I believe he has exhibited some spleen against me in the last number ; he is very angry with me for attempting to clothe the ideas of a short algebraical calculation in the language of words, and professing his inability to understand the Paper (on Cohesion), he thinks it better to attempt to show its obscurity, than to give any extract from the more intelligible parts, or even the heads of the sections. I would rather, however, be severely handled by a man who understands something of the subject, than be treated with affected contempt by a fool, which, by a strange fatality, has hitherto been my lot. My book, however, will certainly be intelligible enough ; you have no idea how many well-sounding periods have been condemned, because they contained too many hard words."

If he was regardless of symmetry and elegance in his mathematical processes, and disposed to conduct his investigations by methods which satisfied his own mind of their sufficiency without reference to the more systematic forms of demonstration or deduction which others required, he was probably, on that very account, more disposed than they were, to reflect profoundly upon the physical principles which were made the basis of his reasoning His lectures on optics, embody, as might be expected, the views which he had previously developed in his well-known Memoirs : but those on the passive strength and elasticity of materials,

[a] An eminent mathematician, afterwards Plumian Professor at Cambridge, whose works first broke down the barrier which separated the writings of English and Continental mathematicians from each other. His treatise on Plane and Physical Astronomy is much the best that has ever appeared in this country. He reviewed the Lectures when they appeared, " and though," says Young, in another of his letters, " he has treated me handsomely enough, he has done his business in a very slovenly way, considering the variety of matter of which his readers had a right to expect some general account." It required in fact a long-continued and careful study to appreciate either the vast amount or the value of the original matter which this work contained.

—on the sources and effects of sound—on the essential properties of matter—on the sources, the effects, the measures and the nature of heat—on electricity in equilibrium and in motion—and on climates—are full of original and instructive speculations, which were in many cases greatly in advance of the knowledge of the age in which they were written. On such subjects, when not attempting to conduct mathematical investigations in ordinary language, he writes with great clearness, vigour and precision.

We shall quote a few specimens.

In speaking of the divisibility of matter, he says :—

" It remains to be examined how far we have any experience of the actual extent of the divisibility of matter ; and we shall find no appearance of anything like a limit to this property. The smallest spherical object, visible to a good eye, is about $\frac{1}{2000}$ of an inch in diameter; by the assistance of a microscope, we may perhaps distinguish a body one hundredth part as small, or $\frac{1}{200000}$ of an inch in diameter. The thickness of gold leaf is less than this, and the gilding of lace is still thinner, probably in some cases not above one ten millionth part of an inch ; so that $\frac{1}{2000}$ of a grain would cover a square inch, and a portion barely large enough to be visible by a microscope, might weigh only the eighty million millionth part of a grain. A grain of musk is said to be divisible into three hundred and twenty quadrillions of parts, each of which is capable of affecting the olfactory nerves. There are even living beings, visible to the microscope, of which a million million would not make up the bulk of a common grain of sand. But it is still more remarkable, that, as far as we can discover, many of these animalcules are as complicated in their structure as an elephant or a whale. It is true that the physiology of the various classes of animals is somewhat more simple as they deviate more from the form of quadrupeds, and from that of the human species ; the solid particles of the blood do not by any means vary in their magnitude in the same ratio with the bulk of the animal; and some of the lower classes appear to approximate very much to the nature of the vegetable world. But there are single instances that seem wholly to destroy this gradation : Lyonnet has discovered a far greater variety of parts in the caterpillar of the willow butterfly, than we can observe in many animals of the largest dimensions ; and among the microscopic insects in particular, we see a prodigality of machinery, subservient to the various purposes of the contracted life of the little animal, in the structure of which nature appears to be ostentatious of her power of giving perfection to her minutest works." [a]

When Young (in one of his Optical Memoirs) spoke of the "luminiferous ether probably pervading the substance of all material bodies as freely as wind passes through a grove of trees," the comparison was ridiculed by his Reviewer as equally amusing and absurd, from its utter want of likeness : yet if we reflect for a moment upon the relations which probably exist between the ultimate material particles of the densest bodies which are known to us and the space which they occupy, we shall not be startled by any hypothesis which may be made with respect to the perfect freedom of transmission of gravity, light, heat, or electricity, even if we assume them to be corporeal and different from each other. A cubic inch of platinum contains 200,000 times as many gravitating atoms as the same space filled with pure hydrogen gas, yet both of these substances are free from any sensible interstices and appear to be equally continuous.

" But besides this porosity," says he, " there is still room for the supposition, that even the ultimate particles of matter may be permeable to the causes of attractions of various kinds, especially if those causes are immaterial ; nor is there anything in the unprejudiced study of physical philosophy, that can induce us to doubt the existence of immaterial substances ; on the

[a] Lectures, p. 608.

contrary we see analogies that lead us almost directly to such an opinion. The electrical fluid is supposed to be essentially different from common matter; the general medium of light and heat, according to some, or the principle of caloric, according to others, is equally distinct from it. We see forms of matter differing in subtility and mobility, under the names of solids, liquids, and gases; above these are the semimaterial existences which produce the phænomena of electricity and magnetism, and either caloric or a universal ether; higher still perhaps are the causes of gravitation, and the immediate agents in attractions of all kinds, which exhibit some phænomena apparently still more remote from all that is compatible with material bodies; and of these different orders of beings, the more refined and immaterial appear to pervade freely the grosser. It seems therefore natural to believe that the analogy may be continued still further, until it rises into existence absolutely immaterial and spiritual. We know not but that thousands of spiritual worlds may exist unseen for ever by human eyes; nor, have we any reason to suppose that even the presence of matter, in a given spot necessarily excludes these existences from it. Those who maintain that nature always teems with life, wherever living beings can be placed, may therefore speculate with freedom on the possibility of independent worlds; some existing in different parts of space, others pervading each other, unseen and unknown, in the same space, and others again to which space may not be a necessary mode of existence." [a]

In the lecture on the Measures and Nature of Heat, after giving a masterly exposition of the popular theory of the day which regarded heat, under the name of caloric, as a separate substance, capable of quantitative measurement, for which different bodies, both aeriform, liquid and solid, possessed different and specific capacities, he proceeds—after showing the difficulties which many phenomena, especially those of friction, present to the acceptance of such views— as follows :—

[a] Lectures, p. 610, 611.

" The preceding discussion naturally leads us to an examination of the various theories which have been formed respecting the intimate nature of heat ; a subject upon which popular opinion seems to have been lately led away by very superficial considerations. The facility with which the mind conceives the existence of an independent substance, liable to no material variations, except those of its quantity and distribution, especially, when an appropriate name, and a place in the order of the simplest elements has been bestowed on it, appears to have caused the most eminent chemical philosophers to overlook some insuperable difficulties attending the hypothesis of caloric. Caloric has been considered as a peculiar elastic or ethereal fluid, pervading the substance or the pores of all bodies, in different quantities, according to their different capacities for heat and according to their actual temperatures ; and being transferred from one body to another upon any change of capacity, or upon any other disturbance of the equilibrium of temperature : it has also been commonly supposed to be the general principle or cause of repulsion ; and in its passage from one body to another, by radiation, it has been imagined by some to flow in a continued stream, and by others in the form of separate particles, moving with inconceivable velocity, at great distances from each other.

" The circumstances which have been already stated, respecting the production of heat by friction, appear to afford an unanswerable confutation of the whole of this doctrine. If the heat is neither received from the surrounding bodies—which it cannot be without a depression of their temperature—nor derived from the quantity already accumulated in the bodies themselves—which it could not be, even if their capacities were diminished in any imaginable degree—there is no alternative but to allow that heat must be actually generated by friction ; and if it is generated out of nothing, it cannot be matter, nor even an immaterial or semi material substance. The collateral parts of the theory have also their separate difficulties : thus, if heat were the general principle of repulsion, its augmentation could not diminish the elasticity of solids and of fluids ; if it constituted a continued fluid, it could not radiate freely through the same space in different directions ; and if its repulsive particles followed each other at a distance, they would still approach near enough to each other, in the focus of a burning-glass, to have their motions deflected from a recti-linear direction.

" If heat is not a substance, it must be a quality ; and this quality can only be motion. It was Newton's opinion that heat consists in a minute vibratory motion of the particles of bodies, and that this motion is communicated through an apparent vacuum, by the undulations of an elastic medium, which is also concerned in the phænomena of light. If the arguments which have been lately advanced, in favour of the undulatory nature of light, be deemed valid, there will be still stronger reasons for admitting this doctrine respecting heat, and it will only be necessary to suppose the vibrations and undulations, principally constituting it, to be larger and stronger than those of light, while at the same time the smaller vibrations of light, and even the blackening rays, derived from still more minute vibrations, may perhaps, when sufficiently condensed, concur in producing the effects of heat. These effects, beginning from the blacken-ing rays, which are invisible, are a little more perceptible in the violet, which still possess but a faint power of illumination ; the yellow-green afford the most light ; the red give less light, but much more heat, while the still larger and less frequent vibrations, which have no effect on the sense of sight, may be supposed to give rise to the least refrangible rays, and to constitute invisible heat." [a]

After noticing some other arguments of a less satis-factory nature, he points out some very striking ana-logies—supposing this second and more philosophical hypothesis were adopted—between the phenomena of sound and heat.

" If heat, when attached to any substance, be supposed to consist in minute vibrations, and when propagated from one body to another, to depend on the undulations of a medium highly elastic, its effects must strongly resemble those of sound, since every sounding body is in a state of vibration, and the air, or any other medium, which transmits sound, conveys its

[a] Lectures, p. 653, 654.

undulations to distant parts by means of its elasticity. And we shall find that the principal phænomena of heat may actually be illustrated by a comparison with those of sound. The excitation of heat and sound are not only similar, but often identical, as in the operations of friction and percussion ; they are both communicated, sometimes by contact, and sometimes by radiation ; for besides the common radiation of sound through the air, its effects are communicated by contact, when the end of a tuning-fork is placed on a table, or on the sounding-board of an instrument, which receives from the fork an impression that is afterwards propagated as a distinct sound. And the effect of radiant heat, in raising the temperature of the body upon which it falls, resembles the sympathetic agitation of a string, when the sound of another string which is in unison with it, is transmitted to it through the air. The water which is dashed about by the vibrating extremities of a tuning fork dipped into it, may represent the manner in which the particles at the surface of a liquid are thrown out of the reach of the force of cohesion, and converted into vapour ; and the extrication of heat, in consequence of condensation, may be compared with the increase of sound produced by lightly touching a long chord which is slowly vibrating, or revolving in such a manner as to emit little or no audible sound ; while the diminution of heat by expansion, and the increase of the capacity of a substance for heat, may be attributed to the greater space afforded to each particle, allowing it to be equally agitated with a less perceptible effect on the neighbouring particles. In some cases indeed heat and sound not only resemble each other in their operations, but produce precisely the same effects ; thus, an artificial magnet, the force of which is quickly destroyed by heat, is affected more slowly in a similar manner, when made to ring for a considerable time : and an electrical jar may be discharged, either by heating it, or by causing it to sound by the friction of the finger.

" All these analogies are certainly favourable to the opinion of the vibratory nature of heat, which has been sufficiently sanctioned by the authority of the greatest philosophers of past times, and of the most sober reasoners of the present. Those, however, who look up with unqualified reverence to the dogmas of the modern schools of chemistry, will probably long retain a partiality for the convenient but superficial and inaccurate modes of reasoning, which have been founded on the favourite hypothesis of the existence of caloric as a separate substance; but it may be presumed that in the end a careful and repeated examination of the facts which have been adduced in confutation of that system, will make a sufficient impression on the minds of the cultivators of chemistry, to induce them to listen to a less objectionable theory." [a]

The discovery of the polarization and subsequently of the refraction of heat, due chiefly to the labours of Professor James Forbes of Edinburgh, have supplied other links in the chain of analogy between light and heat. If light is due to the undulations of an ether, it seems hardly possible not to accept the conclusion, that the phenomena of heat are referable to a similar origin.

The substance of his fiftieth lecture on the Cohesion of Fluids was embodied in an Essay read to the Royal Society, on the 20th of December, 1804, and published in their Transactions for the following year. The investigations which it contains are amongst the most original and important of the contributions which he made to physical science; but being conducted entirely without the aid of figures or symbolical reasoning, are extremely obscure. A long time consequently elapsed before their value was fully appreciated.

This Essay was republished in the Appendix to the second volume of his Lectures, including, amongst some other additions, a running commentary upon some general observations which La Place had appended to an essay on the same subject, which was published in 1806,[b] and in which several of Young's conclusions

---

[a] Lectures, p. 655—657.

[b] Théorie de l'Action Capillaire, published as a Supplement to the 10th book of the Mécanique Céleste; read to the Institut in December, 1806, and published in the following April.

were reproduced inadvertently—as we are bound to conclude—and therefore without any acknowledgment. In a second essay [a] supplementary to it, published in the following year, the author corrects and enlarges his former investigations and recognizes, in terms of respect, though by no means to their full extent, the previous labours of Dr. Young.

The phenomena, whose explanation forms the subject of Dr. Young's Essay, are matters of familiar occurrence and observation. A drop of fluid is placed upon a horizontal surface ; it is not diffused, but assumes a position of repose in a curve surface which holds it together as if enveloped in a sheet. A similar drop is suspended from a similar surface. What is the origin of the power which sustains it and prevents it from bursting ? Mercury in barometrical or other capillary tubes is depressed more or less in the inverse proportion of their diameters, and its upper surface is not flat, but convex, thus entailing the necessity of a very important correction of the indications which barometers afford, more especially when their diameters are small : but if instead of mercury we use water or any other fluid of less than twice the density of the glass, these effects are reversed, the surface being raised instead of depressed and being concave instead of convex. What are the forces which produce these and many other remarkable consequences ? Are we required to look for them in the mutual actions of the fluids and solids on each other, or to call to our aid, in addition to them, some properties of those fluids less obvious to our observation than those which are required for the explanation of their ordinary phenomena ?

Whatever be the forces which a solid surface exercises

[a] Supplement à la Théorie de l'Action Capillaire. Paris, 1807.

upon a fluid in contact with it, it is certain that the
distance to which their action extends is absolutely
infinitesimal. For, however thick or however thin
such a solid may be, it is found by observation that
the elevation or depression of the fluid in contact with
it, is always the same, so long as its substance continues the same. Another consequence of this mutual
action—which constitutes a fundamental proposition
of this theory—is the constancy, under the same
circumstances, of the angle included between the two
surfaces of the fluid—that is, between the one which
is free and the other which is in contact with the
solid—in all forms of the phenomenon. This angle
is 90° when the density of the fluid is twice as great
as that of the solid, a conclusion which Clairaut had
long since indicated: if the density of the fluid be
greater than twice that of the solid, this angle is
greater—if less—it is less than 90°; thus for mercury
and crown glass, it is about 140°, and for water and
the same, about 70°; values which will at once point
out the convexity in one case, and the concavity in
the other, of their respective surfaces in barometrical
and other tubes.

It was Young who first fully explained the principles upon which this angle, which he named the
appropriate angle, could be determined in all cases:
this determination forms an important step in the
formation of a correct theory of the cohesion and
non diffusion of fluids.

The second step is of not less importance and involves considerations of a very refined and difficult
character. What is the origin of the forces which produce an uniform tension in the enveloping sheet of the
fluid, so that the pressures to which it is exposed are

resisted and its particles maintained in a state of equilibrium?

All explanations of this remarkable phenomenon have involved, in their earlier or later stages, some assumptions respecting the internal constitution of fluids in their liquid as distinguished from their aeriform state. In the latter case, the operation of the forces by which the ultimate particles of the fluid are repelled from each other is manifest, and is only counteracted by the external pressure by which its further expansion is confined : but the passage to the state of liquidity, in whatever manner it is effected, is always more or less sudden and violent, attended by a considerable evolution of heat, producing an effect which is more or less permanent and stable, notwithstanding the removal of the causes which produced it. We cannot suppose that the repulsive forces become cohesive or attractive, by this change of state, without supposing the particles to be brought into contact with each other by the compression of the fluid into a smaller space, a supposition hardly reconcileable with their perfect mobility, and also negatived by facts of observation without number ; and we are thus necessarily conducted, as it were, to the assumption of the co-existence of cohesive and repulsive forces, following different laws, but confined to a sphere of action in both cases, which we are obliged, for reasons already stated, to regard as infinitesimally small. Thus, if the repulsive force varies, as in the case of aeriform bodies, inversely as the distance of the particles or any higher power of the distance, the cohesive force being constant and acting within a certain infinitesimal sphere only, or confined to a certain number of the particles of the fluid—which is one of the assumptions which Young has made—

there would result, as he has shown, from the combination of their actions at any point on a curved part of the sheet, a force directed to the concave part of the curve, which would be greater, the greater the curvature. Such would be the nature of the force which would be found to produce an uniform tension of the surface and adequate to counteract the hydrostatic pressures which would otherwise produce motion.

Later investigations of a very refined nature[a]—to which he very properly attached considerable importance —enabled him to assign the amount of the deficiency of the mutual actions of the superficial particles of a fluid thus constituted, and to show it to be one-fifth part of the whole force of a stratum of the fluid equal in thickness to the diameter of the infinitesimal sphere within which the action of the constant cohesive forces were assumed to be confined : the same investigation shows also that the sphere of the repulsive, must be supposed to be greater than that of the cohesive, forces, and that the fluid must be slightly condensed towards its interior parts in order to produce a resistance equivalent to the excess of the cohesion of the surface.

Having thus shown the necessity and justified the existence of an uniform superficial tension of the fluids concerned in capillary actions, he then avails himself of the principle, which Segner of Göttingen had applied to the solution of these problems in 1751. If a curve line, like the elastic curve, be uniformly stretched, the normal force which it exerts, at any of its points, is directly as the curvature. If the curve produced by capillary action was cylindrical, as in the case of a fluid included between two parallel plane surfaces, where

---

[a] In an appendix to his 'Elementary Illustrations of the Celestial Mechanics of Laplace.' Works, vol. i., p. 485.

the curvature is *single*, this principle would be strictly applicable to it: but Segner erroneously applied it to all such surfaces, whether their curvature was single or double; whereas in the latter case, it is proportional to the sum of the greatest and least curvatures of the surface, which is equivalent, as is well known, to the sum of any two of its curvatures that are at right angles to each other. This important correction was made by Young, who thus reduced the difficulties of the solution of the problem to those of analysis merely. Those difficulties however are sufficiently formidable and can only be conquered, even in the more simple cases, by slow and difficult processes of approximation.

In the Memoir presented to the Royal Society he considered the case of a single curvature only : but in an admirable revision of his earlier investigations, which is given in an Article on the cohesion of fluids in the Supplement of the Encyclopædia Britannica, he has extended his solution to surfaces of revolution and has thus been enabled to deduce from it the bases of numerical determinations of the phenomena of ordinary capillary tubes even when their diameters are considerable ; results which he had only partially attained, by less direct methods, in his former Essay.

The principles established in this Memoir, and the results obtained from them, are applied with great success to the solution of several other problems of no small interest and difficulty. Besides the determination of the height of ascent of lighter fluids, such as water, in narrow capillary tubes, he finds the weight of water raised by a circular disc wetted by the fluid and in contact with it, when gently raised above it, until the fluid detaches itself from the solid ; and he finds the relation between the weight of *adhesion* thus determined and the height of ascent in a given tube. These and many other questions, whose solutions are more or less immediately deducible from the same principles—such as the height of adhesion of mercury to gold, silver, tin, and substances which it is capable of wetting, as well as the thickness at which a portion of it will spread out on glass—the strong cohesion of plane surfaces produced by the interposition of a small quantity of fluid which wets them—the repulsions and attractions of floating bodies, both wet and dry, under different circumstances—are treated with the sagacious brevity—we wish we could venture to say perspicuity, which is usual with him, and the results are reduced to numbers, by processes which are rarely developed, but which could not be deduced by methods which are commonly employed without enormous labour.

The publication of La Place's first memoir on the subject, a year after his own had appeared in the most public and generally known scientific record in Europe, and in which some of his results were reproduced, without acknowledgment, very naturally annoyed him. No man could accuse this eminent master of analysis— the author of the greatest work on the Mechanism of the Universe which had appeared since the epoch of the Principia—of seeking to augment his own exuberant stores by appropriating the riches of other writers; and though he was certainly not altogether ignorant of the contents of Young's memoir, he had probably paid no sufficient attention to them. The view also which he took of the subject was very different, if not antagonistic, to that of Young. He assumes the fluid to be incompressible : that there is an attraction of the particles of the fluid for each other, as well as a mutual attraction between the particles of the fluid and those of

the tube or solid, and that these forces are sensible only
at insensible distances ; but he makes no reference whatever to the existence of a repulsive force between the
particles of the fluid, unless—in the ultimate analysis—
the assumption of the incompressibility of the fluid
may be said to involve it. From these principles,
however, not only is the differential equation of the
surface of the fluid deduced, but also many special
results of observation are explained with his usual
skill, clearness, and sagacity, in the formation, evolution, and interpretation of his formulæ.

In an appendix to his memoir, which was republished in the second volume of his lectures and also in
an article in the first number of the Quarterly Review
for 1809, Young has reviewed this treatise of La Place
with a severity, which though excessive, can hardly be
considered as altogether unprovoked and unmerited.

" An ostentatious parade of deep investigation, which leads
almost to nothing, has too often filled the works of the mathematicians of the continent ; and we are sorry to be obliged to
include M. La Place in the number of those, who appear to
have been more influenced on some occasions, by a desire of
commanding admiration, than of communicating knowledge.
We have been sometimes amused, in the perusal of this essay,
with observing that after an expression has travelled, with considerable fatigue, through several pages of Greek, Roman, and
Italic characters, it was transformed, by proper substitution,
into an equation belonging simply to a circle, from which it
would have been just as easy to have set out at once : that a
complicated fluxion, when its fluent had been determined, produced a much simpler theorem, which was a mere mechanical
consequence of the laws of force : and what is of more importance, we have discovered an equation, involving a complete absurdity, when a translation into common language
would have shown that it implied an impossibility and that the
premises from which it was derived, were therefore inadmis-

sible. The point on which M. La Place seems to rest the most material part of his claim to originality, is the deduction of all the phænomena of capillary action from the simple considera- tion of molecular attraction. To us it does not appear that the fundamental principle, from which he sets out, is at all a neces- sary consequence of the established properties of matter : and we conceive that this mode of stating the question is but par- tially justified, by the coincidence of the results derived from it with experiment, since he has not demonstrated that a similar coincidence might not be obtained by proceeding on totally different grounds."

In some observations written upon a loose sheet found amongst his papers, and apparently prepared for a review, Dr. Young gives a still stronger expression to his dissatisfaction with the treatment which he con- ceived he had experienced from La Place.

" We cannot avoid renewing, on this occasion, a complaint which has already been very frequently made by many British philosophers, of an obvious want of candour in our continental neighbours with respect to the originality of scientific investiga- tions and discoveries : we do not ourselves profess to judge with perfect impartiality or infallibility : we have perhaps our feelings and our prejudices as Englishmen, and we wish all possible allowance to be made for the influence which these sentiments may have on our decisions : but we must not therefore refrain from speaking what appears to us to be just and true.

" Whether or no M. La Place had seen the Philosophical Transactions for 1804 before he communicated his first papers to the Institute in 1805, we cannot have any positive means of determining : if he had not seen them, he might and ought to have seen them. The charge of plagiarism may be avoided by proving the negative, but that of originality must fall as far as a coincidence can be shown. But in the second of the papers here noticed (the supplement) M. La Place expressly acknowledges that he had taken an idea from Young's paper, without making any other remark on the identity of almost every other result of his speculations with some of the propositions which Dr.

Young had before advanced. The natural inference which would be made by a reader of this paper is not only that M. La Place had borrowed nothing else from Dr. Young, but that all his other conclusions were original and had not occurred to Dr. Young or to any other person."

It is one of the most embarrassing facts connected with this theory that many of the same conclusions are deducible from very different hypotheses concerning the intimate constitution of fluids. La Place has recognized no molecular forces but those which are attractive, which may follow any law provided that their sphere of action is infinitesimal. Ivory,[a] as was usual with him, has trod closely in his footsteps, adopting both his principles and conclusions, but giving to some of them a more perfect development by calling to his aid an important observation of Professor Leslie [b] on the lateral force produced by the attraction of a solid body upon a fluid. A similar course has been followed by Gauss:[c] but Poisson,[d] with larger views, has combined molecular repulsion as well as attraction in a theory, which has enabled him, with the aid of his admirable powers of analysis, to give a consistent explanation of the most important facts of observation : whilst Young, as

[a] Supplement to the Encyclopædia Britannica : Elevation of Fluids. In the course of this article, after noticing in terms of great praise the formula of La Place, expressing the relation between the pressure and the curvature, in which he had been anticipated by Dr. Young, he adds :—" The labours of philosophers have discovered the facts of capillary action, which have been verified by innumerable experiments : but if the truth is to be told, it may be affirmed that reckoning back from the present time to the speculations of the Florentine academicians, the formula of La Place and the remark of Professor Leslie, relating to the lateral force, are the only approaches that have been made to a sound physical account of the phenomena."

[b] Philosophical Magazine. 1802.

[c] Principia generalia Theoriæ Figuræ Fluidorum in statu equilibrii. Göttingen, 1830.

[d] Nouvelle Théorie de l'Action Capillaire. Paris, 1831.

we have seen, attained the same results, by resorting
to no hypotheses respecting molecular forces, but such
as were required to produce the mutual actions of the
solid and fluid upon each other and to account for the
uniform tension of the envelope of the fluid without
which the equilibrium could not be maintained : a
view of this theory, which seems to be commended to
our acceptance not merely by the facility of its application to the phenomena, but by confining the range
of our hypotheses, more strictly than other methods of
treating it, within the limits prescribed by a just and
legitimate induction from observation.

We have before observed that in the article, on the
Cohesion of Fluids, which was furnished by him to the
Supplement of the Encyclopædia Britannica a year before the appearance, in the same work,[a] of Mr. Ivory's
article on the same subject—though under a different
name—Dr. Young resumed the consideration of some of
the more difficult parts of this theory : availing himself
of the suggestion of Professor Leslie, which has been be-

[a] In writing to Macvey Napier, the editor, on this subject, he says :—
"It is not for my own sake that I wished to interfere with Ivory's Capillary Attraction, because I have very amply shown, in the article which I
have prepared, how much more accurately I have treated the question, even
in a mathematical point of view, than he has done, at least in his paper
presented to the Royal Society, and withdrawn for reconsideration. This
I have stated without reference to any contemporary author, except
La Place, merely as a different mode of considering the subject, as
depending on the general laws of cohesion, and in a way which cannot
possibly give offence to Mr. Ivory. If his reconsideration of the subject
has enabled him to arrive at a more accurate mode of calculation than
mine, I shall modify my remarks accordingly ; but I think, from the
nature of the question, the thing is highly improbable, and La Place has
certainly failed in it." Mr. Ivory's article was printed under the title of
"Elevation of Fluids" more than a year subsequently to that on Cohesion
by Dr. Young : if the proper order of the publication of the articles had
been followed, there is no doubt but the contemptuous allusion to the
labours of Dr. Young on this subject, quoted in a note to p. 208, would
have been duly noticed.

fore alluded to, in tracing more accurately than in his
first memoir and lectures, the elementary actions of the
forces concerned in producing the tension of the enveloping surface and estimating its quantity; and also
engaging in some very remarkable and profound observations on the probable law and range of action of the
cohesive and repulsive forces, and upon the probable
distance of the particles of aqueous vapour and water.
In the same Essay he has also investigated a formula
for determining the angle of contact at the junction of
a solid with fluids of different densities, and has not
only given a much more complete solution of the form
and properties of capillary curves of simple curvature,
but has extended them to those which form surfaces of
revolution, even when they no longer can be considered
—as in tubes of wide diameter—to be small portions of
the surface of a sphere. This essay was written in the
full maturity of his powers; and there is no production
of its author—unless it be the articles on Bridge and
Chromatics in the same, and that on the Tides, in a
subsequent volume—which is more remarkable for the
boldness and success with which it attacks some of
the most difficult speculations of philosophy.

CHAPTER VIII.

MARRIAGE. MEDICAL LIFE AND WORKS.

IN the summer of 1802, during the short peace of
Amiens, the Duke of Richmond consulted Dr. Young
about sending his two great nephews — the present
Duke and his brother—to reside a month or two in
France, for the purpose of acquiring the pronunciation
of the language. As their tutor, Mr. Vincent, did
not speak French, the Duke accepted Dr. Young's
offer to accompany them to Rouen, where he placed
them *en pension* with a French family in which there
were other children to play and converse with. He
availed himself of this excursion to pay a visit to Paris,
where he was introduced to the first Consul at the Institute, who was in the habit of attending and occasionally taking part in the discussions which commonly
take place upon the subjects which are brought before,
that body, whether they be scientific memoirs, or notices
of inventions, or new experiments, or projects of every
description, of which there is never wanting an abundant supply.

In the month of March following he was admitted
at Cambridge to the degree of M.B., at the end of six
years from the date of his first admission to the University. He took the degree of M.D. five years afterwards. On each of these occasions he was required to
hold a disputation in the public schools, which was

preceded by a Latin dissertation on a medical subject.
From the introduction to a memoir, containing Hydrau-
lic Investigations,[a] read to the Royal Society in May,
1808—it would appear that the subject of the last of
these dissertations was the nature of inflammation, and
that in treating it he had occasion to examine atten-
tively the mechanical principles of the circulation of
the blood, which entered into the questions more especially considered in his Croonian lecture on the functions
of the Heart and Arteries,[b] which was read to the
Royal Society on the 10th of November following.
There is no record of either of these Dissertations to
be found among his papers.

On the 14th of June, 1804, he married Miss Eliza
Maxwell. This lady, at that time extremely young,
was the second daughter of J. P. Maxwell, Esq., of
Cavendish Square, and of Trippendence, near Farnborough, Kent, a member of a younger branch of the
family of Sir-William Maxwell of Calderwood Castle,
Lanarkshire. It was a marriage of mutual affection
and esteem, such as he had always looked forward to
as the great object of his professional and other exertions, and secured him a home which was graced by
all the refinements of good manners and a cultivated
taste : it was a singularly happy marriage.

To the members of his wife's family he attached
himself with more than the ordinary affection of a son
and brother-in-law, more especially to her three sisters,
whose accomplishments and agreeable manners contributed not a little to the attractions of their family
residence and his own. One of these sisters, Maria,
was afterwards married to the Rev. J. P. Chambers,
Rector of Hedenham, Norfolk : another, Emily, to

Charles Earle, Esq. : the third, Caroline, is Countess
of Buchan. The most lively letters which Young
wrote, some of which we shall afterwards have occasion
to refer to, were addressed to some one of these ladies.
He was now fairly launched upon the profession of
physic, and apparently with every prospect of success, if
such success depended, in every instance, upon careful
preparatory study, the possession of the most varied
knowledge and an extraordinary capacity for applying it.
His own estimate of the acquirements requisite for a physician was sufficiently high, as appears from the sketch
which he has given of them in the Introduction to his
Medical Literature. But it is well known, from the
experience of others as well as his own, that the highest
qualifications, whether natural or acquired, may fail to
secure professional eminence. Much depends upon the
manner in which a physician approaches the bedside
of his patient; upon the natural expression of a feeling
of sympathy for their sufferings and anxiety to relieve
them : upon the judicious administration of the cordial
of hope : upon the exercise at least, if not upon the
possession, of a decisive and rapid judgment : upon a
thorough knowledge of human nature, and a ready
tact in humouring its caprices : and not a little also
upon the good fortune of achieving some eminent success, which attracts the attention of the world.

The most opposite paths, however, will sometimes
conduct to the same conclusion. The celebrated Dr.
Radcliffe[a] told Dr. Mead, as a great secret, that the
way to succeed in physic was to use everybody ill :—
but Dr. Mead used nobody ill, and succeeded better
than Dr. Radcliffe. The real fact is that the prestige
of a reputation once attained, whether through the in-

Introduction to Medical Literature, p. 2.

fluence of charlatanism, good fortune, or superior merit, is not easily destroyed, and the very eccentricities and extravagances which repel patients of sense and delicacy, tend to confirm the prepossessions of those who are wanting in these qualities, and who are naturally apt to wonder at or admire what they do not understand.

For many years, after his marriage, Dr. Young adhered to the resolution which he had previously announced, of confining his studies and publications to his own profession, as far as the connection of his name with his scientific labours was concerned, but no farther. His memoir on Cohesion was an exception, but it was little more than an expansion of his previous lecture on the subject : whilst two other papers in the Transactions to which we have referred above, though scientific in their treatment and character, were designed to be subservient to important physiological inquiries, and therefore did not absolutely constitute a departure from the principle which he had laid down. But his various contributions, whether original or translated, to Nicholson's journal and other works,[a] including his Theory of the Tides,—one of the most considerable of his scientific labours,—were anonymous, as well as his numerous articles in the Imperial and Quarterly Review, the Retrospect and other periodical publications. It was this voluntary withdrawal of his name from public observation, notwithstanding the variety and importance of his researches, which left nearly undisturbed for many years the impression produced by the intemperate abuse of the Edinburgh Review.

For sixteen years after his marriage, he resided at Worthing between the months of July and October—partly as an agreeable place of retirement, and partly

[a] Works, vol. ii., Nos. 38, 39, 40, 43, 44, 45, 48, 49, 50, 51, and 54.

for medical practice—where he afterwards built a residence of his own. In those days, when continental travel was prevented by the war, the higher classes of society were accustomed to reside during the summer months in quiet and retired watering-places, where they considered themselves safe from the intrusion of the mobs of tradesmen and others, whom the increased facilities of communication have since introduced. Worthing was one of those places which still retained a character intermediate between a village and a town, the approaches to which were not then blocked up by those irregular suburbs, equally injurious to the public health and architectural beauty and order, which have sprung up, as is usual in nearly all our large towns, in the absence of the salutary and necessary interference of the legislature : and the families of distinction who made it their place of occasional sojourn, were in those days enabled to reciprocate visits with the freedom which is hardly compatible with more crowded watering places and more miscellaneous visitors.

It was to this class of visitors that Young was indebted, during his summer residence at Worthing, not only for a fair amount of professional occupation, but likewise for the enjoyment of much cultivated society. He retained through life his fondness for the innocent pleasures of social life, and was always ready to take his part in a dance or a glee, or to join in any scheme of amusement calculated to give life and interest to a party. In a letter to his sister-in-law Emily, now Mrs. Earle, describing his various occupations at this place, he says :—

"I have been dashing through vocal and instrumental music without any reserve or modesty, being determined to keep my-

self in practice for the pleasure of accompanying you. I found
one of Sola's things which I bought of him an excellent exercise ;
and perhaps by the time I see you, I shall be able to play it :
but I have exhibited it once here and twice at Mrs. Burmes-
ter's ; and as for singing, you have no idea what a noise I
made."

The actual practice of every profession must always
tend to dissipate some illusions, by a closer inspection
of the machinery by which it is worked Reputations
which have been unduly magnified in public estimation will sink to their true dimensions ; and the value
of opinions which are founded upon a sound knowledge
of the human frame and of subsidiary branches of
science as well as upon a just induction from facts
and observation, will be distinguished from those
which have no such basis. It is the peculiar misfortune of the medical profession that its members
can rarely dare to confess their ignorance, thinking it
more or less necessary—in order to maintain their
influence with their patients and with the world,
—to speak with equal decision, whether they are
authorised by their knowledge to do so or not; and
the precise localities, or habits, or articles of food,
which one physician will denounce as pestilential,
injurious, or unwholesome, another will recommend
as healthy, salutary or digestible.

" I have told you," says Young, in a letter to the most intimate
of his friends, " that in consultations, however opposite opinions
may be, it is usual to tell the patient that the parties consulted
are perfectly agreed, and it is very unfair to examine the
witnesses separately where so much depends upon opinion. I
was dining at the Duke of Richmond's one day last winter, and
there came in two notes, one from Sir W. Farquhar, and the
other from Dr. Hunter, in answer to an inquiry whether or no
his Grace might venture to eat fruit pies or strawberries. I

trembled for the honour of the profession, and could not conceal my apprehensions from the company : luckily, however, they agreed tolerably well, the only difference of opinion being on the subject of pie-crust."

He had no sooner completed the publication of his Lectures—the result of four or five years of assiduous labour—than his mind was turned to the preparation of another Course, which would bear much the same relation to the medical sciences. He was disposed to think that the study of physic, like that of other sciences, could be as much, if not more advanced, by a careful comparison of the collected observations of others, as by the limited experience of a single practitioner, however varied it might be ; more especially when it is considered that very extensive practice is more or less incompatible with the sacrifice of time which an elaborate discussion of its results would render necessary. In writing to a friend about this period (1807) he says :—

" I believe your pheasants have assisted in bringing my friend Davy into a hundred a-year and the office of Secretary of the Royal Society. It had never occurred to him to offer himself till I suggested it to him one day that he dined with me. The next day he heard of poor Gray's death, and upon applying to the President, he was, after some deliberation, approved, although another person had before been encouraged. If I had not been a member of an *illiberal* profession, I should have liked the situation myself ; but perhaps the public is right in discouraging a divided attention. I purpose seriously to do something in physic, by collecting all that is worth knowing, and comparing it with the general economy of the operations of nature. I do not know who has attempted to do this soberly : Darwin had neither patience nor precision enough ; and I am confident that much more may be learnt and taught in this way than from a routine of old woman's practice, which is all that a fashionable physician obtains. In many other departments of science I have been enabled to draw conclusions from a comparison of the experiments of others, which I should have been much longer in discovering by investigations of my own ; *and why not in physic ? "*

Dr. Young had peculiar qualifications for the execution of such a task. There was no department of knowledge which was not at his command, and facts which would be without significance when presented to ordinary minds, might have been pregnant with meaning by the relations which they exhibited to other branches of knowledge, when brought under the notice of one to whom all such branches were familiar. The advancement of the sciences requires the labours both of masters and workmen ; and whilst the latter are engaged in the fashioning or perfecting or inventing the separate parts of the machine, it is under the directions of the former that they must be put together, and made to work as one whole.

In the month of May, 1807, he made some progress in a canvas for the office of Physician to the Middlesex Hospital ; but though he succeeded in securing the promise of a considerable number of votes, he found the ground so much pre-occupied by Dr. Satterly, who was also supported by the other medical officers, that he had no chance of success, and therefore retired from the contest. The same powerful interest was also pre-engaged for the next vacancy, whenever it should occur ; and though he had good reason to think that he would have succeeded in opposition to it, he did not like to make the attempt, as his colleagues would possess the power of annoying him, if thwarted in their object, by preventing his going out of town in the summer. He soon afterwards engaged in a scheme of lectures, to be given at this Hospital in the two following winters, on the Elements of the Medical Sciences and the Practice of Physic. The plan was no sooner formed than he began to devote all his energies to preparations for it. In writing to a friend, in April, 1809, he says,—

"I have been absorbed in physic day and night,—not altogether in the practice, but more in the theory,—having a course of lectures to prepare for next winter, on which I am to rest, in some degree, my medical reputation."

In the following June we find him engaged in the three examinations required for his admission to the College of Physicians, in preparing for his Lectures, and in writing a medical essay on the Effects of Climate;—

"Amusements," says he, "which, besides the more serious employments of parties, concerts, and dances, really give me very little more spare time than is necessary for visiting my patients."

In reply to the same correspondent, who had remarked upon the misfortune of those, who notwithstanding the possession of the gifts of fortune, have nothing which they are obliged to do, he says :—

"I cannot help thinking it a little unlucky that I have so many motives for exertion when so few would have been sufficient, and that you have so few when you require so many; it might, however, have been much worse than it is; but I often think that I should undergo my *mountainous* labours with somewhat more alacrity if the advantages were as secure as the toil was severe. And yet I cannot always be satisfied with going the shortest way to work. I have been spending a month on some chemical investigations, which I have just completed, merely because I was obliged to give a few lectures on chemistry and pharmacy; but then I consider that I should have no right to give lectures on chemistry if I had done absolutely nothing to prove myself capable of it. Certainly twenty or even fifty pupils would be scarcely an inducement to take all the pains I have taken and shall take in the business, but for the very important advantage which you mention. The longer a person has lived the less he gains by reading, and the more likely he is to forget what he has read and learnt of old ; and the only remedy that I know of is to write upon every subject that he wishes to understand, even if he burns what he has written."

Few persons, who have been much engaged in the study of difficult subjects, will dispute the truth of the last observation.

The Lectures were given during two successive seasons. There were six lectures on Chemistry, six on Physiology, twenty on Nosology and general Practice —including an original classification of diseases—and four on Materia Medica. They were little frequented, as he himself informs us, in consequence of the usual miscalculation which he made, in endeavouring to convey in the space of an hour much more information than his auditors could carry away with them. Many of these lectures were subsequently embodied in his work on Medical Literature, and they would appear to have constituted a very complete and comprehensive view of medical science such as very few of his contemporaries would have been able to produce.

On the 24th of January, 1811, he was elected one of the Physicians to St. George's Hospital—a very important appointment, which has usually been introductory to the first practice in the Metropolis. The vacancy had occurred unexpectedly by the resignation of Dr. Bancroft, and Young was persuaded, by some of his friends to put himself in nomination as a candidate without any previous preparation. The votes of many of his own friends were pre-engaged to Dr. Bond Cabbell, who had failed at a previous contest ; though absent from England at this time, he was again put forward as a candidate by others who acted for him. The result was that one hundred votes were given for Dr. Young, ninety-two for Dr. Cabbell, fifty-one for Dr. Roget, and three for Dr. Harrison.

"There never was," says Young, in writing to Mr. Gurney, "anything like the total number, and the contest has been almost unparalleled : any of the three candidates had advantages which would have secured him in any common case. Local interest and the protracted efforts of a whole family made the Cabbells very naturally confident of triumphant success ; parliamentary influence and the natural wish to serve a man who is likely to be Lord Chancellor, made Sir S. Romilly's nephew very formidable ; and for myself the event speaks. But it is remarkable what a variety of interests I have been obliged to bring into play ; scarcely any one of my friends having procured for me more than two or three favourable answers, so that every one lamented how very little he could do ; yet the aggregate was sufficient for the purpose. Mrs. Young has emerged from death to life by the event of this contest."

He retained his situation at the Hospital for the remainder of his life, even after he had ceased to be dependent upon his profession for such an addition to his income as he deemed sufficient to secure him those comforts and luxuries which his scheme of life required,—those of a gentleman, in fact, who was accustomed to reciprocate visits with the best society though without ostentation and display. He was uniformly attentive to his duties at the Hospital, but he failed there as elsewhere to secure much influence with the pupils,—the numbers attending his clinical lectures, or rather progresses, being generally small compared with those who attached themselves to other teachers. His manners were wanting in warmth and earnestness, and his want of knowledge of the difficulties of students, made him pass over without sufficient notice the very points upon which they felt most desirous of being informed.   It was a current observation amongst the pupils that "Dr. Young was a great philosopher, but a bad physician," and the credence which was given to it, both within and without the walls of the Hospital, continued to give strength to the very prejudice in which it originated—that the highest professional eminence is only attainable by the exclusion of all other pursuits.

A physician of great eminence, distinguished for his classical scholarship and general attainments—who was Dr. Young's successor at the Hospital—has given me very satisfactory reasons for thinking his practice, both there and elsewhere, eminently successful, though not popular.   He lived in an age when what was called *vigorous practice*—partly introduced by our army and navy surgeons—was very generally prevalent; when the use of calomel and the lancet was in the ascendant; when symptoms were rudely interfered with and combated without any proper study of the causes in which they originated;—whether, in fact, they constituted the essence of the disease to be cured or indicated the nature of the remedy to be applied; when the "practical man," as he was accustomed proudly to call himself, stigmatized a just and careful induction from observation and a diligent waiting upon Nature and her operations, as "mere theory,"— preferring his own preconceived notions of the nature of disease, and drawing his own inferences from false facts and blundering experiments.[a]

Such views of medical practice were generally popular with the students, who liked a "royal road"

[a] Dr. J. A. Wilson on Spasm, Languor, and Palsy, p. 67.

to knowledge : whilst the great majority of the medical teachers of the Metropolis—who were not, like Baillie and Hunter and Abernethy, the shining lights of their profession, but young men just entering upon life, with their fortunes and reputations in the future— did not possess the authority, if they had the inclination, to impress upon their pupils the necessity of long continued and systematic preparation and study as the only secure method of thoroughly mastering the principles of the science, the applications of which were to form the business of their lives.   Such a result might have been anticipated from the apathetic indifference which the government of this country formerly showed to all our institutions for education :—London being the only great capital in Europe where the services of men of the greatest professional learning and eminence are not secured, by public honours and rewards, as teachers in its medical schools.

Dr. Young viewed the science of medicine as a branch of inductive philosophy, the principles of which, like those of other inductive sciences, were founded upon observation and experiment, where facts were to be divested as much as possible of every circumstance which was extraneous to the conclusion to be drawn from them, and where the correctness of the conclusion itself was to be tested by repeated appeals to experience—not to the experience of every pretender to the art, but of those only who have been taught to interrogate Nature by the formation, through careful preparatory studies, of those habits of the mind which enable it to appreciate evidence, and to distinguish accurately between the assumption of a conclusion and its demonstration.   It was upon experience thus carefully and scrupulously scrutinized, that Dr.

Young founded his medical practice, not hesitating to employ strong measures when the symptoms of the disease showed them to be necessary, but never rudely thwarting those processes of natural restoration and cure in cases where the same lessons of experience had shown them to be in operation.

The apothecary of the Hospital—a careful and cautious observer—is said to have made the remark that a greater proportion of the patients admitted under Dr. Young were discharged *cured,* or perhaps, in more correct language, *relieved,* than of those who were subjected to a more fashionable and energetic treatment ; a capital fact, which, if it had been properly noticed and studied, would at once have decided the question in dispute. But the statistics of the results of special modes of treatment are rarely collected in our hospitals, though they have been made, it is well known, the means of dissipating many false prejudices and errors in the hospitals of Paris, Berlin, and Vienna. I have been told by one who has examined the records of the Hospital, that the prescriptions which were given by Dr. Young are such as approximate—as nearly as circumstances will enable us to judge—to the best practice of the present day ; and that if he had survived and practised his profession for a few years longer, his claims to dictinction as a physician would have been, in all probability, as fully recognised as were those which were conceded to him as a philosopher and a scholar. It would not be altogether just, however, to the public at large, who may be considered responsible for a just estimate of the claims of those whom they employ, not to state that Dr. Young's manners were not favourable to his success as a practitioner : they were gentle and gentlemanly, but not genial ; he never professed or expressed more than he felt, and resorted to none of those many, and we may add perfectly justifiable, arts by which some physicians recommend themselves to their patients.

His Introduction to Medical Literature, including a system of Practical Nosology, was published early in the year 1813. It is a work of great labour, and bears much the same relation to the medical, that his Lectures bear to the mathematical and physical, sciences. It includes an Introduction on the Study of Physic; Aphorisms relating to Classifications—chiefly extracted from the Philosophia Botanica of Linnæus, the great master of the principles of classification and nomenclature—intermixed with many valuable observations of his own, with a view of adapting them to the medical sciences; a catalogue of about 100 pages of works on medical literature, both general and special, admirably arranged, with notes to direct a student to those works or parts of them which are likely to be most useful. This is followed by much the most important and the only very original part of the work, a System of Practical Nosology and Pharmacology, with most minute references to the best sources of information on every disease or medical agent included in the classification. There is also subjoined a Sketch of Animal Chemistry; Remarks on the Measurement of Minute Particles, especially those of Blood and Pus, by the aid of the Eriometer;[a] and an Essay on the Medical Effects of Climate, which had been published before as an appendix to the Syllabus of his Medical Lectures.

When Dr. Young commenced this undertaking, the nosological arrangement of Dr. Cullen was the one most generally recognized in this country and that

[a] Works, vol. i., p. 343.

which he himself was most disposed to follow. Upon proceeding with his task he found inconsistencies and deficiencies in it which were irreconcileable with every just principle of classification — his genera, orders, and classes being not only wanting in the essential qualities of logical dependence and sequence, but such as to exclude altogether a great number of diseases which found no proper place in his system. It is an objection, however, to all classifications of diseases that their characters are not invariable and persistent; that they change with changes of climate and place, with the habits of society, and even with the lapse of time; but at the same time, it must be allowed, though perfect accuracy may not be attainable, that our general views of the science of medicine will be advanced the nearer we approach to it.

In an age when the systematic study of medicine was so much neglected, it was not to be expected that a work of this nature, so much of which was occupied with speculations apparently so remote from immediate practical applications, would be received with much favour. A contemporary reviewer, who was a fair representative of that large class of mankind who look to the results of science much more than its principles, quotes with marked approbation, in his notice of this work, a sneer of Dr. Fordyce that many ingenious young men were familiar with *enteritis* and *carditis* and *nephritis*, but bring them to the bedside of a patient, and it would quickly appear that they could not tell one *itis* from another *itis*. If it could have been made to appear that the knowledge of the theoretical characters of those diseases was the reason of the ignorance of such persons of their practical symptoms, the observation would have been just; but let a physician, whether young or old—to whom the theoretical and practical characters of these diseases are equally familiar, and who can also reason correctly from the effects which he observes to their causes—be placed in the same situation with one who has facts and the routine of ordinary practice but no principles to guide him; and it is hardly necessary to say which of the two will be prepared to act with confidence and safety in the various phases, sometimes new and unexpected, which all such diseases are apt to assume.

The Sketch of Animal Chemistry, which is given in the Appendix of this work, was translated from the Swedish of Berzelius, by the aid of a grammar and dictionary, without any previous acquaintance with the language; his knowledge of German and of the general structure of languages, aided by a perfect familiarity with the subject and his usual sagacity, was sufficient to guide him. There is found amongst his papers a letter from this illustrious chemist, most gratefully acknowledging this service, and expressing his admiration of the skill and correctness with which the task had been executed. "Tell me," he proceeds, "how is it possible for the same person to possess so deep and comprehensive a knowledge of two sciences so widely different as Natural Philosophy and Medicine, with its subordinate sciences of Anatomy and Physiology? When I reflect that Chemistry constitutes my only pursuit, and that nevertheless I am daily learning how much has been done in that science that has escaped my inquiry, I marvel how you can have had time enough to go over all that you must have required to read in order to produce your Lectures on Natural Philosophy and this Medical Work." The translation is interspersed with many original observations and additions, in one of which he combats the inference drawn by the author, that the crystalline lens—being soluble in water—cannot be muscular ; a conclusion which has been elsewhere noticed.[a]

A new edition of this work was printed in 1823, when the author parted with the copyright for one hundred pounds : he adds—in noticing the fact—the remark, not altogether destitute of truth, that it was too good a book to be worth more ; it was not adapted in fact for popular reading. New references to the later medical journals were inserted, in this new edition, and an Essay on Palpitations was added, which first appeared in the fifth volume of the Medical Transactions of the College of Physicians in London.

In the Quarterly Review we find five articles by Young on medical subjects ; and several more, though shorter, and of a slighter texture, were contributed by him to the Imperial Review at an earlier period. The article on Insanity, in the Third Number of the first of these Reviews, is an essay of great merit, viewing the subject in its moral and metaphysical, as well as its medical bearings ; it was written on the suggestion of his friends, Mr. George Ellis and Sir Walter Scott, and not without some ulterior views to an appointment under the department of Lunacy in the Court of Chancery. His other medical articles, though in all cases giving evidences of a thorough mastery of the subjects upon which he was writing, do not generally possess the additional merit of being interesting to general as well as professional readers.[b]

---

[a] Supra, p. 42.

[b] The subjects of them are, Jones on the Gout, vol. iii. ; Blackall on Dropsies · Adams on Ectropium, vol. xiii ; an article on the Yellow Fever was printed but never published.

The last of his medical publications was 'A Practical and Historical Essay on Consumptive Diseases,' which appeared in 1815. It is a condensed and admirably arranged abstract of everything that has been said and done with regard to consumption. It was written and published within a period of nine months from the time that it was begun, and was undertaken with a view to the possible extension of his practice in a form of disease which is prevalent amongst the higher classes in this country. The work was one of great interest and value, though it failed to accomplish the ulterior object for which it was designed; and at a later period of life, when his circumstances were more independent, he was disposed to congratulate himself that he had thus escaped the danger of lapsing into a species of charlatanism which is sometimes the fate of those who restrict their practice to particular classes of diseases.

CHAPTER . IX.

PHILOLOGICAL ESSAYS.   REVIEWS.

The varied phases presented by Dr. Young's researches make it equally convenient to the biographer and his readers, to depart occasionally from the strict order of time, and to consider them in groups, by which subjects of a similar kind may be brought in some degree into connection with each other. This is the course which I have partially followed in the preceding pages, in devoting separate chapters to his Optical, Mathematical and Physical, and Medical writings; and I shall now proceed, in conformity with the same principle, to notice his philological researches, reserving those relating to the hieroglyphics of Egypt, on account of their great extent and importance, to the following chapter.

More than fourteen years had elapsed since Dr. Young quitted Edinburgh—where he first became known in connection with Greek literature, by the selections from the Anthologia which he made for the second volume of the Analecta of Professor Dalzel, and the notes by which they were accompanied—when an article appeared in the Quarterly Review, which excited more than common attention amongst scholars and men of letters. The subject of it was the Herculanensia, a splendid work, containing several learned philological and antiquarian dissertations relating to

Herculaneum and the ancient condition of the regions
in its neighbourhood. Three of these dissertations,
of very considerable merit, were written by the Rev.
Robert Walpole, an elegant and accomplished scholar,
well known by his Travels in European Turkey and
other works connected with classical literature and
archæology : six of the others were the production
of Sir William Drummond, formerly our ambassador
at Naples, whose critical judgment was not sufficient
to keep under due control the vast mass of curious
learning which his writings usually displayed ; whilst
the remaining dissertation was devoted to the restored
text of a papyrus, which had been unrolled and partially
deciphered by Mr. Hayter and others, under circumstances which are detailed in the article Herculaneum
reprinted in the third volume of Dr. Young's works.[a]
To this was added an elaborate commentary upon it,
written also by Sir William Drummond.

Though Mr. Hayter was, in some degree, indebted
to his reputation as a classical scholar, for the appointment at Naples, which he held for many years, for the
purpose of superintending the unrolling of these papyri,
his powers were found in this, which was the only considerable, instance in which they were brought to trial,
inadequate to the task which he had undertaken,
notwithstanding the assistance he received from several
of the academicians of Portici, who were associated
with him. In almost every part of the deciphered
manuscript, there were more or less considerable *lacunæ*
to be supplied, sometimes extending to two-thirds or
three-fourths of the entire line in which they appeared,
and the only guides to their restoration were the adjoining words or parts of words, taken in connection

with the context of those preceding or following them.
Dr. Young has printed in one page of his Review, a
fac-simile of thirty three lines of a portion of the manuscript, where the deficiencies are the most considerable,
and in another page which immediately follows it, he has
given in two parallel columns, the restored text, first as
proposed by himself, and secondly, by Mr. Hayter and
his colleagues; he has added likewise a list of emendations and substitutions in other parts of the manuscript in which he differs from the editors, and which
he has also embodied in his own exquisite copy of
the entire manuscript—which is now before me—with
the *lacunæ* filled up in a differently coloured ink, so as
not only to produce an intelligible text, which is good
Greek, but also to enable the reader to judge of the
propriety and probability of the restorations which are
proposed, not only with reference to the space which
they occupy, but likewise to the words or portions of
words which precede and follow them. The published
text, which was made the subject of his criticism, was
shown to be neither grammatically correct nor translateable, and even the designation of the subject of
the fragment was changed by the reviewer, upon
grounds which hardly admit of dispute, from being a
discourse *Concerning the Gods*, to one *Concerning Piety
according to Epicurus*. A complete translation of the
fragment, as restored by Dr. Young, was also given in
the Review.

Among many other mistakes which were pointed out
by the reviewer—though in no unfriendly or captious
spirit—which were little creditable to the scholarship
of the editors, there were two which excited more than
common remark. In one case, the following passage
in the text with its *lacunæ*,

καθαπερ κ . . . . . ταινα λεγειν ως . . . αν πολλακις
αηρ λεγη τις εφειν ηρ . . . .

was restored to

καθάπερ καὶ τὸν Πλόυτωνα λέγειν ὡς ἄν πολλάκις
ἀὴρ λεγῇ τις, ἔρειν "Ηρα. . . .

or meaning—*as also, Pluto says, if any one should repeat the word ἀὴρ many times, he would pronounce it*
"Hρα. The quotation which is here attributed to Pluto,
is actually found nearly, though not precisely, in the
same words in the Cratylus of Plato; and though
Sir William Drummond actually refers to it, on account of its resemblance to that in the fragment which
was the subject of his observation, he was not sufficiently startled by the discovery to deprive Pluto of
the honours of authorship which were here for the first
time assigned to him.

In another passage, there are three lines expressly
quoted from a comic drama, called Egypt, by Timocles :
they have been restored and freely translated by Dr.
Young as follows :—

'Οπου γὰρ εἰς τοὺς ὁμολογουμένους θεοὺς
'Ασεβοῦντες οὐ διδόασιν εὐθέως δικὴν,
Τίν' ἀιελούρου βῶμος ἐπιτρίψειεν ἄν;

le even the Gods, whose power all nations own,
crimes of impious men but slowly punish,
at perjured wretch shall dread Grimalkin's altars?"

ιhe same three lines, as having been quoted by
Athenæus, were well known to scholars, and the two
first of them are found complete in the fac-simile copy
of the papyrus. The same copy presents the last in the
following mutilated form :—

τινα . ε . ουρου βω
μος επ_. τριψειεν αν . .
ντ . . εγου . .

In the absence of any knowledge of the corresponding quotation, a competent critic engaged in filling up the *lacunæ* might have concluded, both from the character of the two preceding verses and from the fact of its being expressly taken from a Greek comic poet, that it must have been in Iambic metre; instead of which the Editor produced the following monstrous and untranslateable line :—

τίνα τε δοῦρ' ὃυ βῶμος ἐπιτρίψειεν ἂν ἀντιλέγουσι

If Mr. Hayter had not somewhat imprudently replied to the criticisms of the Reviewer, he might have continued to share the responsibility of mistakes too gross and palpable to be defended, with his Neapolitan colleagues, who had assisted him in the preparation of the text: but the defensive observations which he addressed to Sir William Drummond, as well as the somewhat apologetic and deprecatory remarks which the latter appended to them,[a] were sufficient very seriously to compromise whatever character for good sense and scholarship either one or the other of them might once have laid claim to. Whilst Mr. Hayter, not contented with defending his original emendation, was disposed to contend that even the text of Athenæus, as being confessedly corrupt, would be improved by introducing it, they both of them persevered in putting a manifest quotation from Plato into the mouth of the god Pluto : not to mention many other errors, almost equally indefensible, though not quite so glaring. No subsequent attempt was made to re-establish the character of Mr. Hayter as a scholar,

[a] Observations upon a review of the Herculanensia in the Quarterly Review of last February, by John Hayter, M.A., Chaplain to the Prince of Wales ; to which is subjoined a Letter from Sir William Drummond. 1810.

or to vindicate his conduct with respect to the abandonment of the papyri and of the copies made of them, which were entrusted to his superintendence and care by the Prince of Wales who employed him, when he fled with the Royal Family from Naples to Palermo upon the French invasion in 1806.

The result of the discovery of the Herculaneum manuscripts —originally more than eighteen hundred in number—has signally disappointed the sanguine expectations which it first excited; when the imaginations of every scholar in Europe were haunted by visions of the restoration of the lost books of Livy, of the comedies of Menander and of many of the other choice treasures of ancient literature which the barbarism of the middle ages had destroyed. All the manuscripts in fact were found to be carbonized by heat, and the leaves which composed them glued together by some cementing principle so tenacious as only to give way, in rare cases, to the most cautious and persevering efforts; whilst the greater number were so crushed by the weight of the volcanic matter which had buried them, as to defy all attempts at unrolling them. A great portion also of those which promised better results perished in the various experiments to which they were subjected by adventurers and projectors of all kinds; whilst of more than four hundred which were partially unrolled, legible fragments of not more than eighty were made out, and a worthless Treatise on Music by Philodemus was the only one which had been restored and edited antecedently to the solitary and not more successful effort of Mr. Hayter.

Upon the termination of Mr. Hayter's mission to Naples, a considerable number of the remaining papyri—at that time, however, not more than eighty in number—were sent over to this country, where several of them became the victims of the experiments of a German charlatan : a few of them were entrusted to the Royal Society and placed by them in the hands of Dr. Young, who thus speaks of some experiments to which he resorted with a view of unrolling them :—

"There was one mode of treating the papyri which occurred to him, which promised to be of much use to those who might hereafter be engaged in the operation. This was the employment of the anatomical blowpipe, an instrument which he had many years before been in the habit of using for delicate purposes, in the place of a dissecting knife. The blowpipe served him, like the ῤὶς κάστορος in the epigram, for a knife and a forceps ; for the gum, the goldbeater's skin, and the threads of the Italians. No instrument can be so soft in its pressure as the air, for holding a thin fragment by suction, without danger of injuring it : no edge nor point can be so sharp as to be capable of insinuating itself into all the crevices which the air freely enters. But the humidity of the breath he found to add much to the utility of the instrument : the slight degree of moisture communicated to the under or inner surface of a fold, made it curl up and separate from the parts beneath where the adhesion was not too strong ; while dry air from a bladder was perfectly incapable of detaching it. But the process of separating every leaf in this manner was always tedious and laborious, where there was much adhesion, and sometimes altogether impracticable. Chemical agents of all kinds he tried without the least advantage ; and even maceration for six months in water, applied at first with very great caution, was unable to weaken the adhesion. It is remarkable that the characters were not effaced by this operation, so that the gum which had fixed them on the paper must have wholly lost its solubility, and the rest of its original properties."[a]

The appearance of this Article, equally remarkable for its critical acuteness and vigorous writing, at once placed its author, in the estimation of the public, in

[a] Quarterly Review, vol. iii. p. 19.

the first class of the scholars of the age. The editor of
the Review, in a letter to George Ellis, says, "Young's
article is certainly above all praise. It has had, however, one deplorable effect. ——, who is of the same
college with Blomfield, tells me that the latter, upon
reading it, sent in all haste to Edinburgh, to recall a
review of the Herculanensia, which he had written for
the next number. If this letter arrives in time, we have
lost a triumph." It was not likely, however, that any
production of the very eminent scholar here referred to
could have afforded a triumph to his opponents; but,
like all men of a generous and noble nature, he would
have been the first to welcome a fellow-labourer in a
department of his own field of learning, which had
been made, in this instance, by special and energetic
cultivation, to yield so rich a produce.

Young was intimately associated with the leading
contributors to the Quarterly Review. The principal of
these—after Mr. Gifford the Editor—was George Ellis,
of Sunning Hill, a writer of great wit and vivacity—the
author, not merely of some of the best literary articles
which the Review contained, but also of many others on
the political questions of the day, in which he was sometimes assisted by Mr. Canning and Mr. Huskisson, with
whose views he was thoroughly identified. He was a
man of ardent affections, who felt for his friends almost
as much as for himself; and he had resented, almost
as a personal injury, the treatment which Young had
received from the Edinburgh Review, and was thus
disposed, as much from personal as from party feeling,
not merely to oppose the political and literary dictation
of that powerful Journal, but also to watch with deep
interest the rising fortunes of its rival, in the establishment of which he had taken so considerable a part.

The same number of the Review which was headed by the Herculanensia was closed by Southey's spirit-stirring Life of Nelson ; and these being followed up, in subsequent volumes, by contributions of great interest and ability from Barrow, Walter Scott, Robert Grant, and others, were the means of rapidly extending its popularity and influence.

" It is a consolation to know," says Ellis in writing to Young, " that Brougham, who took advantage of the growing circulation of the Edinburgh Review to disseminate his vile abuse of you, and Jeffrey who permitted him to do so, should be condemned to hear your praises on all sides, and to feel that the publication in which they are engaged is suffering and is likely to suffer by your means."

Young, at different times, contributed eighteen articles to the Quarterly Review. The subjects of nine of them were scientific ; of five, medical ; and of the rest, languages and criticism. Several of those of the first class, and all those of the last, comprehended original researches of no ordinary value, and either have been or will be noticed in the course of this volume : but those relating to medicine, which have been elsewhere referred to, though by no means without merit, were for the most part too exclusively professional to be generally popular, and the exclusion of one of them, on Yellow Fever, from the Review, though it had been accepted and printed, was the occasion, when taken in conjunction with his other engagements, of abandoning his connection with it altogether.

He was much consulted by Mr. Gifford upon many articles submitted to him, more especially such as came within the very comprehensive sphere of his studies ; and we find in the letters which passed between them, amongst many other secrets of authorship, the usual

complaints of the trials to which editors of such
journals are exposed. Some articles were too long and
required pruning; the dulness of others was to be
adapted by a higher seasoning to the public taste; many
were forced upon the Editor by the official or literary
rank of their authors, which he dared not either reject
or retouch; most of them required to be assimilated to
the literary or political views which the Review was
designed to promote; whilst the last and not the least
of his difficulties were the interests of the publisher,
which, though never illiberally urged, could not be
safely or reasonably neglected, though they might be
found to be at variance with the favourite prepossessions
both of editors, authors, and readers.

Young was generally disposed to prefer the rugged
and unknown, to the beaten and familiar, paths of learning.   In a letter to Mr. Gurney, he says—

"I like a deep and difficult investigation when I happen to
have made it easy to myself, if not to all others; and there is a
spirit of gambling in this, whether, as by the cast of a die, a
calculation à perte de vue shall bring out a beautiful and perfect
result or shall be wholly thrown away.   Scientific investigations
are a sort of warfare carried on in the closet or on the couch
against all one's contemporaries and predecessors; I have often
gained a signal victory when I have been half asleep, but more
frequently have found, upon being thoroughly awake, that the
enemy had still the advantage of me, when I thought I had him
fast in a corner, and all this you see keeps me alive."

He loved to grapple, in fact, as we have already had
occasion to remark, with difficult problems in science and
not less so in literature.   A corrupt passage to be restored; a mutilated, rude, or badly spelt inscription to
be completed, or corrected, or interpreted; an alphabet
or a meaning to be extracted from an unknown language by a careful analysis of its different parts, by

connecting what is unknown with what is known, or with
such documents as his various learning could supply,
—were always more or less labours of predilection with
him, where his nice perception and accurate transcription of forms, his intimate knowledge of the principles
of grammar, his patient labour and uncommon sagacity, had full scope for their exercise. His review of
the Herculanensia had made his qualifications for such
tasks generally known; and from that time to the end
of his life, inscriptions from all quarters, especially in
Greek and in the hieroglyphical and cursive characters
of ancient Egypt, were referred to him for discussion
or interpretation. Many copies of such inscriptions,
from Greece, Egypt, and India, are found amongst his
papers, which had been sent to him to be explained,
but which for the most part were deficient either in
sufficiently accurate transcription, or in the detail of
circumstances which alone could give them value.

In the 19th volume of the Archæologia, we find
an interesting notice of a fragment of a very ancient
papyrus, as well as of several curious but somewhat
barbarous sepulchral inscriptions of a late age from
Nubia, which were submitted to him by Lord Mountnorris. In the Appendix to Captain Light's Travels
in Egypt, Nubia, Palestine, and Cyprus, he furnished
restorations and translations of several Greek inscriptions: and when Barrow gave an account in the
Quarterly Review[a] of recent researches in Egypt, more
especially those of Caviglia on the great Sphinx, it was
from Young that he obtained the restoration of the in-

---

[a] The 19th volume, p. 411. Dr. Young complained, however, with some
justice, of the total omission of the criticisms with which his restoration was
accompanied, and to which he appears to have attached considerable value.
The betrayal of his name, in spite of his injunction to the contrary, was
another cause of dissatisfaction.

scription on the second digit of the great paw; "a task," says he, "which he has executed with his usual skill and judgment in clearing away the difficulties of imperfect inscriptions in ancient languages." The most flattering, however, of these testimonies was that which he received from an eminent theologian and scholar, the late Rev. Hugh James Rose,[a] who, in his work entitled "Inscriptiones Græcæ Vetustissimæ," refers in grateful terms to the assistance which he had derived from him in the restoration of some ancient inscriptions, complimenting him upon the variety of his accomplishments in the words of the poet—

"quem tu, Dea, tempore in omni,
Omnibus ornatum voluisti excellere rebus."

In the year 1813 he contributed a very elaborate article to the Quarterly Review, on the Mithridates of Adelung.[b] This was followed, two years afterwards, by another supplementary to it, on Jamieson's Hermes Scythicus, and the Rev. J. Townshend's work entitled, The Character of Moses established for Veracity as a Historian recording Events subsequent to the Deluge.[c] These articles were subsequently incorporated, with much original matter, into the essay under the title of Languages, in the Supplement to the Encyclopædia Britannica.[d] They afford the ordinary proofs of his great industry and power of arrangement, but are not remarkable for views of an original or very striking character, and they should be considered as the results

[a] There are several letters, amongst his papers, addressed to him by Mr. Rose, relating to these inscriptions, and more especially to one of them of great antiquity which was found on the Leucadian promontory, and of which he proposed a very satisfactory restoration.

[b] Quarterly Review, vol. x. Oct. 1813, p. 230.

[c] Quarterly Review, vol. xiv. Oct. 1813, p. 96.

[d] Supplement to the Encyclopædia Britannica, vol. v. 1819. Works, vol. iii., p. 478.

rather of a single effort directed to a special inquiry, than of investigations like those relating to the hieroglyphics of Egypt, to which all the powers of his mind had been long and systematically devoted.

In an essay on Probabilities, in the Philosophical Transactions,[a] he has made the observation that no inference could be drawn, with respect to the relation of two languages to each other, from the coincidence in both of them of the sense of any single word, and no more—that is, supposing the same simple and limited combination of sounds to occur in both, but to be applied accidentally to the same objects, without any common links of connection; and farther, that the odds would be only three to one against the agreement of two such words, and ten to one against the agreement of three of them: for six and ten such words, the numbers expressing these probabilities would become 1700 and 100,000 to 1 respectively. The evidence afforded by results like these, whose irresistible force these large numbers alone can adequately express, are full of interest and instruction, as proving indisputably the existence of a connection—whether through some common primitive language, as Mr. Townshend and others have contended, or through emigration, conquest, commercial intercourse, or other causes—in the vast majority of written as well as many other languages. It is only in the groups of African and South American languages that we fail to discover very manifest traces of influences of this nature.

Dr. Young has divided existing languages into five great families—the Monosyllabic, the Indo-European, the Tataric (subdivided into five subordinate families, the Sporadic, the Caucasian, the Tartarian, the Sibe-

a Works, vol. ii., p. 17.

rian, and the Insular), the African, and the American; a classification which is, with the exception of the first, and in some degree of the second, much too large and comprehensive to present any proper philological connection or marked distinctive character. The bases of a more accurate, but still of a very vague classification, are afforded by a tabulated list, which he has selected from the great work of Adelung, of the words used to express *heaven* or *sky*, and *earth*, in more than 400 languages: for it is obvious that words equivalent to these must have existed in all languages, however primitive and rude, and are such as, from their familiarity and frequent use, were least likely to be modified or altered by intercourse with other nations; and it will be found that the relationships which they indicate in the languages in which they are expressed by words which are essentially the same, however disguised by varieties of form and pronunciation, are very generally, though by no means universally, supported by a further examination of their vocabulary and structure.

The result of later and somewhat more philosophical inquiries has shown that languages are much more intimately related to each other by analogies in their grammatical construction than by community of words; that whilst two or more languages, thus assimilated with each other, may admit of incorporation to almost any extent, no such amalgamation can be effected of those which do not possess this common character, however great may be the intercourse with each other of the nations which speak them, and however numerous may be the individual words which may be interchanged. The comparison, also, of the numeral systems and terms of different languages is full of interest, not merely as regards the practical methods of numeration in which many of them originated, but also as furnishing evidences which are more patent, though not always so decisive, as those which can be derived from other sources, of the intercourse of nations with each other, at some periods of their history, and in many cases of the relations of the languages which they speak.

"The strongest proof," says Young, "of the antiquity of the Chinese language appears to be the great simplicity of its structure, and the want of those abbreviations and conventional implications which have sometimes been called the wings of language. It is natural that, in attempting to express ideas at once by characters, the rude pictures of material objects should first have been principally, if not exclusively traced. Thus the Egyptians had ⊙, ☽, for the *sun* and *moon*, and ⊕ for a country or field; and the Chinese have still 日 月 田 for those objects respectively, the characters having been made square instead of round, which some of them were in their more ancient forms."[a] We shall afterwards find that he was principally guided by the many analogies which appeared to exist between the characters of this singular language and the hieroglyphics of Egypt, to conclude it to be extremely probable, that the expedients to give to the characters a phonetic value, when foreign names and words were to be expressed, were much the same in one language as in the other, and thus to lay the foundations of one of the most remarkable discoveries in modern times.

Dr. Leyden, as quoted by Young, observes that at least twenty different nations employ the Chinese cha-

[a] See Works, vol. iii., p. 509.

racters, and generally with the Chinese significations, though they read them quite differently: and he considers the Cochin-Chinese, the Cantonese, and the Japanese as all essentially different from the Mandarin Chinese, though they all have some words in common. But a question naturally arises in connexion with so singular a system, whether such languages are to be considered different from each other, or the same; whether, in fact, the language which is addressed to the eye or to the ear is the language of the people. The question became one of great interest as affecting the attempts to interpret the hieroglyphics of Egypt. If these hieroglyphics constituted a sacred language, addressed to the eye, and equally intelligible to all the tribes of ancient Egypt, who spoke, as it is well known they did, dialects very different from each other, it would have served, like the Chinese, as a universal language, which all would equally understand, though the inhabitants of different districts would translate it differently to the ear: and further, if they possessed a method of writing their spoken language by alphabetical characters which expressed the sounds of their local language when spoken, the enchorial translation of the same hieroglyphical text might be very different in different regions of the country. Thus the enchorial translation of the hieroglyphical inscription on the Rosetta stone might have been very different in the different copies of it which were directed, in conformity with the decree which it embodies, to be placed in the temples of Upper and Lower Egypt. The importance of these questions will be better understood when they are brought under our consideration by the subject of the next Chapter.

It has often been remarked that the life of a man of

letters or science rarely presents any striking events
which can be separated from the history of those researches which have given him celebrity, and that of
Young offers no exception to the truth of the observation. Though no small portion of his time was occupied with the duties of his profession, they were,
fortunately for his fame, not of so absorbing a kind as
materially to interrupt his other pursuits, or to debar
him from the salutary relaxation afforded by his access
to a large and cultivated society. The following extracts from letters addressed to a sister of Mrs.
Young sufficiently describe his ordinary habits, and
are not altogether without interest from their references to some of the popular topics of the day.

" London, 22nd November, 1814.

" Dearest Emily,

　　" I have long been intending to write to you, but I am
so much engaged in collecting materials for a new medical
work[a] that I have had no leisure to do anything else. It was
not my own wish nor my intention to be so employed; but I
am determined to make a last effort of this kind, which I hope
to complete in the course of a few months, and which I think
will insure me a certain degree of popularity in my profession,
more extensive and more permanent than I have hitherto felt
myself confident in the possession of: but whether I fail or
succeed in this object, I think I shall not hereafter make any
further attempts of the kind.   .   .   .   .   .   .

.   .   .   .

I called yesterday on Gifford, in order to be able to answer
some of your inquiries. The first article in the Quarterly
Review on Brand's Antiquities is by a lawyer named Cohen or
Colquhoun; Mathias I believe by Whitaker; Chalmers of
course by Southey, who has just published his Don Roderick in
a thick 4to of blank verse; the Travels and the Chinese article
by Barrow; Lord Byron by G. Ellis; the Modern Greek by

Treatise on Consumption, see supra, p. 229.

Blomfield; Davy[a] and Adams[b] you know—neither of them was written *con amore*, and they only occupy a private station in the ranks, without disgracing the rest.

"Have you seen the last Edinburgh Review? The first article on painting is by Payne Knight, and is generally admired.[c] It was much discussed last Thursday at Lord Elgin's, where I dined with only West, the President of the Royal Academy, and Ross; besides R. Hay, who came in late in the evening. This was one of the very few dinners that reconcile one to living in London. Lady Elgin, you have heard, is a Grecian; but she has not the manners of a blue-stocking, and she really appears to pursue literature and science with a great deal of zeal and good taste, and without any sacrifice of common sense. She has been reading some of the Greek tragedies, which are reckoned the most difficult works in the language, and she has returned to Homer. I have lent her some mathematical books to take with her into Scotland: she had only read the first six books of Euclid, and asked me what I would recommend her to go on with. West is really a most interesting personage in everything that relates to his profession; in other respects he is very much like any other man of seventy-four: but he was only seven months painting his great picture, which he sold for 3000 guineas, and which produced 13,000 to the British Institution by its exhibition. His present picture is visited daily by 472 people on an average of a fortnight. He paints fifteen hours a day, not requiring any other exercise, and sleeping but seven: he paints without any model, in order to avoid introducing portraits, and to preserve an ideal character of perfection in his figures; but when he has once drawn them, he corrects the attitudes and the lights by comparison with a real figure: for this reason, he said, he never repeated himself. To me it appeared that he did very often repeat the same kind of countenance, and his mode of painting seemed to explain the reason of it, and I ventured to hint something of the kind in an indirect manner. In consequence of his wishing to see me at his house, I called on him last Sunday, and sat a long while with him. He perfectly

[a] Republished in Works, vol. i., p. 575.

[b] Adams on Ectropium, Artificial Pupil and Cataract. Quarterly Review, July 1814, vol. xi.

[c] Review of Northcote's Life of Reynolds. Sept. 1814.

remembered my once having seen him twenty-one years ago, when, as he observed, I was dressed in a different costume. He told me the history of the little Cupid and Psyche which I have :ᵃ he painted it in the year 1760, when he was in his twenty-first year, before he had ever been in England. The very day after his arrival at Rome, Mr. Robinson, Lord Grantham's father, called almost accidentally upon him, and introduced him, immediately to Raphael Mengs, then the first painter there, whom Payne Knight laughs at so unmercifully for studying Corelli's beautiful concerto as a preparation to painting the Nativity.ᵇ Mengs wished to see a specimen of his talents, and gave him some prints of heads from Vandyke to copy in oils. He showed me his copies. And he painted at the same time this little group as a specimen of his own manner, which pleased Mengs so much that he told him he had no occasion to pursue any academical studies at Rome, and advised him not to remain there long for fear of becoming a mannerist, but to travel to all the principal towns in Italy, and to confine his studies to statues and great masters only. He contradicted the report of Raphael's great picture of the Transfiguration having been moved from board to canvas. My friend Merrill, who is a most zealous dilettante, and had lately seen it, was complaining most bitterly of the injury it had suffered from the operation, in the total distortion of many of the finest parts; Lord Elgin added, upon the authority of Visconti, the director of the French Museum, who has lately been in London, that it was found upon examination that the pannel would stand for 100 or 150 years, and that the back-ground only had been slightly repaired, and in a very judicious manner, but that the whole had been a little cleaned.

" West spoke highly of the Americans as a nation possessed of natural talent; and, that he did not speak from personal partiality, he demonstrated by a copy from a large picture of his own, which I had been looking at, without distinguishing which was the original. This was actually the second attempt only of a young man who had been in a counting-house till he happened to attract his master's attention by a very striking likeness

---

ᵃ In the collection of pictures bequeathed to him by his uncle Dr. Brocklesby.

ᵇ Edinburgh Review. Sept. 1814, p. 267.

of Cooke the actor, which he had been amusing himself in painting. His master sent him to Europe to study: his name is Leslie, and he is only nineteen. They have, however, an excellent Academy at Philadelphia, and they have obtained from Paris casts of all the antiques in the Louvre. The collection is open one day in every week for the *separate* inspection of ladies; and West says that the best remarks on the beauty of the antique statues that he recollects to have read have lately been published by a *Quaker lady* of *Philadelphia*: all three characters as little calculated, in the general opinion, to fit her for such an undertaking as can well be imagined.   .   .   .

.   .   .   .

He agreed with me in rejoicing that all the works of art were to remain at Paris; where, he said, they would be of more use to the English than to the French themselves, who were incapable of profiting by them in the same degree; that Paris was no more an unfit residence than Rome, or than any other great city: but that, notwithstanding the perfection of the French collections, which were unique in admitting nothing second rate, the Cartoons of Raphael alone, together with Lord Elgin's statues, would afford more instruction to a student than all the Louvre put together. He said that if Lord Elgin had not brought away the marbles, they would have been utterly lost in another century; as certainly some of the finest fragments of the statues which are now imperfect have been burnt into lime and used for building a house, within these twenty years, by a Greek, who had the knavery to take a large sum from Lord Elgin to let his house be pulled down and the foundation dug up in search of these very pieces. And now I have told you enough of Mr. West, a man who has covered 7000 square feet of canvas, and too much, except that I think all these particulars worth remembering, and therefore worth writing; and if you do not think them worth reading, you are at liberty to pass them over and burn the letter."   .   .   .

"London, 7th Dec., 1815.   Thursday Evening.

"Dearest Emily,

"Being naturally, as you know, of a very loquacious disposition, and being left in perfect solitude by my two runaway ladies, who went off this morning with Major Kater for Hadley,

I have no resource but to gossip a little with you. It is certainly not from idleness that I have not done it before—and you will not easily believe that it is from forgetfulness: you must however admit diffidence among the many reasons; notwithstanding that I have a tolerably good opinion of myself, I know how fastidious you are, and that I ought not to write without being able to send you something worth reading. Your letter I cannot answer, except from recollection, for I scarcely looked at it when Eliza carried it off, and she has never been able to find it again. You said that you could not quite understand my nonsense verses;[a] perhaps you will be able to make them out by means of a nonsensical translation or imitation which I was obliged to hammer out in defiance of the Abbé Weston and to satisfy Taylor Combe's curiosity :—

> Medical men, my mood mistaking,
> Most mawkish monstrous messes making,
> Molest me much; more manfully,
> My mind might meet my malady :
> Medicine's mere mockery murders me.

This is bad enough; but it is much more difficult to execute such alliterations in English than in Latin, and you will say it would be no great loss if it were impossible.

"It was about this time twelvemonth that I gave you an account of my dinner at Lord Elgin's, and of the conversation that passed with West, especially on the subject of the French collections. How little did I then think that I should by this time have discussed the same points with William Hamilton[b] and Canova, immediately after they had been chiefly instrumental in breaking up these collections, and sending back the spoils to the original proprietors! I met them last Sunday at Sir Joseph Banks's.   .   .   .   .
.   .   .   .

Upon the subject of the Louvre, Hamilton said nearly what Lord Castlereagh says in his Note, which has lately been in the papers, with the addition of the real benefit that he thought might be derived from essentially humbling the pride of the French. Indeed Lord Castlereagh's Note states the case very

---

[a] In imitation of the well known and ingenious alliterative verses called Pugna Porcorum, where each word begins with the letter P.

[b] Formerly Ambassador at Naples.

strongly and forcibly; but even supposing it proved that the
measure is just and wise, I cannot help thinking it a real
sacrifice on the part of England. I happened to ask him if
Canova was gone, and I found that he was standing close by,
with his brother, a little abbé. I begged to be introduced
to him, and talked a great deal to him; but I could get nothing
out of him except ' cospetto !' and that an antiquary like me
ought to come to Rome. You may suppose that I chose my
ground, and endeavoured to tell him something that he might
remember me by if we ever met again. This is something like
charlatanerie, but with a stranger, whom one sees but for ten
minutes in one's life, there is no medium between this and insi-
pidity. It seems West is beginning to be reconciled to the loss
of the statues; at least for decency's sake he gave a toast at
the academical dinner, to which Canova was invited, the other
day, ' The Restoration of the Vatican Museum.' Have you
read the Quarterly Review? The last article is of course
Southey's; the African and American I suppose Barrow's; the
Prussian I think Robert Hay's; the others I do not know, but
I shall perhaps hear. I have a long article on ancient languages already printed for the next: I wrote it soon after
Midsummer; it has no great interest nor originality, but looks
respectable enough. I am also about another on yellow fever,[a]
which is wofully dull to write; how it will read I do not know,
but I hope it will not be very long: it has occupied me these
three or four weeks, and made me so stupid that I was fit for
nothing else, and could not even venture to write to you till I
had done the most material parts of it. I have, however, had a
variety of interruptions. One was in making some last experiments on the Herculaneum manuscripts, which I hoped might
be rendered a little more translateable by passing them through
the fire. I found that they underwent the process without difficulty or injury, when well covered with charcoal dust; but the
adhesions remained as obstinate as ever, and I suppose nothing
will ever overcome them. I wished to perform this final experiment in order to determine if I had any chance of making
any material progress in the operation, before I inquired what
Hayter had been doing with the one which I gave up to him
in the summer, especially as he seemed to have been boasting

" This article was printed but never published.

of his great success. I found, however, that he had advanced so slowly as to leave me ample time for consideration before he can possibly want a second manuscript; for in fact he has not detached anything in a legible form, if my intelligence is correct; and I hope hereafter to be able to assist him or his operation in doing something more effectually. I have been also not a little mortified at the blunders of the booksellers and printers who have lost a part of my manuscripts for the Museum Criticum, which was to be engraved on wood, and which I must draw over again. I have had nothing but delay and difficulty in this business. My only motive for choosing this channel for publication was a wish to oblige the proprietor[a] and his learned supporters." .   .   .   .   .

In the summer of 1814, Mr. Macvey Napier, who had undertaken the duty of editing a new Supplement of the Encyclopædia Britannica, applied to him for his assistance as a contributor. The following reply will explain his motives for declining, at that time, to comply with his application.

                                    " Worthing, 9th August, 1814.
" Sir,
        " I have to thank you for your very obliging letter : but, as I had before told a friend of Prof. Leslie in London, I am sorry that it is not in my power at present to comply in any degree with a proposal, which, under other circumstances, would have been far from disagreeable to me : but I feel it a matter of necessity to abstain as much as possible from appearing before the public as an author in any department of science not immediately medical : and even if this objection were removed, I am not sure that I could find time to execute any task of importance in such a way as would be satisfactory to myself. I have therefore only to wish you all possible success in your laudable undertaking, and beg you to believe me,

                " Your obliged and obedient servant,

                                    " Thomas Young."

---

[a] Mr. Murray : the present Bishop of Gloucester was the Editor, and the present Bishop of London one of its principal supporters.

In the early part of the year 1816, a change in his views, induced him to make an offer of his services upon the conditions which are mentioned in the following letter :—

"London, 48, Welbeck Street, 12th Feb., 1816.

" Sir,

"When I had the honour of answering your letter on the subject of the Supplement to the Encyclopædia Britannica, I had no reason to think that I could look forward to any considerable portion of literary leisure : but of late some circumstances have occurred, which have left me somewhat more at liberty than 1 then expected ; and I may have it in my power to render you some material assistance in various departments of your undertaking. I must, however, make one condition, which I fear will create some difficulty : I could not at present allow my name to be published as a contributor to the work ; on the other hand, I could probably furnish you with some articles which you could scarcely obtain from other quarters : I should not refuse to do my best upon any subject of science, and I would consent to acknowledge all my contributions at the end of ten years from the present time. Knowing, however, the importance of names that are familiar to the public, I will not deny that you might fairly offer me a remuneration somewhat less liberal on this account ; and I must therefore beg you to favour me with your sentiments on the subject as soon as is convenient to you. You mentioned to me the article Acoustics as one which you would like me to undertake, but this branch of science might be reserved for Sound. I would also suggest Alphabet, Annuities, Attraction, Capillary Action, Cohesion, Colour, Dew, Egypt, Eye, Forms, Friction, Halo, Hieroglyphic, Hydraulics, Motion, Resistance, Ship, Strength, Tides, and Waves. Anything of a medical nature which you might think desirable would of course be doubly so to me : nor should I be difficult with respect to any other subject that might occur to you. ' L' alte non temo, e l' umili non sdegno.'

"I am, sir,

" Your faithful and obedient servant,

"Thomas Young.

" M. Napier, Esq."

In some of the articles, to which he laid claim, he had been anticipated by arrangements which the Editor had previously made. The subject of Meteorology had been appropriated by Professor Leslie; Attraction and Capillary Attraction and Cohesion by Mr. Ivory. His services, as might have been expected, were thankfully accepted on his own terms, which were that he should receive sixteen guineas a sheet as long as his communications were anonymous, and twenty guineas a sheet, in case he should allow his name to appear. The signature by which his Articles are known · are two consecutive letters in the motto *Fortunam ex aliis*, which he intimates that he had adopted as indicating that his success in his own profession had not been equal to his expectations, and that the value of his scientific labours, though fully appreciated by the philosophers on the continent, had not been estimated with equal justice by his countrymen. It would hardly appear to have occurred to him, while he was giving expression to this feeling, that the very anxiety to secure his co-operation in a great national work was at least a proof that the tide of public opinion had already begun to turn in his favour.

He contributed between the years 1816 and 1823, sixty-three articles to this Supplement, of which forty-six were biographical. Of these contributions that on Egypt was much the most considerable: but the articles on Bridge, Cohesion, Chromatics and especially that on Tides, most of which were reproductions, with very important additions and alterations, of essays which had appeared elsewhere, are hardly surpassed in originality and importance by any works on the subjects of them which have appeared in modern times.

The biographies, though many of them are very brief and compiled from ordinary sources of information, are generally remarkable for great skill in the condensation of his materials and for the easy flow and occasional liveliness of the narrative. They are generally accompanied by a very complete list of the several works of the subjects of his memoirs, with notices more or less ample of those which are remarkable for any important investigation or conclusion. We thus find a notice of nearly one hundred memoirs of Lagrange, of more than two hundred of Lalande, of one hundred and thirty of Fourcroy, of thirty-five of Maskelyne, and of great numbers of those written by Coulomb, Lambert, De La Condamine, and others.

Of the scientific lives, the most elaborate is that of Cavendish, whose memoirs are criticised with the discrimination and minuteness which is due to them as presenting nearly the finest models in our language of scrupulously accurate experimental determinations, and of sagacious yet cautious induction. Their illustrious author did not live to witness the attempt which has been made and vehemently supported in modern times by some writers of the highest eminence both in literature and science, to deprive him of the credit due to his great discovery of the composition of water. An undisturbed possession of more than half a century and guaranteed by a character for honour and veracity which had never previously been impugned, has been found insufficient to protect him from imputations upon his ingenuousness at least, if not upon his honesty. It might reasonably be asked whether the boldest of his contemporaries would have dared to move a finger in derogation either of his claim or of his character?

Young was himself disposed to think highly of his
life of Lagrange, which he had prepared with more
than ordinary labour and care : but we have ventured
elsewhere to dispute the justice of the estimate which
he has formed of the character of that extraordinary
man, which he was disposed to consider as indicative
rather of extraordinary industry, than of great sagacity
and talent.[a] He has done more justice to the works
of Coulomb and Robison, which he was better enabled
to appreciate by the connection of many of them with
his own special studies and investigations : those of
Coulomb, more especially his *Statical Problems relating
to Architecture*, exercised, as he himself informs us, a
most important influence upon some of the most successful of his own speculations.

Of all his biographical sketches that of Porson is
undoubtedly the best.   It is written throughout with
great liveliness and point, and contains some admirable
observations on the real value and importance of classical studies and critical scholarship.   His own early
passion for such studies and the eminence which he attained in them, notwithstanding the variety and absorbing nature of his other occupations, enabled him
thoroughly to appreciate this extraordinary man.   He
enjoyed the privilege also in very early life, as we have
already seen, of sitting occasionally at the feet of this
great master, and he was not indisposed to refer, with
a very pardonable pride, to his own share in critical
conflicts, in which he had participated.[b]   Even the

---

[a] Works, vol. ii., p. 579.

[b] Supra, p. 23. Dr. Young refers, in his sketch, to a party at which he
was present in 1791, when only 18 years of age, where Burney—referring to
a canon of the versification of the Greek tragic writers which Porson had
recently established, prescribing that where an iambic trimeter ends with
a *trisyllabic* word, forming a *pes creticus* as it is called, it must be preceded

beauty and nicety of penmanship, more especially in forming the Greek characters, in which Young as well as Porson so much excelled, formed no slight bond of connection between them: and they were equally well qualified, by their own experience, to form a just estimate of the value of an acquirement or rather of a gift—though some men are disposed to underrate it as mechanical—which not only places every letter of a mutilated manuscript at the command of a copyist, but indelibly fixes attention on the minutest variations of their forms, and thus lays the foundation of those accurate habits of observation which are not less important to a critical scholar than to a man of science. One of his biographers has said that Porson, in speaking of his own Greek writing, "admitted that another person surpassed him not in the stroke but in the sweep of his letters:" but Young himself assures us that this statement was not quite correct; for whilst Porson conceded to him the advantage with respect to the " command of hand" which his system gave him, he preferred the *model* upon which his own was formed. Young himself very modestly adds, that " Porson's hand was more like that of a scholar, whilst his own, as exhibited in the Calligraphia Græca, exhibits more the appearance of the work of a writing-master: holding a middle place between the neatness of Porson and the marvellous accuracy of the country school-master, who made the fac-simile of the Oxford Pindar in the British Museum."

either by a short syllable or by a monosyllable—introduced a very happy illustration of its violation in the verse

Πᾶν ἰκπίπωκας· οὐ λίλειπται κότταβος.

at the very time that Porson—in a state which was unhappily too common with him—was attempting to fill his glass from an empty bottle. Young, with his usual promptitude and courage, suggested the reading κ'οὐδ' ἔνεστι κότταβος, which was equally advantageous to the sense and to the metre.

CHAPTER X.

HIEROGLYPHICAL RESEARCHES.

A TRAVELLER in Egypt, Sir W. Rouse Boughton, had found, in a mummy-case in a catacomb near Thebes, a papyrus written in cursive Egyptian characters, which, though nearly perfect when first discovered, was subsequently very much injured by being accidentally soaked in sea-water. The fragments that remained were submitted, in the spring of the year 1814, to Dr. Young, who appended to a communication made by its discoverer to the Antiquarian Society, a short notice respecting them, which was not otherwise important except as being the occasion of calling the attention of its author to a class of researches upon the sacred and common writing of the ancient Egyptians, for which he afterwards became so famous. Between the month of May—when this first notice was written and sent to the press—and the following November, he subjected the three inscriptions of the well-known Rosetta stone to a most laborious analysis, which ended in a conjectural translation of the second of the three, which was printed as an appendix to his former notice.

Of the three inscriptions upon this stone, the first is in the hieroglyphical or sacred, and the second in the enchorial,[a] characters of Egypt, whilst the third is in

---

[a] The term *demotic* is adopted by Champollion from Herodotus, instead of *enchorial* which is used in the Greek inscription. Young objects to the

Greek; and at the conclusion of the last, it is stated that "*what is here decreed shall be inscribed on a block of hard stone, in sacred, in native (enchorial), and in Greek, characters, and placed in each temple, both of the first and second and third gods.*"[a] We should be authorised to conclude, therefore, that the three inscriptions expressed the same decree, as nearly as was compatible with the genius of the different languages employed and with the sacred and enchorial characters used in two of them, whether those characters were alphabetical, ideographical, or symbolical, or a mixture of all three; and that, consequently, the comparison of them with each other, if carefully made, could not fail to give very important information with respect to the mode in which proper names, or any other words, were written or represented, provided that their peculiar position in the inscriptions, or their frequent recurrence, enabled us sufficiently to identify them.

Unhappily, however, the early portion of the first inscription was destroyed, and many other parts of it mutilated or nearly obliterated; the same observation extended also to many parts of the Greek or third inscription, particularly towards the conclusion; but sufficient of it was preserved not only to make the purport of it intelligible, but also to afford a clue to Porson, and more especially to Heyne, to enable those eminent scholars to restore the whole, or nearly the

use of the former term, on the ground that we have no means of determining the precise nature of the characters thus designated by the historian. See Works, vol. iii. p. 271.

[a] The original Greek, the parts underlined being restored, partly with reference to the extent of the deficient spaces and partly to the context, is as follows :—τὸ δὲ ψήφισμα τοῦτο ἀναγράψαι εἰς στήλην μεγάλην στερεοῦ λίθου, τοῖς τε ἱεροῖς καὶ ἐγχωρίοις καὶ Ἑλληνίκοις γράμμασιν καὶ στῆσαι ἐν ἑκάστῳ τῶν τε πρώτων καὶ δευτέρων καὶ τρίτων ἱερῶν κ. τ. α.

whole, of the deficient parts, without much opening for any material omission or error. The intermediate inscription in the enchorial characters or those in common usage, was nearly complete, with the exception of the beginning of some of the earlier lines.

A fac-simile of the three inscriptions had been engraved by the Antiquarian Society, though wanting in that minute accuracy which is more or less necessary in all cases where the issue of an important critical inquiry may be affected by the most trifling omission, or the most minute variation of form. Young had furnished himself with copies of this engraving when he made his annual visit to Worthing in the summer of 1814, and he there proceeded, by an attentive and methodical comparison of the several parts with each other, to ascertain those portions of the two first inscriptions, and more especially of the second, which corresponded with the Greek.

Silvestre de Sacy, the celebrated orientalist—to whom a copy of the inscriptions upon this stone had been submitted soon after its discovery by the French at the beginning of this century – in a letter addressed to Chaptal,[a] the Minister of the Interior, had pointed out, from their recurrence and position, in the second of the three inscriptions, the groups of characters which expressed the names of Ptolemy, Alexander, and Alexandria ; and Akerblad,[b] a gentleman connected with the diplomatic service of Sweden, a good classical and a first-rate Coptic scholar, who was at that time resident in Paris, pro-

---

[a] Lettre au Citoyen Chaptal, Ministre de l'Intérieur, au sujet de l'Inscription Egyptienne de Rosette. Paris, an x. 1802.

[b] Lettre sur l'Inscription Egyptienne de Rosette, adressée au C. Silvestre de Sacy, Professeur de langue Arabe à l'école spéciale des langues Orientales. Par J. D. Akerblad, 1802. For notices of the labours of Akerblad see Dr Young's Works, vol. iii. p. 30, 44, 79, and 270.

secuted the inquiry much further, assigning the groups of characters corresponding to sixteen other names and words, and determining an alphabet which, though confessedly imperfect, was very generally applicable to the proper names, but which he vainly strove to extend to the whole inscription. Availing himself of the results of their researches, as far as they could be depended upon, Young pasted upon parchment the several portions of the two first inscriptions, as given in the engravings of them, taken line by line or group by group, with those corresponding to them in the Greek text which was written above them. The parchments, with the appended texts, are now before me, and have been prepared with the neatness and minute care for which he was so remarkable. The result was a conjectural translation of the enchorial or Egyptian inscription, both in English and Latin, the first of which was appended to his other remarks on Sir Wm. Boughton's paper, and the second designed for distribution abroad.

In writing to Mr. Gurney, who had heard of the work in which he was engaged, he says —

" You tell me that I shall astonish the world if I make out the inscription. I think it on the contrary astonishing that it should not have been made out already, and that I should find the task so difficult as it appears to be. Certainly the labour of a few days would be sufficient for the comparison of an equal number of lines in any ordinary unknown language, aided by a literal translation, so as to identify pretty satisfactorily all the words that occurred more than once, and to ascertain their meaning : but I have been a month upon this, and have still several passages that occur more than once which I cannot completely identify, or at least understand. But by far the greater part of the words I have ascertained with tolerable certainty, and some of the most interesting without the shadow of a doubt ; but I can read very few of them alphabetically, except the proper names which Akerblad has read before and this is the more intolerably provoking, as there was so much reason to expect a very general coincidence with the Coptic, the names of the three months mentioned in the Greek agreeing very correctly with the Coptic names. I have, however, made so few attempts to obtain an alphabet that I am not yet much discouraged on this head. I have considered the whole as hieroglyphical, and assuredly if it had been truly hieroglyphical I should have succeeded much more rapidly than I have done, because the characters could be easily recognised when they occurred the second time; while in the present inscription they are so carelessly engraved as often to differ exceedingly, besides that the nature of the symbol might possibly have been of some assistance. I have certainly deciphered much more of the Egyptian inscription than Akerblad had done when he published his Essay ten years ago, and as he professed his intention of pursuing the subject, I think he must have done something more; and as he had undoubtedly begun right, I am very desirous of knowing what has prevented his completing the task, and of comparing our ideas, as possibly one may have succeeded where the other has failed. Will you have the goodness to send the enclosed note to Silvestre de Sacy,[a] and tell him at the same time that you will take charge of the answer."

Mr. Gurney was then in Paris, during the short peace of 1814 which followed the first abdication of Napoleon.

In a subsequent letter, written when his labours were concluded, and addressed to the same correspondent, who in a letter from Paris had referred to Champollion's work entitled *L'Egypte sous les Pharaons*,[b] in which the Rosetta inscriptions were said to have been the subject of examination, he says—

"Your first letter disturbed my rest with impatience to see

[a] This letter and the reply to it are given in Dr. Young's Works, vol. iii. pp. 16, 17.

[b] ' L'Egypte sous les Pharaons, ou recherches sur la géographie, la religion, la langue, les écritures, et l'histoire de l'Egypte, avant l'invasion de Cambyses ; par M. Champollion le jeune, professeur d'histoire, bibliothécaire-adjoint de la ville de Grenoble.' Paris, 1814. 2 vols. The work was never completed.

Champollion's work : soon afterwards, however, I had a few lines from Sylvestre de Sacy, mentioning that author, but merely as *pretending* to understand the inscription [a] and not as having published his interpretation. For the present, however, I have done with the subject, and am going to write a medical book : [b] when I shall resume it, or whether at any time, I do not know : but I have certainly every encouragement to pursue it, having already succeeded beyond my late expectations with respect to the hieroglyphics : of these I have deciphered about one half, which is the first step towards any authentic information respecting the ancient history and letters of Egypt. Of the Egyptian, de Sacy has made out three proper names, [c] and Akerblad nine more and five or six Coptic words . I have detected fifty or sixty Coptic words, ten or twelve of them without any doubt, but this makes little more than one tenth of the whole inscription, and I doubt if it will be ever possible to reduce much more of it to Coptic, *especially as I have fully ascertained that some of the characters are hieroglyphics.* I have, however, made out the sense of the whole sufficiently for my purpose, and by means of the variations from the Greek, I have been able to effect a comparison with the hieroglyphics, which it would have been impossible to do satisfactorily without this intermediate step. The repetition of names and titles varies considerably, and in such a manner as to produce a difference between the Greek and hieroglyphics, which was a bar to all further investigation, besides the want of several portions towards the end of the Greek, all of which except one, the Egyptian supplies sufficiently. In general there is little resemblance between the hieroglyphic and the thing represented by it except the numbers under ten ; ⟨glyph⟩ a priest ; ⟨glyph⟩ a shrine ; ⟨glyph⟩ an image, and a few others. God is ⟨glyph⟩ ; in the Egyptian ⟨glyph⟩ . ἀιωνοβίος ⟨glyph⟩; Egyptian ⟨glyph⟩. Vulcan ⟨glyph⟩ ; Egyptian ⟨glyph⟩ . Good ⟨glyph⟩ . King ⟨glyph⟩ . Proper names within a line, as I had conjectured ⟨glyph⟩, and in Egyptian, I had before observed a part

---

[a] Works, vol. iii. p. 17.   [b] His Essay on Consumptive Diseases.
[c] Works vol. iii. pp. 23, 24.

of this character terminating names thus, K . . . . .), without knowing its origin : plurals are formed by three symbols of the same kind, or by three points, as $\mathsf{\Gamma}\mathsf{\Gamma}\mathsf{\Gamma}$ or $\equiv \mathsf{\Gamma}$, gods. If the whole stone could be recovered, we should know much more. The difficulties have been far greater than there was any reason to expect, and I am almost surprised that the labour I have bestowed on them has effected so little in comparison of what it might have happened to effect ; at the same time, in point of public interest, the result is sufficiently striking. My communications will, however, remain anonymous. Notwithstanding what I have heard of Champollion, you will easily imagine that I am not a little anxious to see what *he has done*, and obliged to your kindness in procuring the book."

In another letter towards the end of the same year he says :—

" I have only spent literally five minutes in looking over Champollion, turning by means of the index to the parts where he has quoted the inscription of Rosetta. He follows Akerblad blindly with scarcely any acknowledgment. But he certainly has picked out the sense of a few passages in the inscription by means of Akerblad's investigations—although in four or five Coptic words which he pretends to have found in it,[a] he is wrong in all but one—and that is a very short and a very obvious one. *My translation is printed : it is anonymous, and must for some·time remain so : but everybody whose approbation is worth having will know the author.*"

In the following year, 1816, a revision of this translation was published in the Museum Criticum, a Cam-

[a] Egypte sous les Pharaons, vol. i. p. 23. The author refers to a part to be hereafter published for the result of his examination of this inscription and of the alphabet which he had deduced from it ; an inquiry which he deems to be of no small importance as regards the reading of the various Egyptian manuscripts which are known to be in existence, and also from its possible use in the interpretation of hieroglyphics, with which it may have some connection ; he adds that such an *hypothesis must not be deemed paradoxical.*

bridge journal of classical literature edited by the present learned Bishop of Gloucester, who was at that time Greek Professor. To this translation was added a correspondence relating to it which had passed between himself, Sylvestre de Sacy and Akerblad. In his earlier investigations, Akerblad had begun by assuming the Egyptian language of the age of the Ptolemies—which was used in the second of the three inscriptions—to be identical in grammatical con struction and in a great majority of such of its words, as were not immediately adopted from the Greek, with the Coptic of four or five centuries later; such being the date of the earliest books in that language which have come down to us: and he felt persuaded, therefore, that if he could recover the alphabet, no serious difficulty would present itself, not merely in the restoration, but in the interpretation, of the language. His later investigations, however, had tended to check considerably the sanguine hopes of success in which he had once indulged;[a] the alphabet which he had proposed embracing a small proportion only of the different characters made use of in the inscription, which he found to be more than two hundred in number; it proved in consequence altogether inadequate for its transcription into the Coptic or any other language. Notwithstanding this failure, however, his name should ever be held in honour as one of the founders of our knowledge of Egyptian literature, to the investigation of which he brought no small amount of patient labour and philological learning.

Champollion, as we have already seen, followed in the footsteps of Akerblad, adopting all his hypo-

_____

[a] Works, vol. iii. p. 60. "Je vois," says Sylvestre de Sacy, "qu'il a des doutes sur son alphabet Egyptien, plus que par le passé."

theses, both with respect to the alphabetical character of the Egyptian, as distinguished from the hieroglyphical, inscription, and to the language which, in the present stage of the investigation, it was assumed to express. He had made the history, the topography and antiquities of Egypt, as well as the Coptic language and its kindred dialects, the study of his life, and he started therefore upon this inquiry with advantages which probably no other person possessed: and no one who is acquainted with his later writings can call in doubt his extraordinary sagacity in bringing to bear upon every subject connected with it, not merely the most apposite, but also the most remote and sometimes the most unexpected, illustrations. With the exception, however, of the identification of a few additional Coptic words, very ingeniously elicited from the Egyptian text, he had made no important advance upon what had already been done by Akerblad. Like him also he abandoned the task of identifying the hieroglyphical inscription or portions of it with those corresponding to them in the Egyptian or Greek text, as altogether hopeless, in consequence of the very extensive mutilations which it had undergone.

When Young published in the Museum Criticum, the letters of Sylvestre de Sacy, he suppressed, lest he should compromise the writer, several passages in them, reflecting very severely upon the character of Champollion. In one of these he says:—

" I am of opinion, Sir, that you are more advanced than Akerblad or Champollion, and that you are able to read a great part at least of the Egyptian inscription. If I might venture to advise you, I would recommend you not to be too communicative of your discoveries to M. Champollion. It may happen that he may hereafter make pretension to the priority. He seeks, in many parts of his book, to make it believed that he has discovered many words of the Egyptian inscription of the Rosetta stone : but I am afraid that this is mere charlatanism : I may add that I have very good reasons for thinking so." [a]

He then proceeds to notice a report that some one in Holland had discovered the alphabet of this inscription, and that at Paris, Etienne Quatremère flattered himself that he could read a great part of it, and adds :—

" To say the truth, I cannot persuade myself that if Messrs Akerblad, Etienne Quatremère, or Champollion, had made any real progress in the reading of the Egyptian text, they would not have been in greater haste to make their discovery public. It would be a very rare act of modesty, of which not one of them appears to me to be capable."

This was written in July, 1815. In the following January he returns to his complaints against Champollion :—

" His conduct," says he, " during the reign of three months, has done him little honour, and he has not ventured in consequence to write to me. He must have elsewhere seen by a report which his conduct provoked, and which I had the charge of making, that I was not the dupe of his charlatanism. He is given to play the part of the jay decked in peacock's feathers, but such performances often end very badly." [b]

Without entering upon an inquiry whether the estimate which de Sacy had formed of the moral character of Champollion was well founded or not, it is sufficiently singular that subsequent events were destined to give a somewhat prophetical truth to the

---

[a] Works, vol. iii. p. 51, with the note by Mr. Leitch.

[b] Works, vol. iii. p. 59. He forfeited his appointment as Professor of History at Grenoble, in consequence of the part he took during " the hundred days."

special warnings which he gave to Dr. Young: for it
will be found hereafter to be impossible, upon a fair
consideration of facts and of dates, altogether to
acquit Champollion of the charge of disingenuous
suppression in some instances, and of want of candour
in others, in the controversy which arose between
himself and Young with respect to the discovery of
phonetic hieroglyphics.

Having now abandoned the hope of reading the
enchorial text by means of an alphabet, or of inter-
preting more than the groups of characters which
by their recurrence, succession, or otherwise, admitted
of being connected or identified with the corresponding
words of the Greek translation, there remained two
important subjects of investigation to which Young
immediately applied himself. The first was to perform
the same office for the parts of the hieroglyphical text
which remained upon the stone, as he had already performed for the enchorial: and the second to connect
the parts of the Greek and enchorial text, word by
word, and symbol or character by character, as far
as practicable, with each other, so as to ascertain whether the enchorial characters were or were not derived
from the corresponding hieroglyphics, by abbreviation
or otherwise, with a view to their more rapid transcription for the purposes of ordinary life. If such or any
other determinate connection could thus be established
between them, the study of those hieroglyphical and
enchorial texts, which are known to be translations
of each other, as in the case of the Rosetta stone and,
as was subsequently found to be the case, in innumerable funeral inscriptions and papyri, might be
made to illustrate each other.

Expectations were also very generally entertained

about this period, that a duplicate of the Rosetta stone might be found. It was known from the Greek inscription that many other copies of it had been engraved upon durable materials. Dr. Clarke, the celebrated traveller, had observed a sculptured stone, which might possibly be one of their number, in a wall in the Court of the Institute at Cairo;[a] and Jomard, who had been one of the great Egyptian Commission and who had the principal share in the publication of the results of its labours, informs us, in a letter to Dr. Young,[b] that he and his colleague, Mr. Jollois, had seen a similar trilinguar monument at Menouf,[c] in Lower Egypt, and at the same time refers to the other which had been seen by Dr. Clarke. Very express instructions also had been given, at Dr. Young's suggestion, to Mr. Salt, who had recently been appointed Consul-General in Egypt, to secure these treasures at any cost and to forward them to England.[d]

[a] This stone was afterwards secured by Champollion for the French Museum, and was found to be nearly, if not altogether, worthless.

[b] Works, vol. iii. p. 69.

[c] This stone was afterwards brought by Drovetti, the French Consul at Alexandria to Italy, and finally, after many negotiations, deposited in the Museum at Turin. Dr. Young made repeated attempts to secure a cast of it, but for many years without success. See Works, vol. iii. p. 287. It was a bilinguar and not a trilinguar inscription, in Greek and enchorial, and its value had been to a great extent superseded by other discoveries before it was accurately copied and made known to him.

[d] In writing to his sister-in-law, Mrs. Chambers, on the 7th Dec., 1815, he says, "I met Hamilton at Sir Joseph Banks's on Sunday last, and attacked him immediately on Egyptian affairs; he told me that everything had been done at the Foreign Office which I wished; that Salt had full powers to hunt for all the fragments of which I had shown the importance, and credit for a specific sum to cover his expenses. He had also persuaded the French government to furnish a copy of the magnificent Description de l'Egypte to be sent to Egypt for Salt's immediate use, upon condition that it should be hereafter deposited, with his marginal remarks, in the British Museum. Hamilton is to lend me his copy for a month or two this winter, &c."

" If Salt succeeds," says Dr. Young in writing to Mr. Gurney, " we cannot fail in finding the name of Alexander and all the Ptolemies, wherever they occur, without further investigation, and those of many of the deities."

Of all the proper names originally included in the hieroglyphical inscription of Rosetta, that of Ptolemy alone remains. It occurs four times, and three of them follow in immediate succession, in the following form, under circumstances which enabled Dr. Young to connect them with the Greek text :—

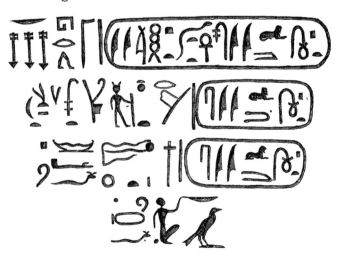

It will be observed that there are three groups of hieroglyphics included within *rings* (the *cartouches* of Champollion), the two last of which are known to express the name of Ptolemy simply, and the first the same name expressed by the same eight characters which are common to all three of them, with the addition of the royal title or motto, which may be translated *living for ever, of Phtha beloved*. Such rings, which are sometimes single and sometimes double, the name generally in one and the motto in the other, but sometimes both of them in one, as in this case, are found everywhere engraved upon the great public and other monuments of Egypt. Though these rings occurred three times in the preceding passage, the part of the Greek text which appeared to correspond to it, presented the name of Ptolemy only twice. Similar discrepancies which occurred in other parts of the several texts—which were not in fact very close or literal transcriptions or translations of each other—added greatly to the difficulty of identifying the name.[a]

"It had," says Dr. Young, "been one of the greatest difficulties attending the translation of the hieroglyphics of Rosetta, to explain how the groups within the rings, which varied considerably in different parts of the pillar, and which occurred in several parts where there was no corresponding name in the Greek, while they were not found in others where they ought to have appeared, could possibly represent the name of Ptolemy; and it was not without considerable labour that I had been able to overcome this difficulty."

Discoveries like these, so difficult in the infancy of a science, appear so simple and so obvious when once made known, that subsequent inquirers are at a loss to conceive in what manner they could ever have occasioned either doubt or hesitation.

These rings were considered in the first instance by Young as indicating proper names, both of persons and places, where the characters expressing them ceased to be addressed to the eye only—as hieroglyphics were commonly supposed to be—but under these special circumstances to the ear, by becoming *phonetic*, whether as representing the ordinary letters of the alphabet or syllables or words. The Chinese, whose language is hieroglyphical, make their characters phonetic by a peculiar mark, when they wish to express a peculiar combination of sounds which conveys no meaning, like a foreign word or name ; and it would obviously be impossible, in any such system of writing, to dispense with some similar expedient, unless certain of the characters were habitually employed as phonetic only, and not as symbols and signs.[a] In examining the enchorial inscription, Young had observed also, as we have already seen,[b] that all the proper, as well as the royal, names appeared to be enclosed between the signs Ϗ and Ϡ, as in the enchorial name of Ptolemy, where they were in the first instance considered by him as representing the end and the beginning of the hieroglyphical ring of the first inscription, thus : Ϗ════Ϡ .

This suggestion, with respect to the circumstances

---

[a] His attention would appear to have been drawn to this provision of the Chinese language with respect to foreign appellations by an article in the Quarterly Review for May, 1816, p. 282. In writing to Mr. Gurney soon after its appearance, he says, "The Chinese article is by Barrow, secretary of the Admiralty, who was with Sir George Staunton and Lord Macartney. I am excessively delighted with it; it gives me a most accurate and perfect idea of the singular structure of that unique language; I had no conception of its nature before : I should almost like to be acquainted with the 214 radical characters, merely as a matter of curiosity." On another occasion (1818) he says, "I was almost tempted last night to begin learning the Chinese language. One of my brothers, who had some business in town, had picked up a Chinese book from some of the Baptist missionaries, which he believed was a portion of the New Testament. From the pages I soon discovered the numerals, from these the number of chapters and that of the verses in the first chapter which agreed with the Gospel of St. John. Having thus obtained the translation, I was very curious to make out the meaning of assemblages of characters within a square which occurred continually, as they reminded me very forcibly of the proper names in the Egyptian hieroglyphics—and they *were* proper names—but not of *persons*, as in Egypt; but they were the names of places—either countries, as some with a gate upon them, or of rivers or towns—the proper names of persons had only a line by their side."

[b] The character which Young, in the first instance, upon very probable grounds, assumed to be the enchorial representative of part of the ring, was in reality the letter *m*, which is very commonly attached as a prefix to proper names in the Coptic language. See supra, p. 264.

under which the rings were used, was ingenious,[a] and became fertile, as we shall see in the progress of these researches, in the most important consequences; for though it was afterwards shown that such rings were confined to the names and titles of royal personages, and that the use of phonetic hieroglyphics was much more extensive than this hypothesis assumed it to be, it gave a definite direction to the inquiry for determining them in the only cases where it was likely to succeed. For if hieroglyphics, in all proper names, were phonetic, whether as expressing letters or syllables, it was obvious that no such ring or cartouche, when the name which it expressed was well determined, would escape examination with a view of testing the correctness of an hypothesis, which had so much probability in its favour. Such a name was that of Ptolemy, as ascertained from its peculiar position and recurrence in this inscription and its relation to the Greek and enchorial text; and it was to the characters which composed it that the principle was first applied, as we shall hereafter see, with almost perfect success.

In the examination of the first inscription of the Rosetta stone, with the view of ascertaining the relations of the parts of it which remain, with those corresponding to them in the Egyptian and Greek text, Young was assisted, not merely by the recurrence of this conspicuous ring of Ptolemy and its attendant groups, but also by other characters which were so clearly ideographic, as to leave no doubt of their meaning.

One of the first of those which he recognised was ![glyph] as meaning a *priest*, from its obvious connection with the pouring out of libations : other signs of this kind were those of *temple, letters, month, statue* : the symbol ⌐ god, its plural ⌐⌐⌐ for gods, and ⚡ for king, constantly recurred, giving well-defined points in the text ; the character 〨,[a] commonly designated the crown of Lower Egypt, which appeared clearly, by its position, to express the preposition *of*, and ⚡ the conjunction *and*, were also of no small use in separating groups from each other.

He was enabled to assign by means of this comparison of the texts with each other, an interpretation, though not without very considerable errors, to nearly one hundred and sixty groups of hieroglyphics, a number which was afterwards augmented to more than two hundred from other sources, more especially from the study and comparison of the funeral rolls. They were published in his article EGYPT, in the supplement of the Encyclopædia Britannica.[b] Though some names of deities and kings were confessedly unknown and expressed by provisional designations, and the grammatical elements of others were not defined, they formed by far the most considerable step in the progress of our knowledge of hieroglyphics, which preceded the determination of the phonetic alphabet by the joint labours of himself and Champollion.

The inspection of this, as well as of most other

---

[a] Subsequently recognised by Young as *n* in the phonetic alphabet, the homophone or equivalent of ᚃᚃᚃ or the wavy line ; it is not only used as a preposition, but also to convert substantives into adjectives : thus νουβ *gold*, becomes ννουβ *golden* by the prefix *n*. The hieroglyphics for several other prepositions and conjunctions were also determined. See Works, vol. iii., Nos. 170, 171, 172, 173, 174, 175, 176.

[b] The list was republished with many omissions and additions, as a species of Hieroglyphical Dictionary at the end of his account of Hieroglyphical Discoveries. See Works, vol. iii. p. 353.

hieroglyphical inscriptions of considerable length, was sufficient to show that a large proportion of the characters which they contained were ideographic, or such as might be considered as representing the objects of which they are more or less clearly delineations; thus offering to the eye, without any knowledge of the language which such inscriptions might be assumed to express, some considerable though not very trustworthy, indication of the subjects to which they referred. No similar assistance was in the first instance afforded by the enchorial manuscripts; for even supposing that any considerable proportion of the characters in which they were written were derived from the corresponding hieroglyphics, their forms were so much altered in passing from one system of writing to the other, that it had hitherto been found very difficult to recognise them, except in very few cases.

The funeral manuscripts, which have been taken in vast numbers, generally from the breasts of mummies in the tombs and catacombs of Egypt, present specimens of writing in different stages of transition from the hieroglyphical characters of the first inscription of Rosetta to others approaching to the cursive or enchorial characters of the second. Very few of such manuscripts—and those apparently reserved for the most solemn commemorations of distinguished persons—are written in the full bold characters of the hieroglyphics of the monuments; others, and many more of them, are written in characters assuming considerable variety of form, but which are all of them copies more or less complete of corresponding hieroglyphics; sometimes their forms are accurately followed, in simple outlines only; at other times more considerable abbreviations, favourable to rapid writing, are admitted, but still keeping up their resemblance to the original hieroglyphics, so as to allow of no doubt of their derivation from them. The last and the most degraded form which they assume is the enchorial—and it was with a view of ascertaining whether these as well as the other characters in the papyri were or were not traceable to the same origin, that Young entered upon the second, and perhaps the most important, stage of his inquiry.

To the first of these several derivative species of writing, Young would appear, from a specimen which he has given from the great Strasburg manuscript— in the last of the plates appended to the article Egypt —to have applied the epithet *hieratic*, classifying under the general designation of *epistolographic* all those that follow it, until they pass, by what he considered almost insensible gradations, into the *enchorial* of the Rosetta stone. Champollion, at a later period, transferred the term *hieratic* to the writing commonly used in the funeral rolls, where the characters are more or less manifest derivatives of hieroglyphics, though very different from the hieroglyphics of the monuments or their linear copies, to which the term had been applied by Young. It was only at a much more advanced stage of these researches, when the much less frequent occurrence of the derivatives of ideographic hieroglyphics in enchorial or demotic texts was ascertained, that a real distinction, beyond the forms of the characters, was established between these different kinds of writing.

In a letter to Mr. Gurney, at the beginning of the year 1816, after referring to various literary and scientific trifles which occupied his attention, "with which," says he, "I have no immediate concern, except as furnishing me with employment which, from habit, is generally to me more an amusement than a fatigue," and complaining of the inconvenience which he had experienced from an act of carelessness, by which part of the manuscripts which he had prepared for the Museum Criticum was lost and which he was required to replace, he proceeds as follows :—

"The printers at Cambridge are models of slow and dignified deliberation. I made it a condition in August last that my paper should be immediately printed. It was accepted; and now, in January, the three sheets are not yet worked off; but it is of little consequence, or rather of none at all. I have had the great Description de l'Egypte for some time on my table, through Mr. W. Hamilton's kindness; [a] and I have been copying out some of the hieroglyphics for future use, but I have not attempted to decipher any of them, meaning to wait for further assistance from Egypt. I much fear, however, from the account which I have received from Paris, that neither of the stones known to be in existence will be of much use; [b] and, unless the fragments of the Rosetta stone can be found, I almost doubt whether much more will ever be done. Certainly I have not yet found either a calendar of months or a chronicle of kings [c] among the hieroglyphics; and I have made out much less than I thought must almost certainly have been intelligible ; in short, very little except the existence of the name of Ptolemy on several of the temples at Philœ, Ambos, and Latopolis. The characters, I believe, are far more numerous than they have been made by those who have attempted to reckon them, and on the whole I have no confidence in being able to do more than fully to illustrate the inscription of Rosetta, and to trace the nature and origin of several of the characters contained in it."

[a] Formerly ambassador at Naples and author of Egyptiaca, who, throughout a long life, has been equally distinguished as a patron and a cultivator of art and literature : he was at that time Under Secretary of State for Foreign Affairs.

[b] Supra, p. 269.

[c] Such chronicles were afterwards discovered at Abydos by Mr. Bankes, and elsewhere.

The great work on Egypt, above alluded to, was
not completed at the time this letter was written,
and the copies of inscriptions to which Young
refers were chiefly those on the great temples of
Thebes, Karnak, Philœ, Edfou, Luxor, Medinet Abou,
Esne, Ombos, Denderah, &c., many of which were
taken from drawings made with more regard to picturesque effect than to minute details, and which were
rarely sufficiently accurate to make them documents
which admitted of much use in a critical inquiry. A
few months subsequently, the last number of the series
appeared,[a] containing—in addition to most accurate
fac-similes of other funeral rolls—by far the most
magnificent and most important that had ever been
discovered, written entirely in the hieroglyphics of the
monuments, and which Young has emphatically called
the Codex Ritualis, as embodying, more fully and completely than any other similar document which was at
that time known, the representations—in the series
of drawings which accompany them—of the scenes
through which the deceased, according to the system of
religious belief amongst the Egyptians, was supposed to
pass, as well as the prayers or invocations addressed to
the different divinities to whom he was successively
presented. They were probably copies of portions of
the Hermetic Books which have been described by
Clemens of Alexandria;[b] and the scenes of the last
judgment, found at the end of nearly all these papyri,

---

[a] See the letters of Jomard, by whom this publication was superintended.
Works, vol. iii. pp. 69 and 71. There is a similar manuscript at Turin,
much more complete and nearly double the size, which Champollion analyzed, and from which Lepsius has printed "The Book of the Dead."—
See Bunsen's 'Egypt's Place in Universal History,' p. 28.

[b] Bunsen's 'Egypt's Place in Universal History,' pp. 9 and 701 where
the passage from Clemens is given.

accurately coincide, even to the number of the judges, with the account which is given by Diodorus of the trial of the dead.[a] This noble manuscript contains more than 500 columns of hieroglyphics, and the drawings or representations under which they are placed are brilliantly coloured.

" I was much struck," says Young, " with the evident relation of some of the figures to the text below ; and having observed the same figures in the margins of several other manuscripts written in the running hand, I was led to examine with attention the corresponding texts, and I found at last a similar agreement in almost all of them. I then made copies of the respective passages in contiguous lines, in such a manner as completely to put an end to the idea of the alphabetical nature of any of them."[b]

The transcription and collation of these texts was a work of no ordinary labour. In one page, are well-drawn copies of the vignettes, and in that opposite to it, are the corresponding texts, three or four in number, placed underneath each other, line by line, character by character, so as to admit of immediate comparison.

[a] The ordinary editions of Diodorus gave this number as more than forty, when all the Egyptian manuscripts give representations of forty-two. Young refers, in a letter to Mr. Gurney written in 1817, with particular pleasure, to the discovery of a manuscript of this author, where the correct number is given :—" Another numerical coincidence has also given me great delight. I had long ago counted XLII personages in the Hieroglyphical manuscripts, whom I had called the Assessor Gods, as being united to Osiris in giving his judgments, and I now find a passage in Diodorus, describing the ceremony of the trial of the dead by 'more than forty judges,' where a good manuscript has *two and forty*. Such coincidences as this tend to reduce the conjectural evidence of history into something like mathematical demonstration, the monuments in question being at least as old as Diodorus. They prove, too, that Diodorus must have known something about Egypt, but he seems to have mixed the accounts of various authors, some better and some worse, and the accuracy of one part of his works by no means renders it impossible, that he may have committed gross blunders in others." See also Works, vol. ii. p. 19.

[b] Works, vol. iii. p. 75, letter to the Archduke John of Austria.

Synonymous groups derived from other manuscripts were occasionally interposed, when they afforded additional illustrations of the objects of comparison, or instructive examples of the interchange of symbols.

The manuscripts in which these various labours are embodied are now before me. One of them, entitled *Formulæ Cultus Egyptii*, contains the collation of the texts of which we are now speaking, derived chiefly from the papyri in the great *Description de l'Egypte*, and others furnished by Mr. Bankes and Lord Mountnorris; another, the *Codex Ritualis Hieroglyphicus*, is chiefly devoted to the great hieroglyphical papyrus of the same work; this is followed by the *Pantheon Hieroglyphicum*, containing an arrangement of the Egyptian deities delineated in that and other manuscripts, with their hieroglyphical titles and their various synonyms, with provisional names assigned to them founded upon their apparent functions, or upon some significant symbol in their hieroglyphical designation;[a] in another very thick manuscript, entitled *Inscriptiones Hieroglyphicæ*, we find exquisite copies, sometimes in colours, of inscriptions from the Egyptian monuments, given in the great French work, with many others derived from obelisks, mummy-cases, the works of Kircher, and other sources. To these may be added, the special works devoted to the inscription of Rosetta, which have been elsewhere noticed; a large and interesting collection of *Excerpta* from ancient and modern authors relating to Egypt; and lastly, a Lexicon Hieroglyphicum, in which nearly 200 hieroglyphics are distributed into

---

[a] The Pantheon in the article Egypt is almost entirely derived from classical and external sources; the Pantheon Hieroglyphicum, founded upon the monuments and manuscripts, is much more complete, more especially as illustrative of the various scenes represented in the ritual of the dead.

classes, as representing the human body and its parts; animals and their parts; vegetables; inorganic natural bodies; fixed structures; instruments or utensils; articles of dress and ornament; imaginary, unknown, or miscellaneous objects. Each of these is subjected to a critical examination, special references to the Rosetta stone and the ritual manuscripts being made with a view to the determination of its probable meaning when used singly or in combination, as well as of its equivalent signs, whether phonetic or otherwise, whenever such were discoverable : some of which will be more particularly noticed hereafter. It is impossible to form a just estimate either of the vast extent to which Dr. Young had carried his hieroglyphical investigations, or of the real progress which he had made in them, without an inspection of these manuscripts. They would appear to have been prepared between the years 1814 and 1818, and to have been the result of labours which, though frequently interrupted by other publications and inquiries, were never entirely lost sight of.

The article Egypt, which was undertaken, as we have seen, for the Supplement of the Encyclopædia Britannica, and written in 1818, though not published until the year following, contained a general view of the results both of his critical and historical labours ; but though it has been pronounced " to be the greatest effort of scholarship and ingenuity of which modern literature can boast,"[a] it should properly be considered as little more than a popular and a superficial sketch of the vast mass of materials upon which it was founded : for not only were those materials in many cases altoge-

[a] Works, vol. iii. p. 86, note, taken from a very able notice of the writings of Dr. Young, in the 'Scotsman' newspaper, and supposed to have been written by Dr. James Brown of Edinburgh.

ther unsuited for a publication designed rather for
general perusal than for special instruction and study,
but the necessity of resorting to costly engravings, at a
period when the art of printing or engraving hieroglyphics was little understood and practised, made it
altogether impossible to do more than refer, by somewhat vague descriptions, to points which could only be
settled by an actual comparison of the characters themselves, or of the groups in which they appeared.

One of the first results at which he arrived was the
relation of the different kinds of Egyptian characters
or letters employed in their hieroglyphical, hieratic or
epistolographic, and enchorial inscriptions and writings.
The most superficial inspection was sufficient to show
that the greatest part of them were tachygraphical
copies of the first; but the derivation of the others, approaching most nearly to the enchorial of the Rosetta
stone, was not quite so manifest. A careful comparison
of texts however, which were obviously copies of the
same original—as in the litanies of the dead—gave indications of this derivation in cases so numerous and
so indisputable as apparently to justify the inference
that they were so in all, and to lead to the conclusion
that unless the typical hieroglyphics were alphabetical, their hieratic or enchorial derivatives could not
be so.

It is now believed that of the existing hieroglyphical characters, which are not more than 1000 in
number, nearly four fifths are ideographic, or symbolical; but at the period of which we are now speaking
—whilst the popular belief, involved in the universal
use of the term *hieroglyphics*, as applied to those signs,
rejected altogether the notion of their being alphabetical under any circumstances—a similar prejudice,
almost equally strong, led men to consider the cha-

racters used in a system of cursive and ordinary
writing as necessarily alphabetical; and we have
already seen that Akerblad and Champollion made
this assumption the basis of their researches. Dr.
Young however showed that neither the alphabet of
Akerblad, nor any modification of it which could be
proposed, was applicable to any considerable part of
the enchorial portion of the Rosetta inscription beyond
the proper names; and the discovery which resulted
from his extensive comparison of texts, that hieroglyphical passed very generally into hieratic or epistolographic and not unfrequently into enchorial, characters,
appeared to him—assuming the correctness of opinions
which no one had hitherto ventured to doubt—to be
decisive of the question which had been raised.[a]

He announced this conclusion in a letter to the
Archduke John of Austria,[b] who, during a recent visit
to England, had interested himself in these inquiries;
and subsequently in another addressed to Akerblad.[c]
Both these letters were printed in the Museum Criticum for 1816, and copies of them were very generally distributed at the time, both at home and
abroad, among all persons engaged in these inquiries,
though the publication of the work in which they
are contained was delayed, from causes which he
could not control, until 1821.

The first of these letters describes generally the pro-

[a] M. Bunsen, in a very unfair estimate of the relative claims of Young
and Champollion, in connection with these researches, observes "that in
1816 Dr. Young even went so far as to deny the existence of an alphabetic
character either in the hieroglyphical or hieratic element:" forgetting the
important limitations which are imposed upon this opinion in several
passages of the very letter which he is criticising, and apparently ignorant
of the very positive conclusions, which are noticed below, which were
announced by Champollion in the Memoir, subsequently suppressed, which
was published at Grenoble in 1821.

[b] Works, vol. iii. p. 74.   [c] Works, vol. iii. p. 79.

cess by which he had arrived at this result; the second gives specific references to plates of different papyri, in the great *Description de l'Egypte*—as documents which were generally accessible—for proofs of its truth.

The conclusion, as we have already seen, was stated in the first instance somewhat too broadly ; but it was farther narrowed, in the article Egypt, which was written nearly two years afterwards, when access to several other funeral rolls, some of which were written in characters, nearly if not decidedly, enchorial, had shown more clearly the difficulties which attended the inquiry. It would have been more correct to say that a sufficient number of characters in the cursive system of writing were derived from the hieroglyphics, to show that it was not alphabetical, according to the ordinary meaning of the term. It appeared, even in the first examination which he made of the Rosetta inscription, that the enchorial characters for a *diadem*, an *asp*, and *everlasting*, were unmistakeably borrowed from the sacred characters ;[a] and though a similar coincidence was not traceable through other parts of the two inscriptions, it seemed to him "not improbable that alphabetical characters might be interspersed with hieroglyphics in the same way that astronomers and chemists of modern times have often employed arbitrary marks as compendious expressions of the objects which are of frequent occurrence in their respective sciences ; but whatever hypothesis could be proposed to account for the fact, no effort, however determined and persevering, had been able to discover any alphabet by which the enchorial inscription could be read into intelligible Egyptian."

[a] Works, vol. iii. p. 133.

In the year 1821 there appeared, at Grenoble, a short memoir, by Champollion, *De l'Ecriture Hiératique des Anciens Egyptiens*, in which the author announced, as an original discovery, that the hieratic characters of the papyri were mere modifications of the forms of corresponding hieroglyphics, adopted for the sake of more rapid and convenient transcription; and further, that these characters are *signs of things and not signs of sounds*.[a] The first of these conclusions, as we have already seen, was substantially the same as that which Young had announced five years before : the second shows also that at this epoch Champollion had either formed no conception of the existence of phonetic hieroglyphics, or, had given it up as altogether untenable, if he had once entertained it.

In the following year appeared the letter to M. Dacier, to which Bunsen has not improperly attached the epithet *immortal*. The memoir, which so recently announced the second of the opinions above referred to, had already been very carefully suppressed, and the plates attached to it, exhibiting a comparison of hieroglyphic and hieratic texts, were afterwards distributed *without date and without the letter-press* which pre-

[a] See Mr. Leitch's notes, Dr. Young's Works, vol. iii. p. 74 and 158, where the following propositions are given from this memoir :—they are taken from a copy presented by the author to Sylvestre de Sacy, "son ancien instructeur," at the sale of whose library it came into the possession of the Duke of Manchester, who kindly allowed Mr. Leitch and myself to consult it.

" 1°. Que l'écriture des manuscrits Egyptiens de la seconde espèce (hiératique) n'est point alphabétique.

" 2°. Que le seconde système n'est qu'une simple modification du système hiéroglyphique.

" 3°. Que cette seconde espèce d'écriture est l'hiératique des auteurs Grecs, et doit être regardée comme une tachy-graphie hiéroglyphique.

" 4°. Enfin, que les caractères hiératiques sont *des signes des choses et non des sons.*"

ceded them. It was a copy of these plates only which was given by Champollion to Young; and we are assured by the latter, in a letter addressed to Sir William Gell in 1827, that he was left in entire ignorance of the date of the publication.[a]

The suppression of a work, expressing opinions which its author has subsequently found reason to abandon, may sometimes be excused, though rarely altogether justified; *but under no circumstances can such a justification be pleaded when the suppression is either designed or calculated to compromise the claims of other persons with reference to our own.* The Memoir in question very clearly showed that, so late as the year 1821, Champollion had made no real progress in removing the mysterious veil which had so long enveloped the ancient literature of Egypt; and even if we allow him to have been altogether ignorant of Young's letters to the Archduke John and Akerblad, printed and circulated, though not published, five years before, it clearly shows that if he had made one step in advance, he had made one step only: but at the interval of little more than a year from this period, during which the Article Egypt had confessedly come under his observation, we find him suddenly pushed forward into the inmost recesses of the sanctuary. From this time forward we hear no

---

[a] Works, vol. iii. p. 443. In his account of some recent discoveries in Hieroglyphical Literature (Works, vol. iii. p. 291), he says, speaking of Champollion's discovery of the derivation of the hieratic from the hieroglyphical characters, "whether he made this discovery before I had printed my letters in the Museum Criticum, in 1816, I have no means of ascertaining. I have never asked him the question, nor is it of much importance either to the world at large or to ourselves. It may not be strictly just to say that a man has no right to claim any discovery as his own till he has printed and published it, but the rule is at least a very useful one."

more of the views which are developed in his first
Memoir: and so successful were his efforts to with-
draw it from circulation and public notice, that, important as this document is in the chronology of the
history of these discoveries, it has been passed over
entirely without notice by nearly every author who
has written on the subject.

Nor is this the only instance in which Champollion
is justly chargeable with a disingenuous suppression
of facts. In his *Précis du Système Hiéroglyphique
des Anciens Egyptiens*, after giving a very partial
account of the labours of his predecessors, and particularly of Dr. Young,[a] on the enchorial and hieroglyphic texts of the Rosetta stone, and on the comparison of those which he found in different funeral
rolls, down to so late a period as 1819, when the
article Egypt was published,—he tells us that at
the same epoch, and without any knowledge of
the opinions of Dr. Young, he had arrived, by a process sufficiently sure, at nearly the same results.[b] We
have the evidence, however, of Sylvestre de Sacy himself, through whom they were transmitted, that he had
given to Champollion Figeac a copy of Dr. Young's
conjectural translation of the enchorial text of Rosetta for the use of his brother; and we know that
copies of his articles in the Museum Criticum, of his
subsequent letters to the Archduke John, and also
of the plates to the Article Egypt, were freely distributed at Paris and elsewhere in 1818, at least a
year before the publication of the latter parts of the
letter-press to which they belonged ; and though
there exists no positive proof that these latter

[a] Page 18.
[b] See *infra*, p. 333, where this account is more fully considered.

documents reached the hands of Champollion, it is
not very probable, considering the interest which
Young's former labours had created amongst all
persons engaged in these researches, that the subject of them could have remained for so many years
absolutely unknown to him: at the same time we
should readily admit that the simple denial of any
person, in the eminent position which Champollion
occupied in the literary world, would have been sufficient to exempt him from question, if other circumstances, which it is impossible altogether to explain away, had not a little tended to invalidate his
testimony.[a]

It has been too much the custom with writers on
the history of hieroglyphical discoveries to estimate
their value, less by a reference to the state of
knowledge at the time they were made, than to a
much more advanced stage of its progress: to compare
in fact the views of Champollion in 1824 and 1830,
or of Lepsius and Birch at a much later period, with
those of Young in 1819, instead of duly considering
the influence which the investigations and speculations of an earlier, thus unfairly weighed against those
of a later, age, have had upon the establishment
of more correct, because more matured, conclusions.
It is this spirit of injustice which can hardly fail
to be observed whenever Champollion or Bunsen, who
has usually followed in his footsteps, have had occasion to notice or criticize the labours of Dr. Young.

To return to the question, from which we digressed,
respecting the relation existing between the different
species of Egyptian writing. Young, as we have seen,
considered the hieratic and enchorial characters as

[a] Works, vol. iii. p. 49.

equally derived in every instance from corresponding hieroglyphics, by a greater or less degradation of their forms; and any person who compares the forms, at least of such of them as correspond to the phonetic hieroglyphics, which are given by Champollion at the end of his *Précis du Système Hiéroglyphique,* will be readily satisfied with the general correctness of his conclusion. The same is true also of many other forms which are not included in that list; but he never was in a condition to assert and never asserted the converse of this proposition, that every hieroglyphic sign had necessarily its corresponding derivative hieratic or enchorial character.

There is no doubt, however, that one of the primary objects of this special branch of his researches was to identify the corresponding hieroglyphical and enchorial characters sufficiently to enable him to reconstruct the deficient parts of the first inscription on the Rosetta stone, by replacing the characters in the enchorial text, one by one, by corresponding hieroglyphics. The conception was ingenious, and if he had been in possession of materials sufficient to enable him to carry the process of identification far enough, the result would have been singularly interesting and instructive, as tending to show more distinctly than by any other means the relations of those different species of writing. It is hardly necessary to say that Young speedily abandoned the attempt to effect the solution of a problem which he found to be impracticable, and which the most learned of our Egyptologers would even now regard with no small alarm.

" The French expedition to Egypt," says M. Bunsen, " brought

to light an important hieroglyphical papyrus, originally found in
the tombs of the kings of Thebes. It was first mentioned by
Cadit (1805); afterwards in the great work upon Egypt compiled under the auspices of Napoleon. The pictured ornaments
showed that it treated of ceremonies in honour of the dead, and
the transmigation of souls. Champollion found a similar papyrus
in the Museum of Turin, in a much more complete state and
about double the size. It was written, like the former, not in
hieratic characters, but in hieroglyphics, the monumental character of the sacred language. Fully appreciating the importance
of this record, he immediately submitted it to close examination
and divided it into three sections. Lepsius recognized in it the
most important basis for deciphering the Egyptian character and
language. He divided it according to the data supplied by the
MS. itself, into 165 sections, and soon perceived that all the
rolls of Papyri in the various European collections devoted to
the same subject contained more or less of these sections.
Champollion assumed its contents to be of a liturgical nature,
and accordingly named it ' The Ritual ;' Lepsius preferred the
title of the ' Book of the Dead,' as it no where contained any
funeral service in the proper sense. On the contrary, the deceased himself is the person who officiates. His soul, on his
long journey through the celestial gates, is giving utterance to
prayers, invocations, confessions which are here recorded. The
first fifteen chapters form a connected, distinct, separate whole,
with the general superscription. ' Here begins the Sections of
the glorification of the Light of Osiris.' This part is illustrated
by a picture of the solemn procession of the corpse, behind
which the deceased appears, offering up prayers to the Sun-god.
The first chapter which is found on several sarcophagi, contains
invocations addressed to Osiris, the lord of the lower world. In
the 9th, Osiris is opening to the deceased, as his son, the paths
of heaven and earth. In the following the Osirian is justified
and ushered into the realms of light. According to Lepsius,
this first section contains the substance of the whole—what
follows is but an amplification of the various acts and adventures of the soul, and some of the sections are frequently repeated word for word." [a]

[a] Egypt's Place in Universal History, p. 25.

The reader who refers to Section VIII.[a] of the article Egypt will find that in these observations and discoveries—the important bearing of which upon the progress of Egyptian learning M. Bunsen has in no respect exaggerated—both Champollion and Lepsius had been long before completely anticipated by Dr. Young. It was Young, as we have already seen, who first instituted the systematic comparison of these funeral rolls and showed that the various sections into which they were divided in various manuscripts—however different in their age or in their style of writing—related more or less to the same scenes represented by the vignettes which headed them, and embraced more or less of the same texts, whether prayers, invocations, or confessions.   It was Young who connected the greatest part of those rolls which he examined, with the great hieroglyphical papyrus of Paris, as the most comprehensive of all those which had come under his observation, and who first came to the important conclusion that they formed a portion of those sacred books ascribed to Hermes or Thoth, of which Diodorus and Clemens of Alexandria speak, which had been transmitted without alteration from the earliest ages.   It was Young also who first applied the epithet Mortuary Ritual to the complete series of those sacred formulæ, a designation which Champollion afterwards adopted, as was usual with him, without acknowledgment, though no part of the work of Dr. Young in which it was mentioned could possibly have been at that time unknown to him.

This identification of texts, in papyri of ages so distant from each other, was undoubtedly the most interesting, if it was not the most important, of all

---

[a] Works, vol. iii. p. 189.

the discoveries in Egyptian literature, which preceded
the determination of the phonetic alphabet. It afforded a means of comparing with each other the
different modes of expressing the same ideas at least,
if not in the same words, in the various characters
which were employed in them, whether they were
hieroglyphical or hieratic; and of identifying equivalent groups or equivalent characters, whether the
latter were used phonetically or not. Such manuscripts and inscriptions likewise, when thus identified
and determined, presented a series of texts, whose
interpretation probably presented fewer difficulties
than most other Egyptian writings—from the pictorial representations, illustrative of the subjects to
which they referred, with which they were generally
headed or accompanied—from the easily recognised
symbols or groups of symbols which expressed the
designation of the various deities concerned in these
scenes—from the frequent recurrence of those phrases
of respect and adoration the meaning of which had
become known to us from other sources,—and, most of
all, from the general sameness and narrow range of the
topics which were introduced into them. By the careful use of the various aids above referred to, combined with a knowledge of the hieroglyphical groups
whose import had been ascertained by the study of
the Rosetta stone and other documents, Young was
enabled to translate conjecturally many passages in
these rituals, and to form a very correct conception
of their general purport in all cases. The Book of
the Dead, which Lepsius has printed, with a translation, from the great Turin papyrus, forms a worthy
termination to a class of researches, which must
be for ever memorable in the annals of the disco-

veries relating to the language and religion of ancient Egypt. The following account, extracted from his manuscripts, referring more especially to some rolls of papyrus sent from Egypt by Mr. Bankes and Lord Mountnorris, will sufficiently establish the correctness of the preceding statement :—

" These manuscripts are arranged in twelve sheets, containing parts of five or six different rolls of papyrus. The first, which is 12 feet in length, contains nine of the twelve, the second and third two, and the fourth and fifth the remaining one. They are all of a similar nature, representing, in the pictorial tablets, homages to the different deities, processions and detached actions, with appropriate hymns subjoined ; and in this, as usual, they agree with all the other Egyptian manuscripts which have hitherto been examined. Some of them agree throughout their extent with each other, excepting, however, the introduction of a *characteristic* phrase, peculiar to each manuscript, as a title of Osiris, which is repeated, and often more than once, in each section ; but in general there are some paragraphs or sections which agree in the different manuscripts, and these may readily be discovered by the identity of the tablets, the text being generally the same where the tablet is the same. The figures in this manuscript are obviously inserted after the text was written.

" The most considerable of the manuscripts hitherto discovered is distinguished by the title of the Strasburg Manuscript, the whole of which is very neatly written or drawn in characters obviously intended for pictures, as distinct hieroglyphics of visible objects "—a kind of writing which may possibly have been called the *hieratic.* The rest of the manuscripts are chiefly in the *epistolographic* character, which is a distant, though a very well-marked imitation of the same forms, rudely copied, character for character.

" In the great manuscript of Mr. Bankes, we find a very entire copy of a series of ten sections, beginning with a homage to Thoth or Hermes, which may be called the *Hermetic decade.*

---

a The linear hieroglyphics of Champollion.

The latter sections, which are wanting in other epistolographic manuscripts, are here quite perfect, though some of the earlier ones have suffered. In the subsequent part of the list there are several detached sections which are found in the Strasburg Manuscript, particularly the head rising out of the lotus, and some of the following tablets. The end, like that of several other of these rolls, contains the chapter devoted to the sacred cow.

"There is also, in sheet V., a list of 22 names of deities, with figures of 10 of them, which are the same, and nearly in the same order, as are commonly found painted on the coffins of mummies and on sarcophagi of stone, particularly that of Apis in the British Museum. These are always distinguished by the relation which they bear to Osiris, which is the same for each deity; and the name of Osiris is always followed by the *characteristic phrase* of the manuscript or monument, which may perhaps have had some allusion to the deceased personage, and who is made to serve without repetition for the whole twenty-two, being written in a column which follows the enumeration of the relations and is followed by that of the names.

"This manuscript, as well as one of the others, exhibits several times the peculiarity of a title of Osiris, which seems to signify sublime and good, being inclosed in a broken ring like a proper name of a man.

$$K \Gamma | \star \unicode{x263A})$$

"In all other instances, the names of the deities are without rings. It cannot be the name of a man concerned in this particular manuscript, because it is found in the Strasburg Manuscript as well as in this, unless it was the same man in both of them; it is, however, observable at Edfou, enclosed in a ring, but the context has not been copied.

"The name of the moon occurs here very distinctly after that of the sun, as the good Lunus; it is several times mentioned in one of the sections, but never with the feminine termination as those of the goddesses generally are; and from this circumstance, as well as from the gender of the Egyptian word, Ioh, there can be no doubt that the moon was a masculine deity among the Egyptians."

Then there follows a more minute and critical exa-

mination of this and the other papyri, section by
section, containing comparisons of synonymous groups
differing only from each other by the use of equivalent symbols, as well as other points which seemed
to be peculiar or remarkable.

We have before spoken of the circumstances which
led Dr. Young, not merely to the identification of the
name of Ptolemy in the first inscription on the Rosetta stone, but also suggested to him the notion that
the rings within which it was there enclosed, and
which appear so constantly upon the monuments,
were designed to indicate that the hieroglyphical characters which they included might possibly be used
phonetically, for the purpose of designating the
names of kings, or persons, or places, whether domestic or foreign, which could not otherwise be expressed;

" a process," says he, " which may be in some measure illustrated by the manner in which the modern Chinese express a
foreign combination of sounds, the characters being rendered
simply ' phonetic ' by an appropriate mark, instead of retaining
their natural signification, and this mark in some modern books
approaching very near to the ring surrounding the hieroglyphic
names."

Thus, the English word *strong* would require three
Chinese characters, *se, te, lung*, to express it, and on the
left side of each of them would be placed the character
kou signifying mouth.[a] Thus 于 *se,* 得 *te,* 龍 *lung,*
without the 口 *kou,* would severally signify *magistrate, to obtain, dragon;* but when this last character
is placed on the left of each of them, their combination would express the name *strong,* such being

a Quarterly Review, May 1810, vol. iii. p. 284.

the only form of it which brings it within the compass
of the Chinese organs of speech, the *r* being replaced
by *l*, as was usual also with the Egyptians.

The Chinese language possesses two hundred and
fourteen primitive characters, some of which are ideographic, or representations of real objects, others symbolical or arbitrary; and it is by their combinations
that they compose a language which is addressed
through the eye to the mind without any necessary
association of sound, and which may, in fact, correspond to different sounds in different provinces of
the empire. If it was assumed, therefore, as was universally the case when these researches began, that
the hieroglyphics were the signs of a similar language,
excluding an alphabetic element—and it obviously
abounded with ideographic characters to a much
greater extent than the Chinese—it would not be an
improbable hypothesis, that some similar expedient
might have been adopted to *phoneticise* the characters
whenever it became necessary to indicate foreign or
other appellations which the customary associations
of sound with such symbols or their combinations were
incompetent to express; under such circumstances,
it was assumed by Dr. Young, that the ring which
enclosed those symbols might very possibly serve the
office of the sign ▯ *kou*, of the Chinese.

There were, however, some conditions necessary
to the successful application of the principle ·thus
suggested for the analysis of groups of symbols,
supposed to be phoneticised by being included within
such rings, which it was not always easy to satisfy.
The first was a tolerably certain antecedent knowledge of the name which these characters were required to express; the second the familiar names in

the spoken language of Egypt, or in the Coptic descended from it, which were used to express the several objects, which the symbols more or less clearly
represented, the initial letter or syllable of which, or
the entire word, whether monosyllabic or not, was
to be made phonetic. This second process, however,
would generally be found impracticable, in consequence
of its being rarely possible, from the paucity of known
Coptic words, to assign the names of the objects
represented by the figurative signs, and also from its
being uncertain whether such names were used for
the same objects in the ancient Egyptian language.
The process of discovery, as we shall see, has generally
been, first to identify the name which the symbols
within the ring expressed, and secondly, when a sufficient number of phonetic symbols has been determined, to apply them either to determine or to assist
in determining, any other phonetic name, the analysis
of which was previously unknown.

Another consequence of this system would be the
probable and almost necessary use of *homophone signs*:
for if several different hieroglyphical characters were
known by names which began, not with the same
letter only, but with the same articulate sound formed
by a consonant and a vowel, they would all equally
admit of being thus phoneticised.[a]

These were the principles which either guided Young
in his analysis of well-ascertained names into their
phonetic elements, or which were, in some degree at
least, resorted to as a test of their accuracy, whenever
he was enabled to determine them conjecturally by the
aid of other considerations; such as those afforded by
the comparison of the hieroglyphics in the rings with

[a] Works, vol. iii. p. 467.

the enchorial characters of the same names, whenever their identity could be determined. He was in possession of the hieroglyphical names of two royal personages, and of two only, those of Ptolemy and Berenice, which were determined with sufficient certainty to enable him to apply his principles to them with tolerable safety. In the analysis of the first he was chiefly guided by secondary considerations, the only considerable error which he made being occasioned by his too exclusive reliance upon the principles above referred to ; in that of the second he was led into serious errors by the same cause.

The train of reasoning which is involved in these speculations is extremely artificial, and such as could hardly occur to two persons engaged independently in seeking for the solution of the problem of reading or analysing the names upon the monuments : but ingenious and refined as the conception was, and memorable as were the conclusions to which it served as a guide, it is now known that very material errors were involved in most of the assumptions upon which it was founded. The rings did not indicate that the characters which they included were necessarily phonetic, with a view of expressing names and appellatives, whether domestic or foreign, which were not otherwise expressible, but were exclusively used as marks of honour to royal personages. The characters, also, within these rings are not more generally phonetic, at least before the age of the Ptolemies, than those which are external to them, inasmuch as ideographic symbols, especially of the names of the deities, were used as well as those which were alphabetical or syllabic : and though it was possible and probable that the phonetic power of a symbol was deduced from the

initial letter or syllable of the word in the Egyptian
language which expressed it, no sufficient proof had
then or has since been produced to show that such was
invariably the case.

We have already seen that in 1821 Champollion
denied altogether the existence of an alphabetic element amongst the hieroglyphics. But in the following year we find him adopting the whole of Young's
principles, and applying them with one modification
only. Like him, he refers to the expedient resorted
to in the Chinese language for the phonetic expression
of foreign appellations ; like him, he regards the rings
as marks of the phonetic use of the characters which
they include, whether of royal or private personages,
whether domestic or foreign ; like him, he supposes
the phonetic power of the symbol to be derived from
the initial letter or syllable of the name of the object
which it expresses in the Egyptian language ; but he
differs from him in considering that such a phonetic
character could express more than a simple letter or the
syllable formed by it when followed by a short vowel ;
and he only notices, for purposes of criticism, those
applications which Young had made of this principle,
where the phonetic power of such a symbol was extended to a syllable, like the Coptic name of the basket
Λ, $\beta\iota\rho$, in phoneticising the hieroglyphical name of Berenice. It would be difficult to point out, in the history
of literature, a more flagrant example of disingenuous
suppression of the real facts bearing upon an important
discovery ; where principles, too peculiar in their character to have occurred independently to two different
minds, are adopted without the least acknowledgment,
though circumstances proved incontestably that they
were neither known nor thought of at a time immediately antecedent to the perusal of the very work in

which they were announced and exemplified; where
the conclusions in one work were passed over without
notice when they were precisely the same as those
which were adopted in the other, but invidiously criticised where an erroneous or somewhat too extended
application of them afforded a handle to lay hold of,
for the purpose of establishing a claim for entire originality. It was in a very different spirit that his illustrious countryman, Fresnel, with much higher pretensions to independent research and discovery, at
once abandoned his claims of priority when he found
that he had been anticipated by Dr. Young.[a]

The ground upon which Champollion rested his
claim, not merely to a principal share in the discovery
of phonetic hieroglyphics, but also to the exclusive
glory of effecting it, was, that Young had taken a
mistaken view of the principle of their phonetization,
when such hieroglyphics no longer, as in ordinary
cases, represented, not sounds, but things; the latter
conceiving, in conformity with the Chinese principle
which he had suggested, though he did not feel it
necessary strictly to follow it, that a symbol when it
became phonetic might represent either a letter or a
syllable, or even a word, if the familiar name of the
object of which the symbol was a figure formed a part
or the whole of the name which was required to be
vocalised: such cases, in fact, being of frequent occurrence in the expression of many royal names, such as
those of Rameses, Thoutmes, and others, when the compound or simple symbolical representation of the deity
becomes a phonetic element of the name, a part of whose
sound it expresses. Champollion contended, on the
contrary, at least in the first instance, that they were
syllabico-alphabetic, such as would be formed by a con-

See supra, p. 165.

sonant and a short vowel—as is usual with the alphabets of the Semitic languages—but not the constituent syllables or parts of words, with more consonants than one. These principles, however, more especially if considered as forming a starting point for subsequent investigations, were in no essential respect different from each other, and the selection of one or the other of them could not fail to be decided by the result of the two or three first applications of them to names previously well known; more especially if such names, like that of Cleopatra, which first came under Champollion's observation, admitted, as we shall afterwards see, of perfect and unambiguous analysis, without the suppression of a single letter.

The Article Egypt, which contained the principal record of Young's researches in hieroglyphical literature, was addressed, as we have before observed,[a] not to learned but to general readers, and it exhibited, therefore, a very imperfect view of the vast mass of manuscript materials which he had collected, and of the patient and skilful analysis to which they had been subjected. These manuscripts were all written before the preparation of that article, and nearly five years before the appearance of Champollion's letter to M. Dacier, and it is obvious, from an inspection of them, that they had received no subsequent additions. The whole of the intervening period, in fact, had been fully occupied in writing nearly seventy articles of the Supplement of the Encyclopædia Britannica, as well as by a great variety of public and other engagements. One of these manuscripts contains a classified dictionary of nearly two hundred hieroglyphical characters, with real or conjec-

a Supra, p. 281.

tural interpretations of their use and meaning, whether singly or in combination with others, which have been derived from the Rosetta stone, from the collation of a great number of ritual and other papyri, from inscriptions on the monuments, and from other sources. M. Bunsen, and other friends of Champollion, have spoken in very disparaging terms of the Lexicon Hieroglyphicum, which is appended to the article Egypt, as uncritical, meagre, and frequently erroneous : but they would probably have been compelled to form a very different estimate, both of the capacity of the writer, and of the real progress which he had made, if the whole of this Lexicon, as well as his collations of the manuscripts, could have been brought under their notice.

We shall subjoin a few extracts relating to some characters, which, from various causes, have been referred to in the discussions which have arisen in the course of these researches, or are otherwise especially deserving of notice : some of them we shall give entire as specimens of others, which are equally copious ; whilst in most cases, we have been compelled to confine ourselves to a few extracts only, from considerations of economy both in space and hieroglyphical printing. It is hardly necessary to remind our readers that the manuscripts from which they are taken were not designed for publication, and having been written in the first infancy of these inquiries, they contain, as might naturally be expected, much that is merely conjectural, and much more that is now known to be altogether erroneous.

No. 179. ▥ This may possibly be something like the article πι, since 2,, which often answers to it in the manuscripts, appears to have some connection with that sound.   But there is no case in which ▥ seems to serve the purpose of an article. Its simplest intelligible use is with ⚘ , for a term of respect following the name of a deity.   ⚘ ▥, which seems never to be inceptive, as its synonym ⬭⸝. ⚯ ▥, (Ros. I., l. 5, 14.) Beloved. ⚷▦⚯, (Ros. I., l. 7), Apis. ⦅⑂⸝⸝ ⚶⚬▥⸗⦆ (Ros. I., l. 7, 11), Ptolemy.   The block possibly π.   The semi-circle τ, but without explanation.   The lion, ⛼ ολε, perhaps an old word, like the ωιλι, which more lately signified ram.   ⬎, μ, which seems to be often indicated, as in ⬏ , ερμα; perhaps μα; and ⎰⎰, ι; or merely μ and ε, as the later Copts wrote; ⎰, may be ος, great; if the Egyptians confounded the c and ος.

▥⸝ No. 91.ᵃ ⊟⸝ (Ros. l. 13); the same. ⊜⊞(Ros. l. 13); it seems here to take the place of ⎰; but this is ⬭, not ▥. ⊔⊜ (Ros. l. 14), uncertain. ⊖▥. No. 201, 152.   A frequent ⬭▥ homage in the great ritual.   Almost all the terms taken singly seem to imply something like greatness or respect, but it is not easy to say how they are connected with each other. ⬭ ▥ should be πτ, and it may have some distinct meaning in ⚯▥. ⎰⎰⚘ ▥ for ⚘ ▥ Tab. III.

The analysis of the name of Ptolemy, which is given in the article Egypt, is chiefly founded upon the relation of some of the principal symbols within the

<hr>

ᵃ The numbers referred to designate the No. in the Dictionary, which the particular symbol referred to occupies.

ring to those which he conceived to correspond to them in the enchorial text of the Rosetta stone; he, therefore, justifies his not assigning a phonetic value to the knot or flower, as he considered it " as not essentially necessary, being often omitted in the sacred characters and always in the enchorial."[a] We find it omitted in some inscriptions which he has copied, where the ring of Ptolemy appears.

Champollion found this character, the knot or flower, as the fourth in order, in the hieroglyphical name of Cleopatra, and he denies the omission of the corresponding character in the enchorial name of Ptolemy, which Young had mistaken for part of the character for *t* which preceded it. The only important misconception, therefore, which occurs in this analysis, was making the *lion* the representative of *lo* or *ole*, instead of simply *l*. Such an error, however, was really not of a kind to embarrass any inquirer, and could not fail to be dissipated by any other application of the principle to a name where the same character appeared in a different combination. The analysis of the name of Cleopatra, as we shall afterwards see, at once settled this question.

In the hieroglyphical form of the same name, the character ⊏ is frequently replaced by ∨, as Young has remarked at the commencement of his manuscript collection of inscriptions from the great temple of Ombos, as given in the great French work on Egypt. In fact, no student of Egyptian literature, who carefully copied inscriptions or manuscripts, could long remain ignorant of permutable signs, which would also become homophonous, in case such permuted signs were found to be phonetic.

[a] Works, vol. iii. p. 156. See also Mr. Leitch's note.

" No 180. ☁. Even if this character sometimes expresses the letter *t*, we cannot derive any very definite sense from the supposition. There is some reason for suspecting that it is a token of respect; thus following the name of Hermes, ὁ μέγας καὶ μέγας. ⫽☁ seems to be its dual; and this dual occurs very frequently where two persons are evidently concerned."_

Then follows a long list of groups in which it appears, with conjectures respecting its probable meaning in some of them.

" No. 183. ⌐. This character occurs too often to have a strongly marked sense: it seems to be sometimes read ος or οι̯, as if *great*, but it is not certain that this is its meaning. In the ring of Ptolemaios, as we have seen, No. 179, it is terminal. It is sometimes a secondary in compound characters, sometimes initial; ⟅⌐ (Ros. I.) *libations*. ⬓⌐ (Ros. I.) *assembly*, probably an epithet. ⌐⫙ (No. 218) *consecrated*. ⟅⌐ (Ros. I.) seems a part of a title of honour, as in the obelisc at Luxor after a name. ⌐⫚ (Ros. I.) seems a term of respect added to a statue. ⌐ʃρϙ (Ros. I.) seems to mean language.

" No. 184, ◀━. Probably synonymous with ⌐, for which it is perpetually exchanged. ⬒ (Ros. I.) seems to be *worship;* θεραπεύειν; *pay attention to.* ⌇⌇⌇ (N. 117) ..... *ments;* this scarcely occurs in the singular. ⌇⌇⌇⌐ is often substituted in the manuscripts. ⌇⌇⌇⎈ This seems a double plural, but it is not incompatible with the former.

" No. 185. ⬓, μ. Seems to relate to place, μα; also to mean *in*, and perhaps *all*. ⬓ (Ros. I.) *belonging to*, stands between temples and Egypt. ⬓ (Ros. I.) *in a month*.

Possibly ⋏, which follows in No. 186, may be a reduplication, and both may mean *all* or *every*. ⊟. No 39, ερμα. ⊒ (Ros I.) *to add.* ⍟ (Ros. I.) *engraved.* (⍓⎮⎮⊒⍭⊡) passim. In the name Ptolemaios ⊐ seems to stand for μα or for μ, as a phonetic character.

" No. 186. ⋏. Possibly *all:* it is frequently confounded with ⊃. ⋏ (Ros. I.) *every* (month). ⋏ (Ros. I.) seems to answer to εκαστω. ⍔⋏ (Ros. I.) *between temples and Egypt as* ⊟ in No. 185. ⊟ *and* ⍟ (Ros. I.) *moreover.*

" No. 58. 🦉 *in.* It seems to be perfectly synonymous with ⊃, and both are often written ⌇ or ∫. ⍔⍔⍔◢ ἐν τοῖς ἱεροῖς (Ros. I.) ⍟ a homage, *perpetual dignity.* The *bird* alone in this and in other instances implies *dignity:* possibly μ did the same.

" No 187. ⍭ A *hundred*, ⲙⲉ. Sometimes also probably *many* or *much*, and often of uncertain degree. It seems to have some connection with ◣ : these signs often occur together, and we have often ⅡⅠ◣ and Ⅱ ⍭, but seldom, if ever, ⅡⅠ without one of these signs. It is frequently exchanged with ◢. Thus ⍔ and ⍔.

There is then added a list of many other groups in which it is used.

" No. 190. ⍮ seems to answer to *lawful*, and in the word *Greek* to be expressed by ⟨ of the enchorial text of the Rosetta inscription ; so that it seems to have a sense, resembling that of divine ⌐ ; perhaps *glorious;* being read ωου or ου.

ノ⟨||丄 (Ros. I.) *Greek.*   The characters seem to be phonetic ; ουει ενεεν, ουεειννιν or ουεινινν, a word which seems to be derived from Ionian.   Expressed by ◖ , that is, ⟪ as a perfect synonym, in Tablet V."

This analysis is noticed in the article Egypt,[a] and is interesting as an example of the application of the principle of phonetization, notwithstanding the error which was made in the selection of the groups of hieroglyphics on the Rosetta stone which corresponded to the word Greek or Ionian.   Champollion denied that Young had either determined the phonetic value of the character ⟋⟍◇ included in this group, or that he had shown it to be a homophone of ᚎᚎᚎ, an assertion which is sufficiently refuted by a reference to No. 253, and by the quotation from the article Egypt, which is given in the Note below.

" No 117. ᚎᚎᚎ , a serrated line is often used to represent a liquid flowing out of one vessel into another : the idea of the fluid has been dropped : for this symbol occurs repeatedly in almost every line of almost every existing inscription, but that of *connection* only is retained, so that it signifies *of* or *to*, and makes an *adjective* of a *substantive*, whether following or

[a] " The word Greek, in Coptic uinin or oueinin, in Thebaic, oueeienin, supposed to be derived from Ionian, seems to exhibit in its form something like an imitation of the sound.   The curl on a stem is sometimes exchanged for the term *divine*, and appears to mean 'glory,' in Coptic oou or oü, which is nearly the sound attributed by Akerblad, to the enchorial character, a little like the Hebrew u ; the feather, as in Ptolemy and Berenice, may be read i or ei, having the three dashes to express them, us usual in the enchorial text; the serpent is *eneh*, 'ever,' and the hat, ⟍⟍ or helmet, which is equivalent to the waved line, ᚎᚎᚎ, and must be read n, so that we have very accurately ouienehn, which seems to be near enough to oueinin to justify us in thinking these characters phonetic."   See also Mr. Leitch's note.   Works, vol. iii. p. 164.

preceding. Thus it seems to answer to ντε, or simply ν, as ννουβ, golden, from νουβ, gold; it appears also sometimes to be phonetic as N; and very often its sense is indistinct; as indeed that of ⲛ is in Coptic. ⫶ⲓⲅ (Ros. I.) *of* the gods, *sacred.*

⸗ (Ros. I.) *upon;* perhaps as making a preposition of the rabbit. ⸗, a combination which perpetually occurs in some manuscripts and inscriptions, and is often left out of the parallel passages of others. It appears to signify . . . *ments,* or . . . *ations,* or . . . . *arious,* as of sundry things connected thereto. ⸗ (Ros. I.) *Institutions* of the country. ⸗ ⸗ (Ros I.) seems to be *sacerdotal — pertinentia ad sacerdotes.* ⸗ (Ros. I.) *ornaments, amplifications.* ⸗ (Ros. I.) *possessions, enjoyments.* ⌇⌇⌇ (Ros. I.) *to him.* In the zodiac at Dendera, *water* is thus represented ⸗ between the fishes. It is not impossible that ⸗ may be another way of representing it, rather than ⸗. But on Tab. II. this symbol ⸗ is exchanged for ⸗ *beloved*, as synonymous in Tablet III. for ⸗.

"253. ⸗ A kind of hat, always represented on the great hawk of the obeliscs, and often on men's heads. It means *of*, and seems perfectly synonymous with ⸗, making an adjective of a substantive, whether preceding or following it, and as a letter it seems to be expressed by N. ⸗ ⸗ (Ros. I.) of the god. ⸗ (Ros I.) for ⸗. ⸗ ⸗ (Ros. I.) *upper and lower* countries. The hat and the cap are in opposition.

"No. 92. ⸗. The feather has sometimes been mistaken for a knife, but this is always straight. It may, however, be intended to represent the wing of an insect; at least the wings of bees are generally represented in the same form; it has also some resemblance to a leaf. When it has any distinct meaning it

seems to signify *ornament.*   ❘ ❘ frequently occurs in passages
where its insertion or omission seems to be indifferent, and it
is scarcely intelligible any otherwise than as a phonetic mark
for I or EE English,   or ❘❘❘ of the enchorial character."

"❘ (Ros. I.) These characters occur very commonly in the
manuscripts as a term of respect, as *great, worshipful, honorable.*
In the Ros. I. ❘ ❘ follows the word *gods,* probably as a redupli-
cative phrase."

Then there follows the analysis of a long list of
groups in which the feathers appear.

" No. 139. ⟁   A plough, or rather, when erect, a hand
hoe, which is represented in the same form. It does not seem
to appear in the proper sense of this representation in any inscription ; but in the Ros I., and apparently elsewhere, very
commonly is used for PHTHAH, the ancestor of most of the
Egyptian deities.

"❘❘⟁⟁⟁ (Ros. I.) beloved by Phthah—ΗΓΑΠΗΜΕ-
ΝΩΙ ΤΩΙ ΦΘΑ.

Young unfortunately translated this group " beloved of Phthah" instead " of Phthah beloved ;" thus
interchanging the significations of ❘❘⟁, μει, " beloved " and ⟁⟁, *Phthah.*

" No. 68. ⌒. This snake seems to be ℈ος or ℈ςο :
it is written in the enchorial ४ or ४, which is not very remote
from the Coptic ⲣ, fei. In some places it means clearly *he,*
him or *it,* which is also ⲣ.   ⟋ (Ros. I.) *to him, apud*
eum, very distinctly ♀ in the enchorial text. ∿∿ (Ros. I.)
probably also *to him, ei.*"

This is followed by many other illustrations.

" No. 245. ✿. This symbol, resembling the shamrock, seems to be synonymous with the shilelah or mace, ⭑, of which Denon has drawn a club or mace of modern date, which is an exact resemblance. ⌐✿⌐✿ (Ros. I.) Θεων Σωτηϱων, dual, *saviour* or *protector gods*. ⭑⌐ (Ros. I.) can scarcely be very different.

" No. 97. ⸸. Possibly a reed, as guiding the bees. Plutarch mentions 3ϱίον, a leaf, as signifying a king. ⸸ (Ros. I.) *king*, alone. 🜚⸸ in the same sense every where, &c &c.

" No. 193. ◯ or ◉. Perhaps connected with the sun, either simply or phonetically as PE from PH, since it seems to signify certainly this. ◯_⸾ is REΣER ΣEMI, &c. &c.

" No. 141. 𐐒. A chain, as a bond of union. Scales are often represented as suspended by such chains. 🝙 (Ros. I.) *with* or *and*. 𐐒_ (Ros. I.) in the same sense.

The examination of the preceding extracts will show that Dr. Young had very sufficiently determined from a careful examination and comparison of texts, and from considerations connected with the grammatical structure of the language in which they are written, the phonetic value of the square, or matt, ▢, to be P; of the semicircle ◠ to be T; of the cerastes or horned snake ⌒ᐟ, to be F; of the reflexed line or back of a seat ⌐, to be S, and the bolt of a door, ◂▸, to be homophonous with it; the three sides of a quadrilateral or the stand of a boat, ▭, to be M, and that it is also homophonous with the divided staff or stake, ⋎, and with the owl ◢; the wavy line, ∿, to be N, and to be homophonous with the hat or crown of Lower Egypt ⤳; the single or double feather to be E, or I, or EE: making altogether twelve phonetic symbols; not to mention others, whose determination, as being more or less syllabic, could not be considered as equally complete and satisfactory.

So completely, in fact, was this principle of phonetization understood, that Mr. Bankes, so well known for his Egyptian collections, to whom Dr. Young had given a sketch of his researches in manuscript, with a copy of the Lexicon of Hieroglyphics, nearly a year before the publication of the article in the Encyclopædia to which it was appended, was enabled by means of them to add another homophone sign, ☪, for the letter N.[a] The correspondence between Young and Sir William Gell, in the years 1821 and 1822, which is published in the third volume of Dr Young's Works, will show the impulse which the course of hieroglyphical literature had received from this Article; but if more testimony were wanting in a case which might really be considered as indisputable—if it had not been disputed—we may refer to the evidence contained not only in the published works of Sir Gardner Wilkinson, but also in a private note-book, written in the year 1821, and communicated by him to Mr. Leitch, in which he makes repeated applications of the phonetic signs discovered by Dr. Young.[b]

The reader of the preceding statements, which admit of the most complete authentification, would learn with surprise that a writer so learned, and usually so candid and impartial, as M. Bunsen, should have ventured to deny that Dr. Young had ever pro-

[a] Works, vol. iii. p. 284.
[b] Works, vol. iii. p. 465, Mr. Leitch's note.

perly conceived the possibility of a phonetic system, but that he had confounded a "certain kind of syllabic system with it;" and further to assert that he was "equally unconscious of the existence of several signs for one sound, the so-called homophone signs, the real key to the hieroglyphic characters, although the hieroglyphic MSS. of the Book of the Dead, which he collated, might have led him to infer it."[a] The first of these charges will be fully refuted by what follows, if it has not been sufficiently so by what has gone before; whilst the reproach which heads the second would probably have been spared, if M. Bunsen had dispassionately studied the works of Dr. Young, and not relied implicitly on the statements of Champollion. It is hardly necessary to add to what we have observed before, that the manuscripts which record the results of these collations are replete with notices of synonymous groups, in addition to those which we have given; and that Champollion at no period of his life was in advance of Dr. Young in a thorough knowledge and appreciation of this great principle of substitution.

But, it may very properly be asked, if Dr. Young had so completely conceived the principle of phonetic hieroglyphics, why was his success in its application to the reading of royal names so limited? He had himself given very satisfactory reasons for thinking, that the rings which appear upon the monuments of Egypt expressed the names of their founders, and not of the deities in whose honour they were built; and he had ransacked the records of classical antiquity for the purpose of identifying them. But it was found to be no easy task to connect such names with the monuments;

[a] Egypt's Place in Universal History, p. 321.

and in the few cases in which they were so connected,
they were generally so disguised by the usual licence
taken by Egyptian artists and workmen in the transcription of foreign names, as not to be very easily
recognised. It was well known also that Greek inscriptions were to be found upon many of the temples; but
either the inscriptions themselves, or the hieroglyphical
rings to which they referred, had hitherto been so
inaccurately copied, as to serve rather to mislead inquiry than to guide it. Thus Mr. Hamilton had
published in his Egyptiaca a Greek inscription on the
temple of Ombos, purporting that it was dedicated
"in the name of the divine Ptolemy Philometer and
Cleopatra and their children, to Arueris Apollo, and the
other gods of the temple, by the infantry and cavalry
of the nome;" but the ring in the plates of the great
Description de l'Egypte, to which his attention was
called in this instance as likely to contain the name
of Cleopatra, was that of a king and not of a queen,
—an unfortunate circumstance, inasmuch as this name
occurs repeatedly in other parts of the temple.

The name, however, of Ptolemy Soter, whose wife was
Berenice, was recognised by him in the Greek inscription on the ceiling of the temple at Karnak; and the
ring of a Ptolemy with which he was familiar, was
combined with a second ring, terminated by the semicircle and oval, ⌒〇, the invariable mark of a female,
and both of them followed by a group of hieroglyphics
which he had ascertained from the Rosetta stone to
mean the Saviour gods [a]—a title which the Greek inscription also assigned to them. He consequently felt
himself authorized to conclude that this was the hieroglyphical name of Berenice, which he accordingly pro-

ceeded to analyse: but it was unfortunate that amongst the characters within this ring,

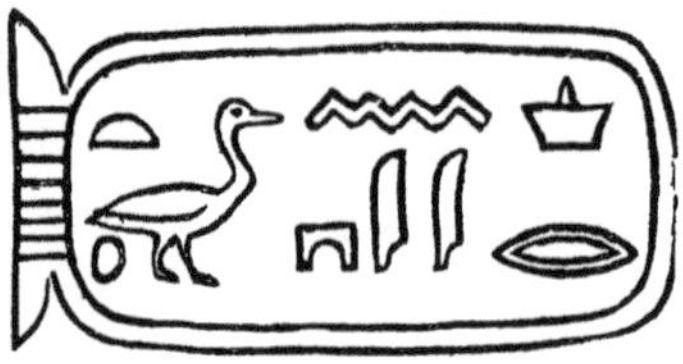

one only, the double feather, was common to those in the name of Ptolemy, though the wavy line was known from other sources to have the phonetic value of N; it was perhaps still more unfortunate that whilst the basket, which is the first of these characters, recalled to his mind its Coptic name *bir*, which is the initial syllable of Berenice or Bereniken, the goose,[a] at its conclusion, suggested upon the doubtful authority of Kircher, its Coptic name of *Kenesöu*, whose initial letters *ke* or *ken* corresponded to those also at the conclusion of the name. Admitting the syllabic values of the first and last of the characters, which this ring contained, as authorised at least, though not required, by the Chinese principle of phonetization, he proceeded, by making the mouth  to be E, the wavy line  to be N, the double feather to be I, and by omitting the footstool as superfluous, to construct the name Berenike.

The warmest advocates of Dr. Young must admit that this analysis, though conformable to the principle which he adopted, was more creditable to his ingenuity than to his judgment; and though it was not calculated to mislead those who continued the inquiry, it was certainly not likely to guide them. As

[a] The *goose* was introduced instead of a *hawk*, or rather *eagle*, by a mistake of the copyist: the phonetic value of the first was S and of the second A.

it was, his enemies failed not to perceive, when the
progress of hieroglyphical discovery had speedily removed all room for doubt or speculation, that it was
the weak point in the application of his system, and
Champollion at once seized upon it as furnishing a
plausible pretext for asserting that Young's principle
of phonetization was not only erroneous but essentially
different from his own.

Young was perfectly well aware that the assumptions
which were made the basis of his principle could only
be verified or corrected by the further discovery of
well ascertained names to which they could be applied;
and it was with a view of assisting in these discoveries that he prepared special instructions to Mr.
Bankes, who was proceeding on a second visit to
Egypt, for the purpose of guiding him in his inquiries. Mr. Salt, to whom Mr. Bankes had communicated these instructions, acknowledges in very
striking terms, in a letter addressed to Mr. W. Hamilton, his great obligations to them, as giving a real
and historical significance to monuments which he
would probably otherwise have passed over without
much observation and remark ;[a] whilst Mr. Bankes was
enabled, partly by means of them and partly by a very
ingenious and complete investigation of his own, to
identify the hieroglyphical name of Cleopatra upon an
obelisk at Philæ with the same name in a Greek inscription upon its base.   It was an engraving of these
inscriptions, with a marginal reference pointing out
distinctly the conclusion at which he had arrived,
which was sent by Mr. Bankes to M. Denon to be presented to the French Institute: and though there is
no reason to doubt that it was this engraving that

[a] Works, vol. iii. p. 284.

really furnished Champollion with the principal materials for his most important discovery, he never
acknowledged his obligations.[a]

The account, in fact, which is given by Champollion
of the recognition and analysis of the name of Cleopatra, would induce a reader to conclude that he had
neither precursor nor assistant in the investigation.

"The hieroglyphical text of the inscription of Rosetta," says
he, "exhibited, on account of its fractures, only the name of Ptolemy. The obelisc found in the Isle of Philæ, and lately removed
to London, contains also the hieroglyphical name of one of the
Ptolemies, expressed by the same characters that occur in the
inscription of Rosetta, surrounded by a ring or border, and it is
followed by a second border, which must necessarily contain the
proper name of a woman, and of a queen of the family of the
Lagidæ, since this group was terminated by the hieroglyphics
expressive of the feminine gender; characters which are found
at the end of the names of all the Egyptian goddesses without
exception. The obelisc was fixed, it is said, to a basis bearing
a Greek inscription, which is a petition of the priests of Isis at
Philæ, addressed to King Ptolemy, to Cleopatra his sister, and
to Cleopatra his wife. Now, if this obelisc, and the hieroglyphical inscription engraved on it were the result of this petition,
which, in fact, adverts to the consecration of a monument of the
kind, the border with the feminine proper name, can only be
that of one of the Cleopatras. This name, and that of Ptolemy,
which in the Greek have several letters in common, were
capable of being employed for a comparison of the hieroglyphical characters composing them, and if the similar characters
in these names expressed in both the same sounds, it followed
that their nature must be entirely phonetic."

[a] See Letronne, Recherches pour servir à l'histoire de l'Egypte, pp. xxx. and
298. It was the copy of this inscription, which was made by Cailliaud, but
without connecting the inscription on the base with the hieroglyphics on
the obelisk, to which Champollion alone refers in his letter to M. Dacier.
M. Letronne claims the merit of having made the suggestion which led
to this identification, independently of Mr. Bankes, and of having communicated it to Champollion : as was usual with him, however, he was not
more grateful to M. Letronne than to Mr. Bankes. See Mr. Leitch's
note, Works, vol. iii. p. 293.

But it should be observed, that it was Dr. Young who first determined, and by no easy process, that the rings on the Rosetta stone contained the name of Ptolemy; it was Dr. Young who determined that the semicircle and oval, found at the end of the second ring ·in connection with the former, was expressive of the feminine gender; and it was Dr. Young who had not only first suggested that the characters in the ring of Ptolemy were phonetic, but had determined, with one very unimportant inaccuracy, the values of four of those which were common to the name of Cleopatra which was required to be analyzed. All the principles involved in the discovery of an alphabet of phonetic hieroglyphics were not only distinctly laid down, but fully exemplified by him, and it only required the farther identification of one or two royal names with the rings which expressed them in hieroglyphics to extend the alphabet already known sufficiently to bring even names, which were not already identified, under its operation.

There were many circumstances also which made this hieroglyphical name singularly adapted for a complete and indisputable analysis: it will be observed that the particular ring known to express the name of

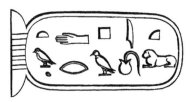

Cleopatra, which came under examination, contained eleven characters, the two last of which, the small semicircle and oval, are, as we have seen, the recognized marks of a female. There remain, therefore, nine

others exactly corresponding to the number of letters in the word Cleopatra.   Of these—the lion, the flower, the feather, and the parallelogram—three appear always, and all of them occasionally, in the hieroglyphical name of Ptolemy, with the several values of the letters L, O, E, and P: amongst the remaining five, there is one repetition—the last character but three and the last—precisely in the same positions as the letter A in KLEOPATRA; if the other three characters, therefore, the quadrant of a circle, the open- hand and the mouth, are phonetic also, they must severally represent the letters K, T, and R, which alone are required to complete the name.

The expression of Greek and Roman names, by means of Egyptian characters, was not only adapted to the genius of the language, into which they were transferred, but partook very generally of those abbreviations and corruptions of form which may be expected in all cases where the transcriber is guided chiefly by his ear.   It thence very rarely happens that the name thus transferred from Greek or Latin to hieroglyphics is complete, letter for letter, as in the very remarkable case of that of Cleopatra on the obelisk at Philæ: other variations of it on other monuments, giving KLEOPTRA, KLEPTRA, KLOPTRA.   The name of Alexander is usually spelt ALKSNTRS, omitting all the short vowels, and in one case ALKSNROS.   Autocrator is presented in the several forms AUTOKRTR, AUTKRTR, AUTOKLTL (L and R being commutable):[a] that of Cæsar, as KAISRS, KAISLS, KAISR: the Emperor Tiberius is with some difficulty recognized as TBLIS or

---

[a] " The old Egyptians " says Dr. Young, " seem to have been as incapable as their school-fellows the Chinese of distinguishing the R from the L." Works, vol. iii. p. 235.

TBRIS: Domitianus as TOMTINS: Trajanus as TRINS: and Augustus (Sebastus) as SBSTS; all these abridged forms of familiar classical names sufficiently justifying the epithet *syllabico-alphabetic* which Champollion in the first instance applied to the phonetic use of hieroglyphics, in a sense which students of the Semitic languages will find no difficulty in understanding.

It may readily be conceived, therefore, how much less certain and instructive would have been the analysis of this hieroglyphical ring, if it had presented the name of Cleopatra, not—as it was in this case found to be—in its complete, but in its abridged and mutilated form, where no limitation on the phonetic values of the characters was imposed by their being precisely equal in number to the letters in the name which they expressed, and where no assistance was derived or derivable from the previous determination of some of them by the analysis of other rings, like that which expressed the name of Ptolemy.

Let us contrast this case with that of Berenice, whose ring, as submitted to Young, contained six characters only, when there were eight letters in the name, and even nine, if it was assumed to be written as it might have been, in the objective case. It was equally probable, therefore, in the absence of all other information to guide us, that our choice would have rested upon any one of the following forms, even excluding others, which inaccurate spelling might have introduced:—

Bereniken	Breniken	Briniken	Brnikn
Berenikes	Brenikes	Brinikes	Brniks
Berenike	Brenike	Brinike	Brnik

It was the first or ninth of these forms which Young adopted, instead of the eleventh; Champollion, who had ascertained the phonetic value of the mouth from the ring of Cleopatra, adopted the tenth, though he had no authority for the phonetic value which he assigned to the goose, which appeared there instead of an eagle, by an error in the copy.

It has been often remarked that the happy accidents which from time to time have led to important discoveries, have usually been reserved to those who are enabled by their genius and promptitude of observation to take advantage of them ; and though we can hardly fail to recognize in the selection, not merely of the ring which contained the name of Cleopatra, but of the same name also unaltered in its spelling by its transcription into phonetic hieroglyphics, a more than usual concurrence of fortunate circumstances, yet, it would be unjust to refuse to Champollion the honour due to his rare skill and sagacity, not merely in this particular application of a principle already known, but in its rapid extension to a multitude of other cases, so as not merely to point out its character and use and some of the limitations to which it was subject, but also to determine the principal elements of a phonetic alphabet. His long study of Coptic literature, both printed and manuscript ; his perfect acquaintance with all that had been written relating to the history, the antiquities, and the religion of Egypt, added to his familiarity with hieratic and enchorial manuscripts, had given him advantages, which no other person, Young hardly excepted, possessed, to enable him to enter upon this inquiry ; and the rapidity of his progress, when once fully started upon his career of discovery, was worthy of the highest admiration. In less than two years from the appearance of the Letter to M. Dacier, his *Précis du Système Hiéroglyphique* was published, a work which will be for ever memorable in the history of hieroglyphical discovery, not merely from the vast range of knowledge which it displays, but from the clear and lucid order in which it is arranged. It was singularly unfortunate that one who possessed so much of his own, should have been so much wanting in a proper sense of justice to those who had preceded him in these investigations, as materially to lessen his claims to the respect and reverence which would otherwise have been most willingly conceded to him.

A letter written by Dr. Young from Paris in September, 1822, to his friend Mr. William Hamilton, gives an interesting account of the extraordinary progress which Champollion was at that time making in deciphering hieroglyphical names :—

" You will easily believe," says he, " that were I ever so much the victim of bad passions, I should feel nothing but exultation at M. Champollion's success. My life seems indeed to be lengthened by the accession of a junior coadjutor in my researches, and of a person too who is so much more versed in the different dialects of the Egyptian language than myself. I have promised him every assistance in his researches that I can procure him in England, and I hope to obtain from him an early communication of all his future observations."[a]

In a similar tone he writes to Mr. Gurney.

" In my own pursuits I have found abundance of novelty to interest me : both the scientific and literary departments of the Institute happening at this moment to be particularly engaged with my late investigations : and a Frenchman having in each of them been engaged in going over my own ground without being fully acquainted with what I had done, and having had to exclaim, *Pereant qui ante nos nostra dixerunt.* Fresnel, a young mathematician of the Civil Engineers, has really been doing some good things in the extension and application of my theory of light, and Champollion, the author of the book you

[a] Works, vol. iii. p. 222.

brought over, has been working still harder upon the Egyptian characters.   He devotes his whole time to the pursuit, and he has been wonderfully successful in some of the documents that he has obtained.

" An Italian of the name of Casati[a] brought over some manuscripts here which were found in a jar at Abydos.   Four are in Greek, like that which Böckh has published at Berlin[b]—the fifth is in the running hand of the Rosetta inscription, and in the same dialect or variety of that hand, so that the introductory part of the manuscript containing the date, with the names of Ptolemy and Cleopatra, is perfectly legible by the help of the Rosetta inscription.   This really is a grand step.   It greatly lessens the impatience that I have hitherto felt for Drovetti's[c] stone at Menouf—about which the people here are as angry as I am.   Champollion has also made out a complete series of the numerals in the running hand by comparing the beginnings of the successive chapters of one of the mummy manuscripts—and he has found a fragment, formerly belonging to the Duc de Choiseul, on which several of the months are distinctly expressed. How far he will acknowledge every thing which he has either borrowed or might have borrowed from me, I am not quite confident; but the world will be sure to remark, *que c'est le premier pas qui coûte*—though the proverb is less true in this case than in most others, for here every step is laborious.   I have many things that I should like to show Champollion in England, but I fear his means of locomotion are extremely limited, and I have no chance of being able to augment them.   His investigations are too voluminous and too minute to be at all adapted for publication, at least without a certainty of loss to the publisher.   Some few things I hope to get from him for our Plates of Hieroglyphics, and if I succeed, I think I shall go on with them immediately, and not wait for Drovetti's stone, nor for Bankes's publishing his inscriptions, but I doubt whether the papyrus can yet with propriety be made public."

We could produce other letters, written at the same

---

[a] Works, vol. iii. p. 234.

[b] This was the manuscript discovered by Anastasy.   Works, vol. iii. p. 305.

[c] Works, vol. iii. p. 217 and 287.

period to his sisters-in-law Mrs. Chambers and Mrs.
Earle, which express the same generous recognition of
the important investigations and discoveries of Champollion, and the same disinterested desire to assist him
by the free communication of whatever documents or
information he possessed. He had himself received from
Fresnel and his friend Arago, whose researches had
long run parallel to his own, the unreserved acknowledgment of the priority of his discoveries, whenever
he was entitled to claim it, and he naturally expected the same honourable treatment from another
fellow-labourer in a class of researches which he had
hitherto almost appropriated as his own. Before he
quitted Paris, however, he had observed that Champollion, when reading to the Institute a paper referring to these researches, abstained from any open
acknowledgment of his obligations to him ; and he
found upon the appearance of his Letter to M. Dacier,
his own labours on the Rosetta stone merely classed
with those of De Sacy and Akerblad,[a] and the only
notice taken of the principles he had laid down and
applied to the determination of the phonetic elements
of the names of Ptolemy and Berenice, was confined
to a singularly uncandid exposition of the errors
which he had made, more especially in the last of the
two.[b]

The *Lettre à M. Dacier* was received with enthu-

---

[a] Sir William Gell, in writing to Dr. Young, soon after the receipt of
Champollion's letter, says, "The Barberini obelisc has been recently re-
erected on the Pincian, and must acquire a great deal of interest from the
new discoveries of Champollion, who, by the bye, after having taken
almost everything from you, puts you down in his book with de Sacy and
Co., though you are the sole inventor and lawful patentee, and De Sacy
did nothing but contradict, instead of forwarding, the discoveries you
made."—Works, vol. iii. p. 230.
[b] Lettre à M. Dacier, p. 15, note.

siasm in Paris, and its author suddenly emerged from
obscurity, poverty and neglect, into the brightest sun-
shine of public and royal favour. De Sacy, who so
many years before had warned Dr. Young to be
cautious in his communications with him, as a person
disposed to appropriate the discoveries of others as
his own, was one of the first to support the exclusive
pretensions of his countryman.[a] Letronne, a man
of candour and real learning,[b] in a work inscribed
to Dr. Young, Champollion, Hyot and Gau, in which
he refers to Champollion's discoveries, even without
mentioning Young as a claimant, incurred the censure
of the enthusiastic admirers of his countryman, because
his recognition of his merits was not sufficiently ample
and unconditional. Even Arago, the steady friend of
Dr. Young, gave way to the current of national feeling;
and we shall find that in his Éloge of Young, he gave
a statement of the controversy between him and
Champollion, which, though characteristic of his usual
epigrammatic point and clearness, is founded upon the
most imperfect and narrow views of the real facts of
the case.

It was with a view of vindicating his just share in
the vast advances recently made in the literature of
ancient Egypt, and of calling attention to the many
important facts connected with them which, when not
mis-stated, had been studiously suppressed in this
celebrated Letter, that Young published, very early in
the year which followed its appearance, "An Account

---

[a] In the Journal des Savans for March, 1825, quoted in the second
edition of Champollion's Précis du Système Hiéroglyphique, p. 38.

[b] Recherches pour servir à l'Histoire de l'Egypte; p. 30. In a letter addressed to Dr. Young (Works, vol. iii. p. 252), he says, "La liberté que
j'ai mise en parlant de certain *charlatan*, de notre pays, monopoleur de
l'Egypte, ne plaît pas à tout le monde : mais c'est-là ce dont je m'inquiète
peu."

of some Recent Discoveries in Hieroglyphical Literature
and Egyptian Antiquities, with the author's Original
Alphabet as extended by M. Champollion, with a translation of five unpublished Greek and Egyptian Manuscripts."

It was in this work that he first abandoned the
anonymous character which he long assumed in publications alien to his profession, and which he continued to preserve from motives which it is not easy
to explain, when his professional were to a considerable extent superseded by other, engagements, and his
celebrity too great to be concealed by the mere suppression of his name. He had now attained his year
of Jubilee, and felt himself fully authorized to
claim for himself the public credit of those investigations, which, though not signalized by any fortunate
coincidences or unexpected facilities, were rewarded
with a success which was not disproportionate to the
long and persevering labour which had been bestowed
upon them.

One of these coincidences, however, more remarkable than the most extravagant romance would appear
to justify us in considering as possible, supplied an
immediate object for this publication beyond the
mere defence of his own claims. An Italian traveller
of the name of Casati[a] brought to Paris, as has
been already mentioned, several manuscripts which
had been found in Upper Egypt. Amongst them
was one, written exactly in the enchorial character
of the Rosetta Stone, which had furnished Champollion with the enchorial name of Cleopatra, and
thus materially assisted him, according to his own
statement, in the analysis of her hieroglyphical name.

[a] Supra, p. 322.

It was a deed of sale, and on the back of the manuscript was written an endorsement of registry, in pretty legible Greek characters. Champollion had furnished Young with a tracing of the enchorial deed before he left Paris; but he omitted the Greek Registry.

Another Egyptian traveller, Mr. George Francis Grey, had purchased from an Arab at Thebes some manuscripts, which he placed, upon his return to England, in the hands of Dr. Young; and the reader may judge of his astonishment when he found, upon examining them, that one of them, written entirely in Greek, purported to be "a Copy of an Egyptian writing," and showed amongst other signatures the names of Apollonius and Antimachus, which he had observed upon the papyrus of Casati, of which it proved to be the antigraph and translation.[a] He lost

---

[a] This discovery is thus noticed in the following letter to Mr. Gurney: "I was afraid I had lost all my boyish eagerness of character, but it was revived yesterday (22nd November, 1822) by a most singular incident in my antiquarian pursuits. George Francis Grey of Backworth has brought back some papers from Egypt: two of them are of *immense value* —one in Greek—the other in the enchorial characters, with Greek endorsement of registry. But the odd thing in the Greek one is that there are sixteen witnesses, and among them are the names of Apollonius, Antimachus, and Antigenes, just where they stand in Casati's manuscript, the preamble of which I have translated in my letter to Bankes. (See Works, vol. iii. p. 236.) The preamble, however, is omitted in the Greek, so that the evidence of identity rests for the present on the coincidence of the names of the witnesses, which in such a multitude is pretty strong presumption. Indeed the other names appear to agree as far as I have examined them. Thus then we have a full equivalent for the lost fragments of the Rosetta stone, which I had *appraised* as worth their weight in diamonds, and if Drovetti's black stone goes to the bottom of the gulf of Genoa I shall care very little about it. I would now scarcely give ten pounds for it. It is odd enough that I have already obtained a little miniature triumph over Champollion in my amusements at Calais. It seems he read the names Antiochus and Antigenes. Grey's MS. has clearly ΑΝΤΙΜΑΧΟΣ ΑΝΤΙΓΕΝΟΥΣ, as I had made them. The Apollonius is so scribbled that it would have been almost impossible to

no time in communicating this extraordinary coincidence to Champollion, begging him to forward to him a copy of the Greek endorsement of the papyrus of Casati, a request which he thought proper either to evade or refuse. " He perhaps," says he, " thought it best for me to try my strength upon the original without any assistance which might have been derived from it with respect to two or three of the names."[a]   An application to M. Raoul Rochette met with a more liberal reception, and a correct copy of the whole manuscript was immediately forwarded to him.

The contents of Mr. Grey's manuscript were not less remarkable than its preservation and discovery. It related to the sale, not of a house or a field, but of portions of the collections and offerings made from time to time on account of or for the benefit of a certain number of mummies, of persons described at length, in very bad Greek, with their children and all their households. The comparison of the manuscripts served to identify more than thirty enchorial names, affording the most important information with respect to the orthographical system of the Egyptian language and showing a more extensive employment of alphabetical writing, to which the alphabet of Akerblad was very generally applicable, than could possibly have been inferred from the inscription of Rosetta.

have deciphered it without a clue, but it is quite manifest when it is once understood.   The title begins Αντιγραφον Γραφης Αιγυπτιας—among other things, *dead bodies* are conveyed by it."   Dr. Young had amused himself, whilst detained at Calais upon his return from France, in writing a letter to Mr. Bankes, with translations of the preamble of this papyrus : amongst the signatures which he had decyphered we find the names Apollonius, Antimachus, and Antigenes.   This is printed in his Works, vol. iii. p. 236.

[a] Works, vol. iii. p. 302.

In addition to this important Greek antigraph, Mr. Grey's collection contained three other similar deeds, written in the enchorial character of the Rosetta stone, each of them endorsed with a Greek registry, and executed within eight, seven and one, years respectively of the date of the deed of Casati, which was 146 years before Christ. They are severally deeds of sale of portions of land, the boundaries of which are very carefully defined. The long legal preamble, descriptive of the members of the royal family and other public functionaries, is nearly the same in all these documents, but is wanting in the Greek antigraph, which merely states, after the date of the transaction, that it was followed, as was found to be the case in the enchorial original, *by the usual form.*[a] A copy, however, of this preamble had been previously found in the Greek papyrus of Anastasy,[b] relating to a sale of land at the same place, which took place about forty years afterwards, and which served as a key to its accurate reading and interpretation in the enchorial deeds. Whilst one papyrus was headed by "In the reign of Cleopatra and Ptolemy, her son surnamed Alexander, the gods Philometores Soteres;" that of the others was, "In the reign of our sovereign Ptolemy and Cleopatra his sister, the children of Ptolemy and Cleopatra, the divine, the gods illustrious, and the priest of Alexander, and the saviour gods." The exact parallels of this phraseology, and nearly all the names except that of Cleopatra, had

---

The phrase is META TA KOINA, or "according to the common forms."

[b] This manuscript, which came into the possession of M. Anastasy, the Swedish Consul at Alexandria, was very carefully edited by Professor Böckh, of Berlin : its deficiencies have been still further supplied by Dr. Young from the Greek manuscripts of Casati and the antigraph of Mr. Grey.

been found in the enchorial inscription of the Rosetta
stone, where they had supplied Akerblad with the
principal elements of his enchorial alphabet, whilst
the enchorial characters in the name of Ptolemy had
proved of no small assistance to Young in the analysis
of his hieroglyphical ring. The elements also of the
name of Cleopatra, which the manuscripts of Casati
and Anastasy supplied in such close association with
those of Ptolemy and Alexander as hardly to admit
the possibility of their being mistaken, were destined
at a subsequent period, as we have seen, to be of no
less important use to Champollion in the analysis of
the hieroglyphical ring of Cleopatra, which proved the
keystone of his subsequent discoveries.

No proofs had hitherto been afforded of the applicability of the enchorial alphabet of Akerblad, nor of any
imaginary extension which it might have received, to
any names or words which were not foreign to Egypt
and the Egyptian language; and whilst the analyses
of Young and Akerblad were confined to Greek words
and names, those of Champollion were extended to the
principal members of the Ptolemaic dynasty in Egypt
as well as to the Roman emperors who succeeded to
their rule. No example had yet been given of the
application of phonetic hieroglyphics either to an
Egyptian deity or to an Egyptian monarch antecedent
to the Macedonian conquest, or to any other name,
whether of person or of thing.

The results of the comparison and interpretation of
these manuscripts formed a great epoch in the history
of the researches into the system of Egyptian writing.
Akerblad, as we have seen, had begun by assuming the
enchorial inscription of the Rosetta stone to be entirely
alphabetical, and appealed, in confirmation of his opinion,

to the sixteen names to which he had applied his alphabet, with partial at least, if not with complete success.[a] Young, who took up the inquiry, was startled by finding more than two hundred different characters in this inscription, which, in the absence of a knowledge of purely ideographical symbols or homophone signs, seemed to render the selection of an alphabet from such a multitude an impracticable task. The names also, to which the alphabet deduced by Akerblad was applicable, were all Greek; and the Coptic words which he endeavoured to form from it were not such as were consistent with the context as limited by the Greek inscription, which was known to be its translation. If this alphabet was applicable in this instance to Greek names and to those only, might not the exclusive employment of it in the expression of foreign vocables be explained upon the same principle as that adopted by the Chinese under similar circumstances? It was this principle, so pregnant with important results, which was now for the first time proved to be erroneous by the multitude of native names which appeared to be expressed phonetically, whilst the very frequent occurrence of the names of Egyptian deities, as component elements of ordinary Egyptian names, such as Amonrasonther, Ammonius, Arsiesis, Petosiris, Petarpocrates, &c., which were expressed by the peculiar symbols of those deities, and not alphabetically, was apparently sufficient to justify the views of Dr. Young, rather than of Champollion, with respect to the occasional use of hieroglyphical symbols to represent syllables, and even words, as well as simple letters. Such a usage, however, probably originating in the

deep reverence with which this remarkable people
regarded the symbolical and other representations of
their deities, can properly be considered as exceptional
only, and as furnishing another correction of those
premature generalizations, of which the history of
these researches gives so many examples.

It was the opinion of Dr. Young, as we have already
seen, that the enchorial characters were derived from
the hieroglyphics, by a gradual and successive degradation of their forms, though he has nowhere asserted
that the two systems were coextensive with each
other; and Champollion, in his *Lettre à M. Dacier*,
has adopted the same conclusion without any limitation whatever.[a] If it was further asserted, as the most
probable consequence of this hypothesis, that not only
was the phonetic system inherent in those two species
of writing, but that its usage was coextensive in one and

---

[a] " Whatever I have said," says Champollion, " of the origin, the
formation and the anomalies of the phonetic hieroglyphical alphabet,
is applicable almost entirely to the phonetic demotic alphabet. These
two systems of phonetic writing were as intimately connected with
each other as the *ideographic sacerdotal system* was with the *ideographic popular system*, of which it was but the emanation, or with the
pure *hieroglyphic system*, from which it drew its origin. The *demotic*
letters are nothing more, in fact, for the most part, than the *hieratic*
signs of the phonetic hieroglyphics themselves. There exists, then,
no other fundamental difference between the two alphabets—the *hieroglyphical* and the *demotic*—than in the form of the signs only, the
value and the motives of that value being entirely the same. I will add
that these phonetic popular signs being nothing else than the hieratic
signs without alteration, there could not of necessity exist in Egypt more
than two systems of phonetic writing : first, the *phonetic hieroglyphical*
writing, employed upon the great monuments, and secondly, the *hieratico-
demotic* writing, which is that of the Greek proper names of the Rosetta
stone and of the demotic papyrus (of Casati) in the Bibliothèque du Roi ;
and it is not improbable that we shall one day find ourselves employed in
transcribing the name of some Greek or Roman sovereign in such rolls of
papyrus into the hieratic of the funeral rolls."—Lettre à M. Dacier, p. 39,
edition of 1822.

the other : it would follow, therefore, from this discovery
of its extensive application to ordinary Egyptian names
in these enchorial rolls of Casati and Grey, that the principle of phonetization did not originate, as both Young
and Champollion had supposed, in the expression of
foreign vocables. The larger and more extended views,
which were thus opened to hieroglyphical research, were
speedily realized. In a letter to Dr. Young,[a] in the
summer succeeding the publication of these very remarkable discoveries, Champollion refers to a mummy-
case discovered by the well known traveller, Cailliaud,
in which the names of the deceased and of his mother,
expressed in the hieroglyphics of the monuments, are
severally reproduced in Greek characters inscribed by
the side of them. The first, which is translated
ΠΕΤΕΜΕΝΩΝ Ο ΚΑΙ ΑΜΜΩΝΙΟC, is expressed
in hieroglyphics by the group ▦ whose phonetic
values, P, T, M, N, composing the Egyptian name Peta-
men, *belonging to Ammon*, were already well known ;
the second, with the well known hieroglyphical characters of the name of Cleopatra, with the two first
letters ΚΛ . . . . . . of her name in Greek by the
side of it, the remaining portion of the name being
nearly obliterated.[b] In neither case were the hieroglyphics of these names enclosed in a ring. The conclusions
founded upon the examination of this monument were
thus in entire accordance with those afforded by the
enchorial papyri, and at once dissipated or corrected

---

[a] Works, vol. iii. p. 368. See also *Précis du Système Hiéroglyphique*,
p. 411.

[b] See Champollion, *Précis du Système Hiéroglyphique*, p. 412 : also a
very able Dissertation by Letronne, entitled, 'Observations critiques et
archéologiques sur l'objet des représentations zodiacales à l'occasion d'un
zodiaque Egyptien peint dans une caisse de momie qui port une inscription
du temps de Trajan.'

many hypotheses upon which great reliance had been placed. The ring was no longer essential as indicating the phonetic values of the symbols which it enclosed; whilst those phonetic symbols were employed to designate Egyptian as well as foreign names, whether of kings, or gods, or ordinary men. The attention of travellers, archæologists, and scholars was now thoroughly roused to a sense of the importance of those views, and to the character of the means by which they might be extended. The documents which were thus accumulated and brought under the examination of those who were capable of appreciating their value, furnished the means of rapidly extending our knowledge of the lost literature of Egypt.

Before we quit the notice of this work of Dr. Young, it is but an act of justice to him to call attention to his exemplary modesty and forbearance in touching upon the subjects of controversy between himself and Champollion. He confines himself strictly to the facts which are patent upon his various hieroglyphical publications, and to just and legitimate inferences from them, appealing in no instance to the unpublished documents which were only partially embodied in his article Egypt, of which we have felt ourselves fully authorized in making use in the preceding narrative. Champollion is treated throughout with the respect which was undoubtedly due to his eminent talents and discoveries, and though a gentle remonstrance is sometimes addressed to him upon the general omission in his Letter to M. Dacier of all notice of his own labours, it is never accompanied by an insinuation that the suppression originated in any motive that was inconsistent with his honour.

Champollion, in the *Précis du Système Hiérogly-*

phique, which was published in the following year, was
far from responding to the generous forbearance of his
rival. He presents himself to his readers as in exclusive
possession of a province which he had long conquered
for himself, every attack or intrusion upon which, from
whatever quarter it might come, was treated as an
act of presumption or resented as an injury. The
chronology of facts connected with these discoveries
is studiously suppressed, and it is Champollion in
1824, with all the knowledge which had been accu-
mulating since the commencement of these researches,
who is weighed against Young at various and much
earlier stages of their progress. We thus find the
imperfect and in some respects incorrect notions of the
relations of the enchorial system of writing on the
Rosetta stone, to the hieratic commonly used in
the funeral rolls, which Young maintained in his
letter to the Archduke John, in 1816, contrasted
with his own more matured views in 1824; whilst he
passes over without notice Young's special researches
in connection with the papyri of Grey and Casati in
the preceding year, which were probably a principal source of Champollion's own knowledge on the
subject. Whatever principle or discovery had been
previously established or made known, is appropriated
without any acknowledgment, and the dates which
would have proved the unquestionable priority of Dr.
Young are carefully suppressed : but no opportunity
is lost of bringing prominently before the reader
whatever error he may have committed, with a view
of showing not only his own superiority, but his
entire independence and originality.

As a further illustration of this spirit of misrepresentation on the part of Champollion, and we may add

likewise of some of his followers, we trust that we shall be pardoned if we venture, even at the expense of some repetitions, to present to our readers the several propositions which he has put forward, as embodying Dr. Young's views on the relations of the different species of Egyptian writing, which we have more than once had occasion to notice. They are as follows :[a]

1. "The writing of the intermediate text of the Rosetta stone is the *same as that of the papyri* (the funeral rolls), which are not hieroglyphic. *The signs of this enchorial text have been degraded in the hands of the people.* It is on this account that we find in this text *forms which are not found in the papyri.*"

2. "The writing of the intermediate text, and that of the papyri, are *purely ideographic*, like that of the hieroglyphic texts."

3. "Though every character is ideographic in the papyri and the intermediate text of the Rosetta stone, he acknowledges that the greater part of the proper names of the intermediate text are susceptible of a species of reading by the alphabet of Akerblad. He concludes from thence that the Egyptians, for the purpose of transcribing *foreign proper names*, were accustomed, like the Chinese, to make use of signs really ideographic, but diverted from their ordinary expression, so as accidentally, as it were, to make them represent *sounds.*"

4. "He thinks the writing of the papyri is in no respect alphabetical, as has been commonly believed."

5. "He adds that the signs of the papyri are only abbreviations of the hieroglyphical characters, properly so called."

6. "Finally, he gives the name of *hieratic writing*, not to that of the papyri, but to certain hieroglyphical texts which I have called *linear.*"

" I ought to say, that at the same epoch, and without having any knowledge of the opinions of Dr. Young, I had arrived. by a method sufficiently sure, at nearly the same results.[b] But it

[a] Précis du Système Hiéroglyphique, p. 17.

[b] It is impossible to reconcile this assertion with the propositions which he announced in his Grénoble Memoir of 1821. See Mr. Leitch's note, Works, vol. iii. p. 157.

will be seen in the course of this work how much the results which I publish to-day differ from those which I have stated above, and that I have abandoned my first views the moment that indisputable facts showed that they were unfounded."

He then proceeds to comment on the preceding propositions, as if they expressed the final and deliberate conclusions to which the researches of Dr. Young had conducted him, and to contrast them with his own later and more matured views on the relations of the different species of Egyptian writing. "The second and fourth of the preceding propositions," he adds, "are entirely destroyed by the general results of this work."[a] But we have had already occasion to observe,[b] that the propositions in question, though enunciated as fully established by Champollion himself in 1821, were never maintained by Dr. Young, and it was chiefly by the researches of the latter that the erroneous conceptions connected with them had been corrected, and their true character established.[c]

The real purport of his argument was, that so large a proportion of the characters employed in the cursive Egyptian writing were manifest derivations from the hieroglyphics, that the first could not be entirely alphabetical, as Akerblad, and even Champollion in his earlier Egyptian studies, had contended, unless the latter were so also; that the alphabet of Akerblad was applicable generally to the proper names of the Rosetta inscription, which were all Greek, but no farther; that it was probable, therefore, that the Egyptians, like the Chinese, made characters, which were otherwise ideographic, phonetic, for the purpose of express-

---

[a] Précis du Système Hiéroglyphique, p. 19.   [b] Supra, p. 285.
[c] Works, vol. iii. pp. 74 and 129.

ing foreign names. These were the considerations which guided Young in all his subsequent investigations; and though many of the assumptions upon which they were founded were shown in the course of their progress to be erroneous, they are not less remarkable for their sagacity and logical coherence, than for the great results to which they led.

We have elsewhere had occasion to notice the results which followed from the discovery of the papyri of Casati and Grey, which opened out new views of the extent to which the alphabetical element prevailed in enchorial texts. Champollion and Young were engaged simultaneously in the prosecution of the researches connected with these papyri, and had some opportunities, as we have seen, of personal, though not of unreserved, communication with each other; and though the particular circumstances which placed the most important of these documents in the possession of the latter enabled him to take precedence in the publication of the results to which they led, there is no reason to suppose that his great competitor was not equally competent to deduce from them similar conclusions. It is not our object to underrate the merits of the great contributions which were made by Champollion to our knowledge of hieroglyphical literature, but to protest against the persevering injustice with which he treated the labours of Dr. Young; and we feel more especially called upon to do so, in consequence of finding that an author who, like M. Bunsen, occupies so high a station amongst men of letters, should have supported with all the weight of his authority some of the grossest of his misrepresentations.

There are two points, and two points only, in the

discovery and establishment of which Champollion
admits that he was anticipated by Dr. Young. One
was the derivation of the hieratic character of the
funeral rolls from the hieroglyphics of the monuments : the other that the rings or cartouches contained the names of persons, like that of Ptolemy
on the Rosetta stone. But in order to reduce as
much as possible the value of the concession which
he thus reluctantly makes, he refers the original
discovery of the first to Professor Tychsen of Göttingen, and of the second to Zoëga[a]—confounding, in both
cases, a vague and unsupported conjecture with a
complete demonstration.

We have elsewhere discussed at such length the
third of the six propositions which Champollion puts
forward as representing the views of Dr. Young—
though it opens with ascribing to him opinions which
we know that he never maintained—that we feel it
to be hardly necessary to refer to it again. With singular injustice, it has sometimes been attempted to
estimate the relative claims of these great rivals by
the numerical results of the phonetic elements which
they respectively determined : forgetting who it was
that first proposed the principle employed in deducing
them, and who it was that first applied it : forgetting
also that the only important limitations which Champollion imposed upon the extent of the principle, involved in these determinations, was not antecedent to,
but consequent upon, its application ; and also that a
single successful exemplification of its use was really
a sufficient guide in other cases, wherever well-known

---

[a] See Works, vol. iii. p. 450.　M. Bunsen more correctly ascribes this
conjecture to Barthelemy, though Zoëga, the most eminent Egyptologist of
his day, approved of it as probable. Egypt's Place, &c., vol. i. p. 313.

hieroglyphical rings or names were at hand to which it could be applied.

" Of the nine letters, which I insist that I had discovered," says Young in a letter to M. Arago,[a] " M. Champollion himself allows me five, and I maintain that a single one would have been sufficient for all that I wished to prove ; the method by which that one was obtained being allowed to be correct and to be capable of further application. The true foundation of the analysis of the Egyptian system of writing, I insist, is the great fact of the original identity of the enchorial with the sacred characters which I discovered and printed in 1816. . . . Whatever deficiencies there might have been in my original alphabet, supposing it to have contained but one letter correctly determined, they would and they must have been gradually supplied by a continued application of the same method to other monuments which have been progressively discovered and made public since the date of my first paper."

The letters which passed between Dr. Young and several of his friends, more especially Sir William Gell, will show that, after the publication of the work which has given occasion to these criticisms, he to a great extent abandoned the more popular and attractive departments of Hieroglyphical literature to Champollion, resuming however, from time to time, his study of the enchorial manuscripts. The vindication of his claims became, however, somewhat of a national question upon the appearance of an article on the subject of them in the Edinburgh Review for December, 1826, written with considerable spirit and ability—but not without several errors—by Dr. James Browne, a young advocate of Edinburgh. These inaccuracies were pointed out in a letter, gratefully acknowledging the general correctness of the statements

---

[a] Works, vol. iii. p. 464.

which it contains, which Dr. Young addressed to the author, who attributed in his reply the most considerable of them to Mr. Jeffrey, the well-known editor, who introduced several alterations, without possessing a sufficient knowledge of the subject to enable him to do so with safety. A subsequent article, by the same writer, corrected some of these mistakes, but others were allowed to remain, out of deference to an authority which it was not safe or prudent to dispute.

In 1827 he printed, in Brande's Philosophical Journal, a letter addressed to the Cavaliere San Quintino, of Turin, containing some valuable criticisms on several plates published under his superintendence by the Hieroglyphical Society, together with some additional remarks in vindication of his own claims to discoveries which the friends and countrymen of Champollion persevered in attributing exclusively to him.[a] These remarks gave some offence at Paris, where the hieroglyphical labours of Dr. Young were little known, except through the partial representations of them which were given in the publications of his rival.

Whilst asserting, however, his own rights in very decided terms, he failed not in this, as on every other occasion, to do full justice to the admirable sagacity, the deep and extensive research, of Champollion, at the same time that he ventured to insinuate that his conclusions were, in some instances, in advance of the documents upon which they were founded, and that it would be premature to accept them as established without further and more conclusive evidence.

In the summer of 1828, he visited Paris for the last time, on his way to Geneva. He was now one of the

[a] Works, vol. iii. p. 444.

eight foreign Associates of the Académie des Sciences, and he took his seat for the first time in that illustrious assembly. He was everywhere received with extraordinary honours—

"I am only afraid;" says he in writing to Mr. Gurney, "that I shall be too fond of Paris and its inhabitants, in preference to my own cold-hearted countrymen, and that, instead of making this my last visit to the continent, as I supposed it would be, I shall be tempted to make a biennial or quadriennial visit, like old Sir Benjamin Truman, whose history you used to tell me; but I suppose this impression will wear off again."

This cordial reception would appear to have warmed his heart, even towards Champollion, of whose conduct he had so much reason to complain, and a reconciliation was effected between them, which on his part at least was obviously sincere.

"My principal object was Champollion, and with him I have been completely successful, as far as I wanted his *assistance:* for, to say the truth, our conferences have not been very gratifying to my *vanity:* he has done so much more, and so much better than I had any reason to believe he would or could have done; and as he feels his own importance more, he feels less occasion to be tenacious of any trifling claims which may justly be denied him; and in this spirit he has borne my criticisms with perfect good humour, though Arago has charged me with some degree of undue severity and wanted to pass the matter over as not having been published as mine; but to this I could not consent, and supposing that Champollion might have been unacquainted with the remarks, I thought it a matter of conscience to carry them to him this morning before I allowed him to continue his profuse liberality in furnishing me with more than I want: but he still continues his good offices. He devoted seven whole hours at once to looking over with me his papers and the magnificent collection which is committed to his care, and which beats every other museum in the world beyond all comparison, though it has cost only 20,000*l.* I doubt not he felt a pleasure in the display, but he must be so much accustomed, to admiration and to more than I gave him, that I am certainly not the less obliged to him on this score. He is going to Egypt in a few weeks at the king's expense, with a party of a dozen artists and savans. He is to let me, in the mean time, have the use of all his collections and his notes relating to the enchorial character, that I may make what use 1 please of them : and he is to employ a cheap artist to copy at my expense all the manuscripts on papyrus that I want, and to give me permission to publish any or all of them If you see Col. Leake, pray tell him that the council of the R.S.L. must' not retard my proceedings from their economy, for that their honours will be pledged to the production of what is really of importance."

This promise, however, of renewed activity in a class of investigations which he had for several years to a great extent abandoned, was destined to be disappointed. The malady which proved fatal in the following year manifested itself in a gradual decay of strength before he reached Geneva, and he shortly afterwards returned to England, not altogether a confirmed invalid, but with many indications of his speedily becoming so. His last hieroglyphical work was the correction of the sheets of his Enchorial Dictionary appended to Archdeacon Tattam's Grammar, the advertisement of which he wrote on his death-bed : it gives, however, melancholy proofs of his diminished powers in the partial forgetfulness of some of his own discoveries.

Before he left Paris, he had promised to furnish Arago with a statement of the precise dates of the several steps which he had made in his hieroglyphical investigations. There was no person who had so good a right to make this demand; for he had been the first to recognise the importance of his optical researches, and had on every occasion maintained his credit with the most generous friendship. The reply to this request was forwarded to Arago from Geneva,[a] and contains a singularly clear and dispassionate statement of the principal, though by no means the most important, points in the controversy upon which the attention of the public had then been fixed for several years : and whilst it vindicates his own claims with equal moderation and good sense, does more than justice to the merits of Champollion. This statement, however, would not appear to have satisfied the mind of his correspondent, or to have proved sufficient to counterbalance the national feeling with which the question was generally regarded. In the Eloge which he was required to pronounce, a few years later, upon Dr. Young, as Sécretaire Perpétuel de l'Académie, the decision is given against him upon grounds which are singularly narrow and unsatisfactory. It is contended that his principle of phonetization contained a mixture of truth and error ; that it was essentially distinguished from that of Champollion in attributing to the hieroglyphical symbols the power of vocalising syllables, and even words, as well as letters ; that he left it in a state in which it was not applicable to other names, or capable of determining the correctness of a phonetic analysis when made, referring to his mistake of the ring of Cæsar (Autocrator) for that of Arsinoe : he even denies his knowledge of the existence of homophone signs. The answers to these criticisms have been given before, and it is not necessary to repeat them ; but they originated in a neglect of the chronology of a series of progressive researches, where the final structure is alone regarded in its complete and finished state, the foundations upon which it rests being entirely overlooked.

---

[a] Works, vol. iii. p. 464.

It was not the only instance in which the passion of this powerful and eloquent writer for signalising what he considered the great epochs in discoveries in various departments of science has led him to erroneous and unjust decisions, when their progress has been more indebted to continuous and patient labour, guided by just principles of reasoning and philosophy, than to any sudden outbreak of genius which has superseded the rules which ordinary men must be compelled to submit to.

Before I conclude this chapter on the lost literature of Egypt, I wish to express my obligations to the valuable labours of my friend, Mr. Leitch, not merely in editing the last volume of Dr. Young's works, in which his hieroglyphical writings and correspondence are contained, but likewise for the able and learned notes with which they are accompanied. Though I have been greatly assisted by the perusal of these notes in putting together the preceding statements, I have pursued as much as possible an independent course, by referring to the unpublished documents in my possession, which were not sufficiently known to Mr. Leitch, nor even to myself until I was required to study them in connection with the publications which had been founded upon them. It was only after this perusal that I became fully aware how very imperfectly the published writings of Dr. Young represented either the extent or the character of his researches—or the real progress he had made in the discovery of phonetic hieroglyphics, many years before Champollion had made his appearance in the field.

CHAPTER XI.

COMMISSIONS. BOARD OF LONGITUDE.

ABOUT the year 1810, Mr. Seppings, a master ship-wright in Chatham Dockyard, proposed several improvements in marine architecture, which excited very great attention.

The principal timbers and plankings of our ships were formerly disposed at right angles with each other. Thus the ribs were at right angles to the keel or back-bone; the planks, both within and without, at right angles to the ribs; the beams which supported the decks at right angles to the outer framework; the carlings at right angles to the beams; the ledges at right angles to the carlings; and the planks of the floors at right angles·to the beams, or parallel to the sides. By this arrangement of the timbers, the bolts which secured them to each other were generally found at the angles of a parallelogram, a figure which could collapse, or tend to collapse, without bringing into operation the strength of its sides either to resist their compression or extension; but if diagonal beams are introduced and bolted into the sides at the opposite angles, the system becomes thenceforward firm and immoveable.

It was with a view of giving greater stiffness and strength to the whole framework of the ship, that Mr. Seppings introduced a series of triangular braces between the ribs, and replaced the diagonals in every

parallelogram wherever it was found. The inner planking of the sides he entirely removed, filling up the space
between the inner and outer skins of the vessel—which
had formerly been a nursery for the most offensive
vermin and a receptacle for impurities—by short timbers closely wedged together, so as to form a compact
and continuous mass of great strength and durability,
such as was water-tight even if the external planking
had been removed. The decks also were made to
contribute to the same object by diagonal planking;
other arrangements were everywhere made upon the
same principle; and all the beams of the ship were so disposed and so firmly held together by bolts and braces,
that even the most trivial displacement could not take
place without bringing into action the most powerful
antagonistic forces to resist it.

The effect of these improvements was to reduce,
almost from feet to inches, that arching of a ship, when
first launched, which is produced by the sinking of
the vast masses fore and aft, under the operation
of those violent pressures, some of them acting at an
enormous leverage, to which no adequate resistance had
hitherto been opposed, and which were sometimes found
to be so considerable, that when the back of the ship
was not actually broken, she not unusually became a
cripple for the short remainder of her existence. At a
subsequent period, Mr. Seppings further proposed the
substitution of round for flat sterns, by which, in our
larger men of war, he not only gained a vast increase
of strength in the framework of the ship, but provided
an armament at a most important point, where she
had hitherto been the most vulnerable.

These improvements, obvious as many of them were,
were not liked by many of the officials and master

shipwrights of our dockyards, with whose habits and perquisites they interfered;[a] whilst many of the old captains and admirals, whose magnificent stern drawing-rooms were thus invaded by 32-pounders, were furious in their opposition. So violent, in fact, was the resistance made to their introduction, that the Admiralty felt it necessary to consult men of science on the expediency of the changes which were proposed, and Mr. Barrow, afterwards Sir John Barrow, one of the Secretaries of the Admiralty, was directed to request Dr. Young, amongst others, to report upon them.[b] He was at first disposed to decline the commission, as at variance with the resolution he had adopted of appearing ostensibly before the public in no investigation which was not connected with his professional studies; but he was finally induced, from a sense of public duty, to undertake the investigation. The subject of carpentry, and the mechanical principles which determine the strength or weakness of combinations of timbers, had been considered in his lectures in connection with much larger and more philosophical views than in any other work which had appeared in this country, some articles by Professor Robison in the Encyclopædia Britannica alone excepted.[c]

[a] In a letter addressed to Dr. Young in the course of these enquiries, Mr. Seppings says, "I have no wish to excite in yours or any one's breast the sense of pity for the situation in which I have been placed, in consequence of the principle I have recommended. Though my task has been, and is, very arduous, I may say that I have been excommunicated by those in my own profession : indeed, they have passed judgment without making themselves masters of the principle. All this I can forgive, as it accords with the old adage, 'Two of a trade can never agree;' but I should want the spirit of a man were I to pass over the conduct of a certain person who has followed me step by step, that would hardly have been commendable had I been guilty of a crime." The person alluded to was high in office, and used all his influence to thwart the adoption of these improvements.

[b] See the latter's Works, vol. i. p. 535.   [c] Works, vol. i. p. 535.

The substance of the Report which he addressed to
the Admiralty on this subject was embodied in a Memoir read to the Royal Society on the 24th March,
1814, and which is published in their Transactions for
that year. It contains a most searching inquiry into
the whole subject, analysing the causes which produce
the arching of ships, estimating the various pressures,
whether longitudinal, lateral, or vertical, to which they
are subject, the mechanical effects of those pressures,
and the best disposition of the timbers to resist them,
with a special discussion of the efficiency of the arrangements which Mr. Seppings had proposed for this purpose. The general conclusion of his investigations
was greatly in their favour, though he was enabled by
his more profound knowledge of mechanical principles
to point out some defects, and many contingencies to
which a ship might be exposed which they were not
competent to meet. Dr. Young was not easily seduced
into enthusiasm, and though his approbation of the
main points of the new system was very decisive, it
was upon the whole too cold and limited by too many
conditions, to satisfy the wishes of the more ardent of
its admirers.

The leader of the malcontents was Sir John Barrow,
who had noticed these improvements in several articles
in the Quarterly Review, in terms of the most emphatic
approbation. He was an extremely vigorous and popular
writer, and though his scientific knowledge was very
limited, he possessed a remarkable capacity for making
difficult subjects plain, and had succeeded not merely
in making the new system familiar to the public, but
in raising greater expectations of its efficiency than experience was likely altogether to justify. As might
have been anticipated, he was equally dissatisfied with

the amount of approbation which Dr. Young bestowed upon it, and with what he considered the needless obscurity in which his opinions were expressed :—

"We have perused Dr. Young's remarks," says he, "with care, and we may add with pain; for if we understand them rightly, which we are by no means sure that we always do, the tendency is, if not to deprive the author of the merit of the invention, at least to diminish the value of it. He cannot, we think, disapprove of the principle; yet so many conditionals, hypotheticals, and potentials are employed, that if approbation be meant, either of the principle or its application, it is at any rate 'damn'd with faint praise.' Dr. Young will not infer from this that we undervalue science, or that we do not cordially agree with him that no assistance which can be afforded by the abstract sciences should be withheld from the service of the public. Far be it from us to think otherwise ; our regret arises from seeing ' abstract science ' misapplied, in raising doubts on points of practice which common sense and experience are best able to determine, and which no calculus can reach."[a]

The Lords of the Admiralty would appear to have been still more embarrassed than their Secretary by the scientific character of this Report. "Though science," writes an innocent official, and a violent opponent of these changes, "is much respected by their Lordships, and your paper is much esteemed by them, it is too learned."

Whilst it may readily be admitted that abstract science is useless if not combined with good sense and experience, yet the converse of this proposition is at least as correct, if not more so ; it may in fact be affirmed that no great public works can be safely entrusted to practical men, however great their ability, if they are deficient in a sound knowledge of mechanical principles and their application. Our naval administration for the last half-century has dearly paid the penalty of its neglect or indifference to the scientific attainments of its advisers.   At one time, we find them getting rid of the Board of Longitude as an inconvenient incumbrance upon their independence; at another, they sacrifice the Naval College, in which a body of master shipwrights was in a successful course of scientific training, almost simultaneously with the act which entrusted the construction of our ships of war to a man who was notoriously wanting in scientific qualifications.   The appointments also of the engineers of the same body had been too commonly much more determined by considerations of party patronage than of merit; and the public service, which should have commanded the talents of men the most distinguished for scientific and practical knowledge, has sometimes presented a picture of inefficiency which no lover of his country could contemplate without pain.

In the year 1816, Dr. Young was appointed secretary to a Commission for ascertaining the length of the seconds pendulum, for comparing the French and English standards with each other, and for considering whether it would be practicable and advisable to establish throughout the empire a more uniform system of weights and measures.   The three reports, with their appendices, which this Commission made in 1819, 1820, and 1821, were drawn up by Dr. Young, who subsequently embodied a detailed account of their proceedings in an article in the Supplement of the Encyclopædia Britannica.[a]

The operations for ascertaining the length of the seconds pendulum were entrusted to Captain Kater, an engineer officer of great ingenuity and mechanical skill,

---

[a] Works, vol. ii. p. 427.

whose happy use of the principle of the commutability of the centres of suspension and oscillation was considered a most important step towards the accurate practical solution of this problem. All the known resources of art and science were brought to bear upon this measurement; and apart from theoretical corrections which later researches have shown to be imperfect or erroneous, it is not probable that the accuracy of the determination which it afforded will ever be surpassed. It assigned a length of the seconds pendulum, in terms of the parliamentary standard yard, of 39.13860 inches, the pendulum being supposed to be swung *in vacuo*·at the level of the sea in the latitude of London, the temperature of its mass and of the air being supposed to be 62° of Fahrenheit. It was shown by Dr. Young, in a subsequent Memoir in the Philosophical Transactions, that the correction applied for the reduction to the level of the sea was too great by at least one third, and the length which was ultimately adopted when cleared of this error was 39.13929 inches. The most eminent men of science of the day, including Dr. Wollaston, a member of the Commission, a man eminently cautious and dispassionate in forming his conclusions, expressed their entire confidence in the correctness of this last result.

So general, in fact, was this conviction, that the Imperial Legislature attempted to invest it with an absolutely immutable character. In an Act introduced in 1824 by Sir George Clerk, one of the members of the Commission, it was declared that the length of the seconds pendulum—under the conditions above mentioned—bore to the length of the imperial standard yard not only the proportion of the numbers 39.1393 and 36 to each other, but that if ever the latter should be lost or destroyed, *it shall be restored to the same length* by making it bear to the length of the seconds pendulum the precise proportion of those numbers. The course of events was destined very speedily to bring the authority of this enactment to a trial. In 1835, the standards of length, weight, and capacity were destroyed in the burning of the Houses of Parliament; and, in 1837, a new Commission was appointed to restore them. But the progress of scientific inquiry, in the interval which had elapsed between the first and second Commission, had shown that nearly all the theoretical corrections which Captain Kater had applied to the reduction of his observations were imperfect or erroneous. Bessel had shown that the formula used for the reduction to a vacuum was very defective; and Colonel Sabine had established the same fact by very decisive experiments; Dr. Young had not only shown, as we have seen, that the reduction to the level of the sea was erroneous, but also that it might be materially affected by local circumstances,[a] and Colonel Sabine had given reason for thinking that such circumstances, whether geological or otherwise, were not obscurely indicated in the neighbourhood where the pendulum was swung; and Mr. Baily, who repeated and varied all the observations with his usual perseverance and skill, discovered other anomalies and possible sources of error, which threw additional doubts upon the perfect accuracy of this and similar determinations. Without attempting to assign the precise amount of the error, it was morally certain that Captain Kater's value was too great. The lost standards of length and weight have since been restored by Mr. Sheepshanks and Professor Miller, under the authority of a Commission, which has recently made

a Works, vol. ii. p. 99.

its report,—not by following the directions of the Act, but by a very careful comparison of the best copies of those standards which were known to be in existence. The pride of philosophy was destined to encounter a similar rebuke, in the attempt made in France to found, upon imperishable bases, the determination of the length of the metre, as one ten-millionth part of a quadrant of the earth's meridian. An arc, of nearly one-seventh part of the length of this meridian, between the parallels of Dunkirk and Iviça, one of the Balearic Islands, was measured, with every precaution which the most advanced resources of art and science could supply, to obtain a result from which every appreciable source of error was eliminated. This was extended both ways, by the aid of well known formulæ, to the pole and the equator : and upon this determination the length of the metre was assigned. A subsequent revision of the calculations made manifest an unquestionable mistake of at least 34 toises, and many others would in all probability be discovered if the operation were repeated. The standard metre, therefore, the authority of which continues to be recognised, is no longer an integral part of the earth's meridian, as it was once proudly assumed to be ; and it cannot be restored to that character without disturbing the integrity of the whole existing metrical system of France.

The Commissioners of 1816, in their Report, deprecated any great or violent changes in the standards of weights and measures already in use, as well on account of the great derangement which such alterations would produce in the ordinary transactions of commerce and trade, as from the conviction that no peculiar advantage would accrue from having such standards commensurable with any invariable quantity existing in

nature. The only alteration they proposed—which
was in our measures of capacity—was hardly consistent
with this very wise recommendation. The gallons,
and their multiples and submultiples, which were then
in use for the measurement of corn, ale, and wine,
were all of them different from each other; and little
doubt could be felt with respect to the expediency of
reducing them all to the same capacity. Instead, however, of retaining the corn gallon as the common basis
of such measures, the change of which would produce
by far the greatest derangement in existing contracts
and arrangements, they proposed an *imperial* gallon,
different from them all, upon the trivial ground of its
holding, when filled, a quantity of distilled water,
weighing exactly 10lbs. avoirdupois, at the temperature
of 62° of Fahrenheit. With a view of giving a practical value to this philosophical fact, the same imperial
gallon was made the basis of a clause of the Act which
embodied this Report, providing—when the correctness
of such a measure is disputed and a recognised standard
is not at hand—a reference to a magistrate, who is required to verify it by weighing its contents in rain water
at the temperature of 62° Fahrenheit, against the statutable weights. It would be a curious inquiry to ascertain, if such an experiment ever has been or ever
should be tried, what would be the degree of confidence
to which such a determination would be entitled—
whether, in fact, there are any measures, however accurate, which would stand the test of such an inquiry
when conducted in the presence, or by the agency, of
such a tribunal.

The same Commissioners not only declined to
recommend the decimalisation of our coinage and of
the primary units of weights and measures, but ex-

pressed their preference of the duodecimal and other scales which are prevalent amongst those in use, as admitting of much greater subdivision or more frequent bisection. Their successors in 1837 came to an opposite conclusion, which public opinion has already sufficiently confirmed, and which cannot fail before long to receive the sanction of the Legislature. Circumstances, however, were not then wanting which appeared to justify recommendations of so contradictory a character : at the one period an impression prevailed that the decimal system had failed to become popular in France, where a foolish reactionary decree of the Bourbons had forbidden the use of it in all the minor transactions of trade ; at the other, the metrical system in its integrity was known to be in full operation both in France and in Belgium. At the one period, all departures from ancient practices were looked upon with suspicion ; at the other, they were welcomed as conformable to the spirit of the age. The very same influences which would then have opposed the general acceptance of such a change, would now be employed to recommend it.

In the year 1814, Dr. Young became a member of a Committee of the Royal Society, appointed at the request of the Secretary of State for the Home Department, to investigate the degree of danger which might result from the general introduction of gas into the metropolis, and more especially from the erection of large gasometers in crowded neighbourhoods. A recent explosion of a gas-seasoning house, at Woolwich, had produced general alarm, and it had not yet been sufficiently ascertained under what circumstances coal-gas was capable of explosion, or through what length of tubing, if any, its flame would run back into the reservoir. The chemical part of this inquiry was chiefly conducted by Mr. Tennant and Dr. Wollaston ; and the results at which they arrived were not only satisfactory, as tending to remove all apprehensions of danger—supposing reasonable precautions to be taken —but also as clearly showing that the flame of gas in a small tube is not transmissible ; a most important fact, which became, in the hands of Sir Humphry Davy (who was abroad at the time, and took no part in the proceedings of this Committee), the origin of the safety-lamp : and it may be truly said that science has rarely made a more valuable gift to the cause of humanity.

Dr. Young communicated to this Committee an investigation of the probable force of the explosion of coal gas, founded upon the same principles which are involved in the usual estimate of the explosive force of gunpowder. It was a problem of a very high order of difficulty, the elements of whose solution were of a very hypothetical and uncertain character. The conclusion at which he arrived was, that the explosive force of coal gas—with the requisite admixture of atmospheric air—was somewhat less than one-thousandth part of the same mass of gunpowder. Such questions were then full of interest, though they have ceased to be so now. Some of the dangers which were most seriously apprehended have been shown to be unreal, and the precautions are now well understood which are necessary to protect us from others ; thus affording an additional proof that the most powerful and apparently dangerous of natural agents may be made of benefit to mankind, if we diligently strive to study and master the conditions which a wise and bountiful Providence has attached to the use of them.

In November, 1818, Dr. Young was appointed

superintendent of the Nautical Almanac; and Secretary of the Board of Longitude, under the provisions of an Act of Parliament, by which its constitution had been recently remodelled. The Admiralty warrant, by which he was appointed, assigned him a stipend of three hundred pounds per annum in the first of these capacities, and of one hundred in the second ; an amount of remuneration hardly adequate for the discharge of such laborious and responsible duties, but which he considered sufficient to justify his appearing henceforward before the public in his proper character of a man of science, without regarding the possible loss of professional income which might result from his doing so.

His selection for this office would appear to have been due to the very general confidence reposed in his industry and capacity. He had written no special memoirs on astronomy, and had taken no part in the questions of the day which related to the promotion of that science ; but the results which followed from his appointment showed that the opinion entertained of the universality and soundness of his attainments was not misplaced, and we shall find him discharging the new duties which devolved upon him, including a very extensive astronomical correspondence, with a mastery of the subject as complete and technical, as if the study of the science had formed the chief business of his life.

The Nautical Almanac had been projected by Dr. Maskelyne in 1765 : though limited in its objects, as its name indicated, to the promotion of the interests of navigation, and not intended as an Astronomical Ephemeris, it had attained an unequalled reputation for accuracy—the places for the sun and moon, and the principal fixed stars, as well as other fundamental ele-

ments of astronomy, which were given in it, being
founded upon the system of observations which Brad-
ley, the most illustrious of practical astronomers,
had first introduced, and which Maskelyne himself,
though not his immediate successor, had continued
and perfected with equal perseverance and skill
for nearly half a century. His own successor at the
Observatory, Mr. Pond, succeeded also to the charge
of the Almanac. He was an observer of remarkable
tact and delicacy, with a very clear understanding,
which enabled him to reason correctly upon the general
instrumental results of his observations; but his mathematical knowledge was very limited, and he was not
equal to that larger and more philosophical discussion
of his observations which was requisite to give them
their complete astronomical interpretation.[a] His feeble
health and gentle disposition disqualified him also for
the task of sufficiently controlling the subordinate
parties employed in the preparation of the Nautical
Almanac, and the consequence was, that errors were
allowed to creep into it, which seriously compromised
the character of a publication which had hitherto been
deemed to be altogether unimpeachable.

It was chiefly with a view of relieving the Astronomer Royal from the responsibility of this charge—
which under ordinary circumstances would appear to
be a natural incident of his office—that a new Board of
Longitude was formed, including some new, but un-

---

[a] Schumacher, in his correspondence with Dr. Young, makes frequent
references to Mr. Pond's want of sufficient theoretical and technical knowledge to enable him to treat his observations properly : such also would
appear to have been the opinion of Bessel and the other astronomers of
Germany. Mr. Sheepshanks, however, a most competent judge, and other
English astronomers, have been accustomed to speak of him with great
respect as not merely a skilful, but an eminently philosophical observer.

paid members, in addition to those who formerly composed it. When Dr. Young succeeded to the office of superintendent, under the general direction of this Board, he lost no time in making every practicable arrangement to prevent the recurrence of errors in the Almanac, which might not only be the means of endangering the safety of our ships, but which had already lessened the implicit faith which had so long been reposed in it. In all other respects, however, he continued to adhere strictly to the system which had been followed by his predecessors, considering it as designed for nautical rather than for astronomical purposes.

It is not easy, however, to define the precise limits which separate the wants of the navigator from those of the traveller and astronomer. A scientific and well educated captain may be placed under circumstances which will require him to act in all these capacities, when he visits unknown regions ; and observations, which are impracticable at sea, made at the various points at which he touches, may not only furnish important geographical determinations, but, by enabling him to ascertain or test the rates of chronometers, may increase materially the correctness and efficiency of those which are required for the security of his ship. It was not, therefore, without some show of reason, when the Nautical Almanac made its appearance under new auspices, that some discontent should have been expressed at the somewhat limited character of the information which it continued to supply. Astronomy also had begun to be much more generally cultivated. Several private and some public Observatories had been recently established at home : whilst those on the continent at Berlin, at Konigsberg, at Altona,

Milan, and elsewhere, were placed under the care of men
equally distinguished for their theoretical and practical knowledge, who were daily enriching astronomy
by new researches, as well as by the publication of
astronomical Ephemerides which put to shame our
own contributions to the science.

Mr. F. Baily was one of the first to call public
attention to a fact so humiliating to our national
pride. In early life he had made himself known by
publishing an admirable treatise on Life Annuities,
which still continues to be regarded as of classical
authority ; and he had recently abandoned pursuits in
which he had realised a large fortune, for the cultivation of astronomy in which he was destined to earn a
reputation for learned research and practical industry
which was second to that of few of his contemporaries.

In a preface and introduction to a collection of very
useful Astronomical Tales, published in 1822, he complains that it was not easy to refer to a single table of
English origin which was used in the computations of
the National Almanac, and he contrasts the meagre-
ness of the contents of that publication with the much
more ample information furnished by the foreign
Ephemerides. As a proof also of the inert acquiescence
of its editors in continuing to retain without inquiry
whatever had been once introduced into it, however
antiquated and useless, he refers to a note upon the
telescopes which are proper to be used in observing the
eclipses of the satellites of Jupiter, as being, among
others, "common refracting telescopes of from fifteen
to twenty feet," though such instruments had been
superseded by achromatic telescopes for more than fifty
years. He omitted to notice, however, as in candour
he was bound to have done, that Dr. Young expressly

referred the note to its author Dr. Maskelyne, who had
introduced it when such telescopes were common, and
that it was retained rather as an historical fact than
as a direction for the instruction of seamen.

To these observations of Mr. Baily, which were very
temperately urged, a short and somewhat ungracious
reply was inserted by Dr. Young in the Journal of the
Royal Institution, in which they were characterized as
"superfluous and frivolous." Mr. Baily, who was in
general sufficiently cautious in forming his opinions,
but very resolute and sometimes stern in defending
them—when he believed them to be well founded—
was prompt in his rejoinder. A movement party for
the reform of the National Ephemeris was gradually
formed amongst English astronomers and astronomical
amateurs of which Mr. Baily was the acknowledged
leader, and which gained strength from day to day : and
though the most distinguished of their number were
somewhat repelled by the unguarded vehemence of
some of those who took part in it, so powerful was the
combination that no reasonable doubt could be entertained with respect to what would be the final issue of
the contest.

Though Dr. Young continued steadily to resist all
changes in the form of the Nautical Almanac, he was
prepared to make some concessions to the demands
addressed to him by those whose opinions he respected,
and who at the same time paid a reasonable deference
to his own. Several tables, more especially those of
the moon's distance from the principal planets, the
want of which in the Nautical Almanac had been
complained of and not unreasonably, were already included in the Danish Ephemeris, and arrangements
were made by Dr. Young with the editor, Schumacher

of Altona, an astronomer of great modesty, industry, and learning, for a very early communication of a large number of copies of these tables, which were made saleable by the Admiralty bookseller at very moderate prices.[a]   On the recommendation also of Sir John Herschel,—who was a member of the Board of Longitude,—a supplement to the Nautical Almanac was published at a later period, containing other tables of great use to working astronomers in the reduction of their observations, more especially as auxiliary to the new arrangement of the formulæ of reduction which Bessel of Konigsberg had recently introduced in the Preface to his Tabulæ Regiomontanæ, and which has proved of such eminent service to Astronomy.[b] Professor Airy, who had recently succeeded to the charge of the Cambridge Observatory, and who had already given examples of that rare combination of practical and theoretical knowledge with habits of systematic order and arrangement, for which he is now so justly celebrated, had joined in some representations upon the expediency of uniting in one book all the information which astronomers as well as navigators were likely to require.

"If every practical astronomer," says Young in reply to him, "were like you, I should think it right for the Admiralty to consider the importance of saving your time almost as much as that of nautical men.   But when I see people who possess nothing of science but a few fine instruments and a good deal of leisure, affecting to call themselves astronomers and to dictate

[a] Only fifty copies of these tables were thus disposed of, whilst the sale of the Nautical Almanac exceeded 7000. Dr. Young appealed to this fact as confirmatory of his argument, that the Nautical Almanac contained all the information which practical seamen required.

[b] The principle of this distribution of the elements of correction had occurred also to Mr. Baily, who ceased to pursue the investigation when he found that he had been anticipated by Bessel.

to the public what ought to be done for the promotion of astronomical science, I do certainly feel a disposition to rebel against their authority;" and again, "with respect to the N. A., I hope I so expressed myself as professing a readiness to be convinced by you and not to adopt your opinions without having vanquished my own doubts. I am most anxious for your assistance in recommending whatever you think right, and I trust you will not condemn me, if I am not always persuaded."

A general cause of complaint against Dr. Young's administration of his office was founded upon his reserving his lists of occultations and various astronomical investigations for publication, under the title of Nautical Collections, in the Journal of the Royal Institution, which was edited by Mr. Brande, instead of including them in a supplement or appendix to the Nautical Almanac, such as was always appended to the Connaissance des Tems. "When I see," says Dr. Brinkley in a letter to him, "the valuable articles contained in the Journal, I cannot but think they would be better placed in a supplement to the Nautical Almanac. I doubt not but the reasons are good for not adding such a supplement, but I am ignorant of them. I really believe that the supplement to the Connaissance des Tems has done more service to astronomy than any other publication whatever." All persons engaged in the cultivation of particular branches of science will be ready to acknowledge the great importance of concentrating, as much as possible, in a cheap and easily accessible publication, the current information relating to it : it is this character which has caused the Astronomische Nachrichten, which Schumacher instituted and conducted for so many years with so much regularity and ability, to exercise the most important influence upon the progress of astronomy.

In the year 1828, the Board of Longitude, which had

been reconstituted ten years before, and which for nearly three quarters of a century had formed the only ostensible link which connected the cultivation of science with the Government of this country, was dissolved. The third reading of the Act of Parliament for that purpose, took place, upon the motion of Mr. Croker, in a house of five members only, one of whom, Mr. Davies Gilbert, was President of the Royal Society and an official member of the Board at whose obsequies he assisted, but who had not the courage, whilst pronouncing its eulogy, to resist an act of barbarism which was neither called for by any just considerations of expediency nor of rational economy. The Admiralty was authorized to assume the functions which had hitherto been discharged by the Board—and Dr. Young, as superintendent of the Nautical Almanac, assisted by Mr. Faraday as a chemist, and Colonel Sabine as a practical observer, were appointed as its advisers, whenever their assistance was required, upon questions which concerned the scientific interests of navigation and astronomy.

Such an act was not likely to check the agitation which prevailed amongst astronomers, as, independently of other and more serious objections, it tended to give additional authority to Dr. Young, who had so long resisted their demands. A memorandum, very temperately worded, but strongly supported, was presented to the Prime Minister, the Duke of Wellington. A Report on this Memorandum was made by Dr. Young, in February, 1829. Though his health was at that time rapidly declining, his observations were written with his usual precision and ability, giving way in one instance only to feelings of personal resentment, if a stronger term may not be used, which had been provoked by attacks of unusual violence and bitterness; it is hardly necessary to add that he adhered substantially to the views which he had pre-viously maintained. His death, which took place about two months afterwards, put an end to the contest. It was followed, as is well known, by a Committee of the Astronomical Society appointed under the authority of the Admiralty, upon whose report the Nautical Almanac was entirely reorganized, and assumed the form which it has ever since retained.

Upon a review of the origin and progress of this controversy, which was carried on with so much acri-mony and for so many years, it is difficult for the warmest admirers of Dr. Young altogether to justify the line of conduct which he pursued. Of the two grounds upon which he chiefly rested his defence,—expense to the Government, and the interests of navi-gation,—the first was absolutely unworthy of notice, and the second could hardly be compromised by the embarrassment produced by placing in the hands of seamen more than they required, when the most simple instructions would direct them what to look for. Neither was he much more fortunate in another argu-ment which he put forward, that astronomers had no special claim for such public aid in their researches, as an ample and carefully prepared Ephemeris would afford them. It is precisely in those cases, where private enterprise must necessarily fail, or where no effectual co-operation can be otherwise secured, that it becomes the duty of a government to interpose; for, by such in-terference wisely and judiciously exercised, the great body of the people will be taught to regard the machinery of government not as designed for the interests of parti-cular classes and parties, but as essentially necessary to the attainment of much higher objects, the promo-

tion of science, of education, of the public health, and
of rational progress in whatever concerns the good of
the community.

Dr. Young contributed to the Astronomical and
Nautical Collections in Brande's Quarterly Journal
several important articles on Refraction. He had
observed that the series employed for expressing the
refraction in terms of the density failed at the horizon,
because the sine of the altitude was a divisor of the
co-efficients, and it occurred to him that this inconvenience might be avoided by expressing the density
in a series in terms of the refraction. The series
which was thus obtained, though not always very con-
vergent in extreme cases, is convenient for obtaining a
tolerably accurate result from any proposed theory of
the law which governs the relations of the height,
temperature, and density of the atmosphere, being
capable of determining the refraction by the aid of a
small number of its terms. He was accustomed to
consider this principle of reversing the ordinary form
of exhibiting the series for refraction as one of the
happiest ideas that had ever occurred to him in a physical investigation.

These papers gave rise to a very acrimonious controversy between himself and Mr. Ivory, who was engaged about the same time in the same class of
researches. Mr. Ivory, whose temper was somewhat
morose and jealous, was a worshipper of La Place and
the French School of analysts, to whose methods he was
the first to give a very general currency in this country ;
and he was too apt—as in his Memoir on Cohesion of
Fluids, to which we have before referred—to make the
physical principles on which his investigations were
founded in some degree subordinate to the analytical

elegance and completeness of the methods which he employed. As an analist however, and in the direct applications of analysis to physical questions, he had few superiors. With such prepossessions, it was not surprising that he should have failed to recognize, in this as well as in other instances, the importance of Dr. Young's conclusions, in connection with the inelegance and apparent insufficiency of his methods; and should have been disposed to dispute the correct‑ ness of the assumptions upon which his series were founded; to doubt their convergency, at least for very low altitudes, and to maintain generally that such series were only resorted to in the infancy of analytical science.[a] Dr. Young replied to these imputations by showing that his method was applicable not only to every hypothesis respecting the distribution of heat in the atmosphere to which the methods of La Place, Bessel and Ivory were applicable, but also to others which they did not venture to investigate, in consequence of considering them beyond the powers of the analysis which those methods required.

Formulæ or series for refraction, though founded upon very different views of the constitution of the atmosphere, may give—when their constants are sufficiently determined by observation—results which are nearly coincident for considerable altitudes and within moderate limits of temperature : it is only when we approach the horizon, or for extreme heat or extreme cold, that the considerable discrepancies begin to appear. Thus, whilst the formula which Dr. Brinkley proposed gives results, for extreme cold, even near the horizon, which have been found, in some remarkable observations, to be nearly correct, those given

a Works, vol. ii. p. 39.

by that of Dr. Young, under similar circumstances, are much too small. Other sources of discrepancy have their origin in the different- methods which are adopted for ascertaining the temperature. Are we to trust to the indications of the thermometer within or without the observatory, or are we to make use of both? Dr. Young would trust to the first,[a] Dr. Brinkley to the second, and Bessel would take account of both of them; whilst the difficulty in a well constructed or well regulated observatory would be evaded by making the difference between them as much as possible disappear. It is in the searching discussion of questions, like these, apparently so trivial and so unimportant, that those minute quantities are involved, the detection and accurate determination of which will form the basis of the most important results of the astronomy of the future; of the values in fact of the standards by which we shall be able to measure the dimensions of the remotest portions of the universe which are penetrable by our telescopes.

[a] Works, vol. ii. p. 73.

CHAPTER XII.

OPTICAL DISCOVERIES.—SECOND EPOCH.

In the interval of twelve years which elapsed between the publication of his Reply to the Edinburgh Review and the appearance of Fresnel's first Memoir on Diffraction in 1816, the name of Dr. Young was ostensibly connected with no important experimental or theoretical optical investigations. In fact, his previous labours upon the subject seemed to have been absolutely forgotten, and it would be difficult to point out a single allusion made to them in any optical work or memoir published during that period, either at home or abroad. In the intermediate period La Place had published his celebrated Memoir on the double refraction of Iceland spar : Malus had discovered the polarization of light by reflection, and was engaged in a brilliant series of researches connecting his discovery with the optical properties of crystalline bodies, when a premature death brought his labours to a close : Brewster was enriching every department of experimental optics with the most remarkable speculations and discoveries : Arago had found out the colours of crystalline plates produced by polarized light, and though less fertile than some of his contemporaries in the number of his contributions to the science, he was second to none of them in the critical sagacity with which he analysed their labours : Biot was combining theoretical and practical researches with a success and ingenuity which seemed to promise him the first place amongst optical discoverers, when it was his misfortune to waste his energies and compromise his reputation in the proposition and obstinate maintenance of his theory of moveable polarization : at a later period, the labours of Fresnel,—who—though treading generally in the footsteps of Young, required no foreign aid either to guide or support him,—was destined to give unity and system to the vast mass of facts and theories which his predecessors had accumulated and prepared. "Of the splendid constellation of great names just enumerated," writes Sir John Herschel shortly after the most important of this vast series of investigations had been brought to a conclusion, "we admire the living and revere the dead[a] far too warmly and too deeply to suffer us to sit in judgment on their respective claims to priority in this or that particular discovery ; to balance the mathematical skill of one against the experimental dexterity of another, or the philosophical acumen of a third : so long as 'one star differeth from another in glory,'—so long as there shall exist varieties or even incompatibilities of excellence,—so long will the admiration of mankind be sufficient for all who merit it."[b]

But in the mean time Young, though he engaged in no continuous optical investigation and preserved strictly the *incognito* which he considered to be due to his profession, was neither an idle nor an unconcerned observer of what was passing around him. The Memoir[c] of La Place, which took the lead in the series of researches above referred to, was published in

---

[a] Malus and Fresnel were then dead.

[b] Article Light, Encyclopædia Metropolitana, §. 780.

[c] " Sur la loi de la Réfraction extraordinaire dans les Cristaux Diaphanes."—*Journal de Physique* for 1809.

the beginning of the year 1809, and in it its illustrious author had brought the Newtonian theory of
emission and the principle of least action in the form
which Maupertuis had given to it, to bear upon the
explanation of the extraordinary as well as ordinary
ray in Iceland crystal; and he had obtained results
which appeared so completely to represent the phenomena, that it was considered by himself as well as by
the great body of men of science both in France and
elsewhere—who bowed implicitly to his authority—as
a crucial test of the sufficiency of the received theory
to explain them.[a]

It was this Memoir which became, soon after its
appearance, the subject of a remarkable Article which
Young contributed to the Quarterly Review,[b] in which
he showed or rather asserted that one of the two mechanical principles upon which its conclusions were
founded was misapplied and the other an arbitrary
assumption;[c] whilst he himself partially deduced the
course of the extraordinary ray from assumptions respecting the unequal elasticities of the ether, which
transmits the undulations, in the direction of the axis
of the crystal and in a plane at right angles to it, which
were perfectly legitimate inductions from observation
and which subsequent investigations have fully confirmed.

---

[a] " La découverte d'Huygens," says Biot, " liée par M. La Place aux
principes de la mécanique, est aujourd'hui la base de toutes nos recherches
sur la double refraction."—*Traité de Physique*, tom iii. p. 365, 1816.

[b] Quarterly Review for November, 1809.   Dr. Young's Works, vol. i.
p. 220.

[c] " Les calculs de M. de La Place," says M. Fresnel, " n'ont point
éclairé la question théorique : car ils ne montrent pas pourquoi la force ré-
pulsive qui émane de l'axe, varierait comme le carré du sinus de l'inclinai-
son du rayon extraordinaire sur celui-ci ; et il est bien difficile de justifier
cette hypothèse par de considérations mécaniques."—*Mémoires de l'Institut*,
tom. vii. p. 47, 1827.

The law of sines was determined by Huygens upon the principles of the undulatory theory, by the aid of Fermat's principle of the *law of the least time*, where the time of transmitting an undulation, from a point without to a point within, a different refracting medium, was required to be a *minimum*: and as the paths without as well as within, the medium are straight lines, it was the sum of the quotients formed by dividing the exterior and interior path, by the velocities with which they are respectively described, which was required to answer this condition and which was found by him to furnish the law which had been so long recognized as established by experiment.

The principle of *least action*, as stated by Maupertuis, required the sum of the products of the space and velocity, without and within the refracting medium, to be a *minimum*; but as we have already seen that the velocities of the propagation of the rays of light through different media, according to the Newtonian and the Huygenian theories, are in the inverse proportion to each other, it follows that the principle of *least action*, upon the first hypothesis, gives precisely the same result as that of *least time* upon the other, and that they must lead, therefore, to the same construction for determining the position of the extraordinary ray in a doubly refracting crystal, whatever be the position of the incident ray with respect to its axis.

Inasmuch as these two principles can only give coincident results by assuming other results which are in direct contradiction to each other, it seems necessarily to follow, that, even assuming them to be generally true, there are some circumstances connected with the solution of this problem which limit the application of one of them. This limitation, which is rather insinuated than proved in Young's Review of La Place's Memoir, is very clearly and fully stated in a passage of a Life of Fermat, inserted by him, with a special view to this question, in the Supplement of the Encyclopædia Britannica, which is reprinted in the second volume of his Works.[a]

The solution which Huygens gave of the problem of double refraction, assumed the coexistence of two media within the crystal, one propagating its undulations according to the ordinary law, and the other transmitting them with different velocities in different directions, so as to produce a spheroidical wave, whose axis of revolution was coincident with the axis of the crystal. If we further conceive the existence of a third imaginary spherical wave, whose centre is the point of incidence, spreading itself with the same velocity as if it was propagated in the medium external to the crystal, and if from the point where the incident ray produced would meet this imaginary wave, we suppose tangent planes to be drawn to the spherical and spheroidical waves respectively, which are really propagated within the crystal, then the lines joining the point of incidence and the two points of contact respectively, will represent the courses of the ordinary and extraordinary ray. It is hardly necessary to add that it is precisely to the same construction that we are conducted by the theory of La Place.

But the important question arises—upon what grounds are we justified in assuming the coexistence within the crystal of spherical and spheroidical waves of equal intensities, producing rays of light whose courses are found by observation to be determined by the preceding construction. It was this very coin-

cidence, as being too remarkable and too complicated
to have resulted from a false hypothesis, which
induced its illustrious author to assume that it was
true.

" Newton," says Young, in the first of his Memoirs on Light,
" has advanced the singular refraction of Iceland crystal as an
argument that the particles of light must be projected cor-
puscles, since he thinks it probable that the different sides of
these particles must be differently attracted by the crystal, and
since Huygens has expressed his inability to account in a satisfactory manner for all the phenomena. But, contrary to what
might have been expected from Newton's usual accuracy and
candour, he has laid down a new law for the refraction, without
giving a reason for rejecting that of Huygens, which Mr. Haüy
has proved to be more accurate than Newton's ; and, without
attempting to deduce from his own system any explanation of
the more universal and striking effects of doubling spars, he
has omitted to notice that Huygens' most elegant and ingenious
theory perfectly accords with those effects in all particulars, and
of course derives from them additional pretensions to truth." *

Dr. Wollaston was induced by these observations of
Young, to subject the construction of Huygens to a
more accurate examination than it had hitherto received, by bringing to bear upon the enquiry the
ingenious method which he had recently devised for
the determination of the refractive indices of liquid
and crystalline bodies. His examination fully established the accuracy of the Huygenian measures.

" I think the result of these comparisons," says he, at the
conclusion of his investigation, " must be admitted to be highly
favourable to the Huygenian theory ; and although the existence of two refractions at the same time in the same substance
be not well accounted for, and still less their interchange with
each other when a ray of light is made to pass through a
second piece of spar situated transversely to the first, yet the

* Works, vol. i. p. 166.

oblique refraction, when considered alone, seems nearly as well explained as any other optical phenomenon. For since the theory by which he was guided in his enquiries affords (as has lately been shown by Dr. Young) a simple explanation of several phenomena not yet accounted for upon any other hypothesis, it must be admitted, that it is entitled to a higher degree of consideration than it has hitherto received."[a]

Whatever disposition, however, Dr. Wollaston may have felt to view this theory with favour, he was restrained from adopting its conclusions by the habitual caution of his character, or rather, by the want of that bold and enterprising spirit of speculation which is more or less essential to those who make great revolutions in science.

It was the kindred science of sound which had suggested to Young his principle of interference, and he was under a similar obligation to the same science for the suggestion of the principle which formed the first step in the solution of the great problem of double refraction. Amongst the vast treasure of acoustical facts which are recorded in the works of Cladni, there is one which states that the velocity with which sound is transmitted in the direction of the fibres of a block of Scotch fir is to that with which it is transmitted transversely to them, in the proportion of the numbers 5 and 4.[b] It is a question which naturally springs out of such an observation, to determine the velocity of the transmission of sound in any other direction, or the curve surface which bounds the simultaneous undulations which are thus propagated in every direction through a substance thus constituted. Is it not a spheroid, whose axes are in the direction and in the proportion of the greatest and least

[a] Philosophical Transactions, 1802.
[b] Dr. Young's Works, vol. i. p. 228.

velocities of propagation? But if the fibrous structure of a mass of wood produces such an effect upon the vibrations or sounds transmitted through it, why may not a similar effect be produced by the internal constitution of a doubly-refracting crystal upon the luminiferous ether which transmits the undulations which constitute light? For, inasmuch as the facts of ordinary refraction, interpreted in conformity with the undulatory theory, compel us to admit that the elasticity of this ether is less within a refracting body than without it, the very existence of different refracting powers in the direction of the axis, and transversely to it, in a doubly-refracting crystal, would lead us naturally to the conclusion, that the ether in this case is so modified by the peculiar crystalline structure, that its elasticity in these directions is also different. Upon this assumption, Young proceeds to show that, under such circumstances, the curve surface which bounds the simultaneous undulations in all directions within the crystal will be a spheroid, whose axes coincide with the directions, and are proportional to the square roots, of the greatest and least elasticities.

The principle which is involved in this investigation is the same as that which is made the foundation of the subsequent and much more complete investigation of Fresnel,[a] when all the conditions, which the solution of the problem was required to satisfy, were before him : which is, that in a medium constituted as the ether within a doubly-refracting crystal was assumed to be, a particle infinitesimally displaced would not be urged back in the direction of the displacement, unless such displacement took place in the direction of the principal axis of elasticity, or transversely to it. If the

[a] Mémoires de l'Institut, tom vii. p. 47.

forces which this displacement brings into operation
be estimated in these axial directions, and then further
resolved in the direction of the wave's motion,—such
being the forces which alone are concerned in its propagation,—the whole elastic force of propagation will
be obtained, and the increment of the velocity corresponding to it will be proportional to its square root.
It may then be easily shown that the expression which
represents this increment is proportional to that of the
perpendicular upon the tangent plane to a spheroid,
which is therefore the surface which in this case bounds
the simultaneous undulations. It is hardly necessary
to observe that the velocity of propagation in any direction is in all cases proportional to the corresponding
diameter.

Great as was the sagacity shown by Dr. Young in
giving to this acoustical observation of Cladni its analogical interpretation in the constitution of the luminiferous ether within a doubly refracting crystal,—
the existence of biaxal crystals being at that time unknown,—and clear as was the conception shown in the
investigation of the machinery by which undulations
would be propagated in such a medium, it must nevertheless be allowed that the solution given by him was
incomplete, even when viewed with reference to the
form in which the question was presented to him.
For, whilst it sufficiently accounted for the propagation of the extraordinary, it failed to show the existence of the ordinary, ray; in other words, the whole
of the incident light should appear, from the investigation, to be absorbed in the extraordinary ray. It is
well known that Huygens felt the difficulty of accounting for the resolution of the incident into the
ordinary and extraordinary ray by the operation of

the same medium; and it was for the purpose of evading it that he assumed the coexistence of two media within the crystal, one of which transmitted the ordinary and the other, the extraordinary, ray.

Attention, also, had not yet been sufficiently called to the important observations of the same illustrious philosopher on the action of a second crystal, with its principal axis placed at right angles to the first, through which the bifurcated ray is transmitted, when it is found that its separate branches are no longer subdivided, but the ordinary ray of the first becomes the extraordinary ray of the second, and conversely.[a]

The same observations, when subsequently made by Newton, exercised, as is well known, no inconsiderable influence upon his views of the theory of light. The affections impressed upon the two branches of the divided ray were attributed by him to a species of polarity in the luminous molecules,—a remark which induced Malus, when he discovered a similar affection produced, under certain circumstances, in reflected light, to give to it the name of *polarization*. It was subsequently shown that the two branches of the divided ray in Iceland and in other doubly-refracting crystals were always equal in intensity, and that they were polarized in planes which were at right angles to each other. No solution of this great problem could be considered as complete which did not embrace both these and all other effects which the action of the crystal produced upon the incident ray.

In a Review, also written by Dr. Young, in the following year, of the second volume of the *Mémoires de Physique et de Chimie de la Société d'Arcueil*, in which an abstract of the celebrated memoir of Malus first

---

[a] Traité de la Lumière, cap. v.

made its appearance, he speaks of the phenomena of polarization announced in it, as

" being conclusive with respect to the insufficiency of the undulatory theory in its present state for explaining all the phenomena of light.[a] But we are not therefore by any means persuaded of the perfect sufficiency of the projectile system ; and all the satisfaction that we have derived from an attentive examination of the accumulated evidence which has been brought forward, within the last ten years, is that of being convinced that much more evidence is still wanting before it can possibly be decided."[b]

More than five years afterwards, we find him, in a letter to Sir David Brewster, expressing the same opinion :—

" With respect to my fundamental hypotheses respecting the nature of light, I become less and less fond of dwelling upon them, as I learn more and more facts like those M. Malus discovered, because, though they may not be incompatible with those facts, they certainly give no assistance in explaining them. But this observation does not extend to my laws of interference as explanatory of the phenomena of periodical colours, since almost every new case of the production of colours, which has lately been discovered, ranges itself as a simple consequence of these laws, and is as regularly deducible from them by calculation, as the motions of the planets are deducible from the laws of gravitation."[c]

The colours produced by polarized light, when passing through certain crystalline plates, were first discovered by Arago in 1811, though it would appear that Sir David Brewster was engaged upon an extensive series of observations of a similar kind about the same period, though the results of them were not published

---

[a] Malus was of opinion that the phenomena of polarization were equally irreconcileable with both the theories. See his letter to Dr. Young. —Works, vol. i. p. 248, note.

[b] Works, vol. i. p. 248.   [c] Works, vol. i. p. 360.

before 1813. To Biot, however, is due the chief merit of having generalized the facts connected with these remarkable phenomena, and of expressing the general law by which they appeared to be governed. It was in the notice of the Memoir[a] in which these last investigations were contained, which is given in the Quarterly Review for 1814,[b] that Dr. Young made a very important step in advance, by showing that these phenomena "are reducible, like all other cases of *recurrent* colours, to the general laws of the interference of light."

The solution of this problem, which is one of no ordinary complexity, requires the determination of the lengths of the paths and of the relative velocities with which they are described, of the ordinary and extraordinary ray through a thin plate of a doubly refracting crystal, cut in any direction with respect to its axis. In Iceland spar, where the ratio of the greatest and least refractive densities is nearly that of the numbers 10 and 9, the two rays may make a considerable angle with each other, and the velocities of their transmission may also differ considerably so as to make it difficult to secure a plate sufficiently thin to exhibit the phenomena advantageously ; but if the ratio in question approaches nearly to equality, as, amongst many other crystals, in sulphate of lime, in the form of Muscovy talc,[c] where its terms are as 175 to 176, the ratio of these velocities can never be expressed by smaller numbers than these and their

---

[a] Mémoire sur de nouveaux Rapports entre la Reflexion et la Polarization de la Lumière.—Lu à l'Institut, Juin 1, 1812.

[b] Works, vol. i. p. 269.

[c] This is a biaxal crystal, a circumstance which does not, in this case, very materially modify the phenomena ; it was, at this time, conceived that even in such crystals, one of the two rays followed the ordinary law of refraction.

angular separation is necessarily very small. Under such circumstances, therefore, the ordinary and extraordinary rays, when they emerge parallel, would be superposed and in a condition to interfere, provided the modifications which the crystal produces upon them, are such as would allow them to do so. The thickness also of such a plate of such a substance must be at least 175 times the length of an undulation, in order that one ray may lag behind the other by a single undulation: and inasmuch as a retardation of several undulations may take place, as in the analogous case of Newton's rings, before the overlapping of the different colours, produced by interference, obliterates their distinctive characters, it would be allowable for us to expect the occurrence of such phenomena, even with plates of a thickness so considerable as to come far within the limits of mechanical subdivision.

It remains to trace generally the course of the portions of the two rays which are not transmitted at the second surface but reflected back into the crystal. These reflected portions are found to be subdivided, like the ray first transmitted, into two others, following the same laws as the first, and forming therefore four reflected rays following different but nearly coincident paths. If the letters O and E be taken to represent the paths of the ordinary and extraordinary branches of the ray transmitted at the first surface, and o and e, e and o be the paths of the reflected rays respectively, then we may represent the entire paths of the four systems thus formed—after leaving the first surface of the crystal and returning to it again,—by Oo, Ee, Oe, and Eo respectively; it is obvious that the two last will reach the first surface simultaneously inasmuch as the direct and reverse portions of their entire paths are equal, and the retardation or accelera-tion of the ordinary branch of the ray in one direc-tion will be equal to the acceleration or retardation of the extraordinary branch in the other ;[a] but the paths represented by Oo and Ee are described throughout, one by the ordinary and the other by the extraordi-nary ray ; one of them will therefore lag behind the other, and at their emergence at the first surface, whether combined or not combined with the light reflected from it, they will be in a condition to inter-fere. The phenomena should apparently represent the reflected rings of Newton's scale in the first case, and the transmitted rings in the second, whilst in the general result they should be found to be mixed and confounded with each other, and, if in a condition to interfere, would tend to neutralize each other.

The principle involved in these investigations, which Young embodied in very complicated formulæ and applied numerically to the principal cases enume-rated and classified by Biot, was the true key to the explanation of these and similar phenomena. Its appli-cation, however, required very important limitations. It failed, as Arago observed, in showing under what circumstances the interference of the rays can take place, and why we see no colours unless the crystalized plates are exposed not only to light previously polar-ized but also modified after emergence by being trans-mitted through or reflected by what has been termed an *analysing* plate ; and it was not until a much later period that all these limiting conditions were fully determined.[b]

---

[a] In a biaxal crystal both branches of the ray are extraordinary, though different from each other, a circumstance which does not materially modify the explanation in the text.

[b] In a letter from Fresnel to Young in January, 1825, when speaking

It was about two years after the publication of the
Review, in which this theory was proposed, that the
same able observer, in conjunction with Fresnel, made
the important discovery that rays polarized in opposite
planes would not interfere. Every day, in fact, in that
remarkable period—when so many great observers were
endeavouring to outstrip each other in the career of
discovery—was making known modifications and phenomena of polarized light, which no existing theory
was yet competent to explain. It was polarization
which still continued to cast a dark cloud over the
hopes and fortunes of the undulating theory.[a]

Whilst Young was thus engaged, occasionally only
and at distant intervals, in endeavouring to connect
his own views of the nature of light with some of the
rich harvest of results which, chiefly through the
labours of Brewster, had followed the discoveries of
Malus ; and whilst Biot was labouring with unwearied
energy and not without apparent success in a similar attempt, by means of his theory of moveable
polarization, to reconcile them with the old established doctrines which were sanctioned with the authority of Newton and which continued to receive the
support of the great body of his contemporaries, a
young officer of engineers, inferior to none of those

of their respective shares in these discoveries, he says :—"You first
observed and demonstrated that the colours of crystalline plates proceeded
from the difference of the velocity of transmission of the ordinary and extraordinary rays, but it remained to establish the direction of the polarization of these rays within the plate ; it was necessary to explain why
their interferences produced no colours unless the emergent light was
analysed with a plate of Iceland spar, or by any other mode of polarization ; and why it was also necessary that the light should have received a
previous polarization before it passed through the crystallized plate.—
Works, vol. i. p. 405.

[a] See Dr. Whewell's observation.—Dr. Young's Works, vol. i. p. 248,
note.

who had preceded him in experimental and mathematical skill, and inventiveness,[a] had recently made his appearance upon the scene, who was destined in the course of a few years to connect these scattered and apparently incongruous phenomena by a consistent theory, and to give a new aspect to the whole face of optical science.

The first Memoir of Fresnel on Diffraction, which we have had elsewhere occasion to notice, had already been presented to the Institute, and had been referred, in the ordinary course, to a commission for examination. Arago, who was the reporter of this commission, was so much struck by its merits, that he sought the friendship of the author, and became associated with him for the remainder of his life in common labours, both experimental and theoretical, for the promotion of optical science. It was from Arago that Fresnel first learnt that the ground which he had marked out as his own had been already almost entirely occupied by Dr. Young, and it was under his auspices and advice that the Memoir was revised and enriched with new experiments and modes of observation, including one of great interest and importance of which he was himself the author.[b]

In a letter which accompanied the presentation copy of his Memoir, Fresnel assures Dr. Young, that when he first presented it to the Institute, he was not aware that he had been anticipated by him, or that he had

[a] I adopt this term from Dr. Whewell; there is no other term which adequately expresses the peculiar power and resources which some of his later writings display, more especially his *Mémoire sur la Loi des Modifications que la Réflexion imprime à la Lumière polarizée.*

[b] By making the internal bands of diffraction disappear, by the introposition of a thin piece of transparent glass instead of an opaque screen.— See Dr. Young's Works, vol. i. p. 379; and Annales de Physique et de Chimie, for 1816.

produced as new, explanations of his experiments which had been given many years before.   After referring to some few points in his Memoir, of no great importance, which Young had not noticed, or which he had exhibited under a somewhat novel aspect,—and also to some difficulties which he could not explain, such as the loss of half an undulation under certain circumstances, and the black spot (in reality due to the same cause) in the centre of Newton's rings seen by reflection,—he modestly adds :—

" When we believe that we have made a discovery, it is not without regret that we find that another has made it before us ; and I will frankly confess to you, sir, that such was the feeling I experienced when M. Arago shewed me that there were only a small number of observations really new in my original Memoir. But if anything could console me for not having had the advantage of priority, it is that it has brought me into contact with a philosopher who has enriched physical science with so great a number of important discoveries, a circumstance which has not a little contributed to increase my own confidence in the theory which I have adopted." [a]

The discussions which arose out of this Memoir, and the ample references to Dr. Young's writings which it contained, were the means of calling the attention of men of science in France both to the undulatory theory and to its author.   Arago, as we have seen, adopted it with the ardour which belonged to his character, as well as Humboldt, his most intimate friend and adviser :[b] Ampère, a man of great candour and of eminent

---

[a] Dr. Young's Works, vol. i. p. 378.

[b] In a letter to Young, acknowledging his election, in conjunction with Gay Lussac, as one of the foreign members of the Royal Society, he says—" *Quant à vous, Monsieur, vous savez, j'espère, le cas que l'on fait dans ce pays-ci de vos expériences neuves et ingénieuses sur la route de la lumière. M. Arago a fait récemment des observations très fines qui se lient merveilleusement bien à ce que vous avez découvert sur ces ondulations.*"

philosophical attainments, was also disposed to regard it with favour. But La Place, who was naturally regarded as the Jupiter Olympius [a] of the Institute, and whose opinions were commonly received as abso‧ lute decrees, was violent in his opposition, and Poisson, who took the next rank to La Place as a mathema‧ tician at least, if not as a philosopher, followed in his train. Biot, in addition to his instinctive reverence for the same great man,[b] and his passionate admiration of the optical writings of Newton, was not a little influ‧ enced in his opposition by his anxiety to uphold his own views. He had once noticed the adverse theory, in a considerable work[c] which he had recently published, merely for the purpose of refuting a fundamental ex‧ periment which had been brought forward as decisive in its favour;[d] and Arago, in a letter to Young, stig‧ matizes in indignant terms the "contemptible argu‧ ments by which he supported his opinion."[e]

[a] See the curious reference to La Place in Arago's *Histoire de ma Jeunesse*, p. 17, in the first volume of his Works which are now in the course of publication.

[b] See Dr. Young's Works, vol. i. p. 220, note.

[c] *Traité de Physique Expérimentale et Mathématique*, vol. iii., *ad finem*.

[d] The suppression of the internal bands in diffraction by stopping the light on one side of the object.

[e] In a letter to Sir David Brewster, written shortly after a visit to Paris, in 1817, Dr. Young says—"I suppose M. Biot had the candour to tell you that he had read none of my papers whatever : he promised me that he would do it in the course of the summer, but I dare say he has not found leisure. M. La Place has now arrived at so happy a pre-eminence in science that he thinks it sufficient to assert, where others would assign their reasons, and having once asserted he is not very impatient to retract. He told me in July, as he had often declared before, that the Huygenian theory was incapable of determining the relations of the angles of incidence and refraction ; and when I could hardly help smiling at the absurdity of the assertion and endeavoured to prove to him how easily and necessarily the law was deduced from the hypothesis, he begged me to send him a short demonstration in writing ; I did so, and instead of either admitting it, or endeavouring to point out its deficiency. he now tells me that it is only an "*aperçu*," a sketch or a presumption. (See his letter, Dr. Young's Works, vol. i. p. 374.) With respect to M. Poïsson, when we know how

The same two distinguished men, Arago and Biot, became severally the representatives of the supporters of the opposite theories. The battle was renewed in the hall of the Institute, whenever a new experiment was brought forward or a new Memoir read in favour of one or the other. In 1822, a remarkable Memoir by Fresnel,[a] in which the theory of the colours of crystalline plates was freed from nearly all the difficulties which had hitherto embarrassed it, was referred by the Institute to Arago and Ampère, who reported upon it in terms of approbation so emphatic and unconditional, and showed so pointedly and decisively that the theory of moveable polarization was not reconcileable with the results of observations which this Memoir recorded, that Biot objected to its reception as irregular, in consequence of its appearing to compromise the opinions of the Institute as a body. The Report was subsequently modified, but not sufficiently so to meet the objections which he made to it;[b] and in the debate which ensued, Arago attacked the *rival* theory of Biot, which was really at issue on this question, with so much vehemence both of language and argument, that the friendship between them which had been cemented by common dangers and sufferings in extending Mechain's meridian from Barcelona to Formentera, as well as by various and important common investigations and labours, was permanently dissolved. In the face of

repeatedly and how deeply he has committed himself in praising and in imitating some of M. La Place's least successful speculations, we cannot be surprised at his bearing him out on this point. He praises, for instance, both the theory of capillary attraction and that of oblique refraction as among the highest efforts of human genius, while to me they both appear worse than nugatory."—Works, vol. i. p. 372.

[a] This was the date of the Reports : the Memoir had been presented three years before.

[b] Annales de Chimie.   For 1821, p. 225 and 258.

such opposing influences, the reception of the various Memoirs which Fresnel presented to the Institute in rapid succession was not generally encouraging, and some of the most considerable of them remained un-published for many years, and only became known to men of science by imperfect abstracts of them in the Annales de Chimie, and other journals. In a letter to Dr. Young, written in 1823, seven years subsequently to his first appearance as an author, after referring to several other Memoirs, he adds :—

" All these Memoirs, which I have presented in rapid succes-sion to the Academy of Sciences, have nevertheless failed to open me its gates. It is M. Dulong who has been nominated to fill the vacant place. The members of the *Section de Physique* have not placed me on the same rank with him ; they have put him the first and me the second. You see, sir, that the theory of undulation has brought me no good fortune ; but this does not disgust me ; and I console myself in my unhappiness by studying optics with a new ardour."

The increasing sense, however, not only of his own merits, but also of the correctness of the views which he advocated, became too powerful for the opposition to withstand, and he was elected a member unani-mously before the end of the same year.

In the course of the summer of 1816, Young re-ceived at Worthing a visit from Arago, accompanied by Gay Lussac. The circumstances of this visit, which was itself a very significant indication that he was now rapidly becoming famous, are thus noticed in the well-known Éloge, with which Arago subsequently honoured his memory, as one of the eight foreign members of the Institute :—

" In the year 1816 I visited England, in company with my learned friend Gay Lussac. Fresnel had recently made his début in the career of the sciences, in the most brilliant manner, by his Memoir on Diffraction. This work, which, in our opinion, contained a capital experiment irreconcileable with the Newtonian theory of light, became naturally the first subject of our conversation with Dr. Young. We were astonished at the number of restrictions which he imposed upon our commendations of it, when at last he declared that the experiment which we valued so highly was to be found, since 1807, in his Lectures on Natural Philosophy. This assertion appeared to us unfounded, and a long and very minute discussion followed. Mrs. Young was present at it, without offering to take any part in it—as the fear of being designated by the ridicule implied in the sobriquet of *bas bleus* makes English ladies reserved in the presence of strangers; our neglect of propriety never struck us until the moment when Mrs. Young quitted the room somewhat precipitately. We were beginning to make our apologies to her husband, when we saw her return with an enormous quarto under her arm. It was the first volume of the Treatise on Natural Philosophy. She placed it on the table, opened the book, without saying a word, at page 387,[a] and showed with her finger a figure where the curvilinear course of the diffracted bands, which were the subject of the discussion, is found to be established theoretically."

There were many circumstances in this visit which were particularly gratifying to Young, and he refers to it with great satisfaction in a letter to his sister-in-law Emily, who was at that time, with other members of her family, at Paris :—

" Do you know that I almost fancied you would have heard of me at the sitting of the Institute which you attended ; for I am told that my theories of light have been the subjects of some very warm discussions among the members on some public occasions. They have certainly attracted much more notice at Paris than in London ; and Humboldt the traveller writes to me warmly, wanting me to come there. To show you how far

[a] The reference apparently should be to page 467, and the figure 445. It is more probable that the discussion referred to the propagation of the external bands in diffraction, in hyperbolic curves, as the screen is moved farther and farther from the object, a fact which Fresnel considered to be both new and important ; it was, however, as Young remarked, known to Newton. See Works, vol. i. p. 281.

politeness will go : I had a visit on Sunday week from Gay Lussac the chemist, and Arago the astronomer, who came down from town on purpose to spend an evening with me, and told me, as a motive for their visit, 'On se seroit moqué de nous si nous étions retournés sans vous voir.' They promised to come again a few days hence, on their return through Brighton, and I hope they will stay a longer time."

If Young was able to communicate important information to his visitors, he was not less fortunate in that which he received from them in return. Amongst other facts of great interest and value, such as the equality of the intensity of the colours of thin plates formed in reflected and transmitted light—which it was not easy to explain upon any theory—he was now informed of the decisive experiment by which Arago was enabled to show that rays of light polarized in opposite planes will not interfere with each other. It was the knowledge of this experiment, and of other apparently anomalous facts relating to polarization, which not only rendered it necessary to revise his investigations with regard to the periodical colours of crystalline plates, but likewise served to stimulate him to a still more earnest effort to find out the principle of this mysterious affection of light, which all theories had hitherto failed to explain.

The result of his reflections on this subject was announced in a letter addressed to Arago on the 12th January, 1817 :[a]—

"I have been reflecting," says he, "upon the possibility of giving an imperfect explanation of the affection of light which constitutes polarization, without departing from the genuine doctrine of undulations. It is a principle of this theory that all undulations are simply propagated through homogeneous mediums, in concentric spherical surfaces, like the undulations of sound, consisting simply of the direct and retrograde motions

[a] Works, vol. i. p. 383.

of their particles in the direction of the radius, with their conco-
mitant condensations and rarefactions.   And yet it is possible to
explain in this theory a transverse vibration, propagated also in the
direction of the radius and with equal velocity, the motions of
the particles bearing a certain constant direction with respect to
that radius ; and this is *polarization*."

He recurs to this suggestion in the Article Chromatics, in the Supplement of the Encyclopædia Britannica, which was written—as appears from the first
rough copy of it contained in a large manuscript
volume now before me, every page of which is accurately dated—between the 4th September and the 8th
of October, 1817.   It contains a condensed review of all
his former optical theories, correcting and enlarging
them, as might be expected, to meet the new views
which were opened to him by recent discoveries, and
more especially those connected with the polarization
of light, and with the colours and other properties of
crystalline bodies.   After showing that the theory of
emission, whether as interpreted by M. Biot or in any
other manner, was incompetent to account for the phenomena of polarization, he then proceeds to suggest
some very refined considerations connected with the
possible constitution of elastic mediums, by which
vibrations may be generated which are transverse to
the direction of their propagation.

The conception, however, of such vibrations, and of
such a mode of propagation, was at that time opposed
to the prepossessions of philosophers of every school.
Even Fresnel himself, as he himself assures us, when
the notion of transversal vibrations occurred to him, in
1816, as offering the only legitimate explanation of the
important observation which he and Arago had made,
that two rays polarized at right angles always give the
same quantity of light by their union, hesitated to adopt

or announce it until he could reconcile it better to his mechanical notions. " M. Young, however," says he, " more bold in his conjectures, and less confiding in the views of geometers, published it before me, though perhaps he thought of it after me :" and it is stated by Dr. Whewell,[a] from personal knowledge,

" That Arago was wont to relate, that when he and Fresnel had obtained their joint experimental results of the non-interference of oppositely-polarized pencils, and that when Fresnel . had pointed out that transverse vibrations were the only possible translation of this fact into the undulatory theory, he himself protested that he had not the courage to publish such a conception ; and, accordingly, the second part of the Memoir was published in Fresnel's name alone. What renders this more remarkable is, that it occurred when Arago had in his possession the very letter of Young, in which he proposed the same suggestion."[b]

[a] History of the Inductive Sciences. Vol. ii. p, 418.

[b] It is observed by Fresnel, in his Memoir on the Colours of Crystalline Plates, to which we have before referred, " that a remark in a letter of Dr. Young, dated on the 29th April, 1818, which M. Arago communicated to me, helped to raise in my mind a doubt of the existence of longitudinal vibrations. Dr. Young inferred from the optical properties of crystals of two axes, discovered by Sir David Brewster, that the vibrations of the ether might probably resemble those of a stretched cord of indefinite length, and be propagated in the same manner. There is undoubtedly a great analogy between this definition of luminous waves and that which I have given above, but I do not believe that Dr. Young has shewn in what manner to reconcile such a mutual dependence of the molecules of the ether with its fluidity, and to conceive the production in it of such vibrations to the exclusion of vibrations in the direction of propagation. Now, it was this difficulty which had embarrassed me up to the present time, and hindered me from resting satisfied with my first idea. I ought, nevertheless, to acknowledge, though he may not have given this explanation, that Dr. Young is the first who has announced positively the possibility of such a property of an elastic fluid. I am ignorant whether this learned philosopher has published his views on this subject, or whether they have assumed a definite form in his mind, but I have thought that the publicity about, I hope, to be given to them, cannot be disagreeable to him."— (Annales de Chimie, t. xvii., p. 184, for 1831). This important letter, to which reference is made in the text, was not found amongst the other letters of Dr. Young, which Arago most kindly entrusted to my care ; it probably remained in the possession of Fresnel, to whom it was communicated.

Apparently, and not unreasonably, dissatisfied with the theoretical considerations which he was able to produce in favour of transversal vibrations, Young proceeds to state that:—

"If we assume as a mathematical postulate, in the undulatory theory, without attempting to demonstrate its physical foundation, that a transverse motion may be propagated in a direct line, we may derive from it a tolerable illustration of the subdivision of polarized light by reflection in an oblique plane."

He then shows in what manner, when polarized light is reflected from such a plane, the law which Malus discovered, *of the square of the cosines,*[a] for determining the relative intensities of the reflected light, may be deduced from it; and at a subsequent period, when the important experiments contained in Sir David Brewster's celebrated Memoir On the Laws of Polarization and Double Refraction in regularly-crystallized Bodies, were brought under his observation, under circumstances which have been elsewhere noticed,[b] he pointed out, in a letter appended to the Memoir, as the only interpretation compatible with the facts, that the direction of the polarization must be determined by the direction of the greatest and least refractive densities of the crystal, and not by that in which the ray is propagated.

The tendency of all these speculations was manifest. Polarization was connected with transversal vibrations ; its phenomena were otherwise altogether inexplicable. It was further connected with the direction of the greatest and least refractive densities of a doubly refracting crystal, and therefore with the phenomena of double refraction, which Young had shewn to be dependent on them. Brewster's great dis-

[a] Works, vol. i. p. 335.   [b] Works, vol. i. p. 373.

covery of biaxal crystals, and the accurate experimental analysis of their properties which had been made by himself and Biot, had opened extended views of the action of crystalline bodies upon light, and greatly increased the number of phenomena which the future theory, if ever it was to be found out, would be required to explain. Both the rays in crystals of this species, forming much the most extensive class of such bodies, were in reality extraordinary, though observation had failed to make the discovery. It was at this point in the progress of these researches that Young suggested that an ellipsoid or some almond-shaped surface (*amygdaloid*) might represent the form of the wave surface in biaxal crystals in the same manner as the spheriod in those with one axis; and it is sufficiently remarkable that if, instead of resting satisfied with a mere suggestion, founded on a somewhat vague analogy, of what the form of this surface might be, he had applied the principles of his former investigation to the effect which would be produced by three axes of elasticity, all of which were unequal instead of two of them only, as in crystals with one axis, he could hardly have failed to discover the characteristic property of the wave surface in such cases, and thus to reduce the determination of its equation and the properties of the surface itself to a question of pure geometry only. His own resolution also of a polarized beam, upon the hypothesis of transversal vibrations by oblique reflection into two others, and the deduction from these of the law which Malus had discovered, would have been another step to conduct him to the explanation of the origin and polarization of the two branches of the bifurcated ray. Near as were these approaches to the true and complete theory, and com-

pletely master as he had shown himself to be of the
position from which a first and successful assault upon
it could be made, he was diverted from the attempt
by other and more pressing occupations,[a] and thus left
to his younger and more enterprising successor a discovery which will make his name for ever memorable
in the history of optical science.

It was a most important observation of Arago, to
which we have before referred—that the intensity of
the colours of thin plates is the same, or very nearly
so, when seen both by reflected and transmitted light
—which set Young upon an enquiry into the possible
physical causes of a result apparently so different from
that to which the ordinary reasonings in this and
some similar cases would have led.   He had long perceived the necessity of the conservation of the *vis viva*
in the estimation of the intensity of light, as following
the square and not the simple power of the energy of
the elementary particles of the ether, as measured by
the amplitude of their vibrations; and by supposing
the inertia of the particles of the ether, within and
without the refracting or reflecting body, to be different
from each other—without attempting to assign its
cause—he was enabled, by following out the analogical
effects of particles of this ether, within and without
this body, impinging upon each other, to shew, upon
extremely probable grounds, that the relations between
the light reflected and transmitted would be nearly
such as Arago had observed.   The same principles are
further applied to determine the intensity of reflected
light under different circumstances, and to give results

---

[a] He had written and prepared for the Encyclopædia, in the course of
little more than one year, the articles Bridge, Carpentry, Chromatics,
Cohesion, Egypt, all of them remarkable for laborious and original research.

which are not very discrepant from observation. The same principle was confessedly made by Fresnel,[a] the foundation of his most ingenious researches on the intensity of the reflected and refracted ray of polarized light, under all circumstances of incidence with respect to the plane of polarization.

It required a somewhat- different, though an analogous, machinery to account for the loss of half an undulation, under various circumstances; but the attempt which he has made, though by no means so satisfactory as in the former cases, is equally remarkable for its sagacity and fertility of illustration.[b] It is in researches like these, where we have no *à priori* knowledge of the constitution of the luminiferous ether or of the influence of crystalline bodies upon its properties to guide us,[c] that we are left to speculation alone— controlled however by just mechanical principles whenever analogy will enable us to appeal to them—in devising hypotheses which experiment may possibly hereafter enable us to verify. It was in-framing such hypotheses that Fresnel displayed all the peculiar resources of his genius.

At the close of an admirable exposition of the undulatory theory, which was given in his great work on Optics, shortly after the completion of this great series of discoveries, Sir John Herschel has awarded, as is usual with him, the honours which are due to its

---

[a] Annales de Chimie, tom. 17, 1821 ; Note sur la coloration des lames crystallisées, p. 191.

[b] Article Chromatics.—Works, vol. i. p. 330.

[c] The late Professor McCullagh, of Dublin, whose investigations in connection with some of the most refined and difficult questions of the undulatory theory, have gained him a just celebrity, was accustomed to insist upon this absence of a principle, like that of gravitation, as constituting the real difficulty which will probably long continue to check the progress of theoretical optics.

authors with a justice and propriety which all, persons
who have carefully followed in the train of their discoveries will be ready to confirm :—

" Such is the beautiful theory of Fresnel and Young ; for we
must not, in our regard for one great name, forget the justice
which is due to the other ; and to separate them and assign to
each his share would be as impracticable as invidious, so intimately are they blended together throughout every part of this
system—early, acute, and pregnant suggestion characterizing
the one ; and maturity of thought, fulness of systematic development and decisive experimental illustration, equally distinguishing the other."

With such praise, coming from such a quarter, Young
was very naturally highly gratified.   After quoting it
in a letter to Mrs. Earle (November, 1827), he says :—

"I think he has divided the prize very fairly ; and I dare
say poor Fresnel, if he had lived, would have preferred his
share of the honour as much as I do mine.   It was before I
knew you that mine was earned ; and acute suggestion was then,
and indeed always, more in the line of my ambition than experimental illustration.   But surely one that is conscious that
such things may be said with some truth, or who imagines it,
has no farther temptation to be President of the Royal Society,
even if he could."

The health of Fresnel, which had always been delicate, began rapidly to decline soon after the completion
of the last of his Memoirs.   Mr. Macvey Napier, the
editor of the Supplement of the Encyclopædia Britannica, who had obtained an Article on Chromatics from
Dr. Young, and had been promised another on Polarization by Arago, was anxious to obtain an exposition of
his later theories from Fresnel, and thus to combine in
one publication, in the illustration of one department
of science, the labours of three of the greatest theorists
and experimentalists of the age.   In a letter addressed

to Dr. Young, at the close of the year 1824, Fresnel expressed a willingness to execute this task, though he never accomplished it :—

"I could produce," says he, "in a small compass, an Article sufficiently interesting (*bien nourri*), in expounding the views which I entertain on the principal phenomena of optics, which for some years have been sufficiently definite ; but it will be a fortnight before I can begin, and a month before you can receive it."

And, in conclusion, under the depressing influence of his fatal malady, he adds :—

"*Je vous prie de m'excuser mon brouillon ; je suis accablé par la fatigue et le besoin de sommeil.*" [a]

It was in reply, not long afterwards, to another letter from Young renewing his inquiries, that he declined the execution of his task, on account of the serious nature of his illness. His correspondent would appear to have referred to the notice which his own labours were likely to receive in the exposition of their common optical theories which was thus expected to be forthcoming, and to have insinuated that he had *planted the tree, whilst Fresnel had gathered the fruit.* There is something very touching in the mixture of the querulousness of the invalid and of the noble candour which was proper to his character, which is observable in his comment on this comparison. After complaining that sufficient attention had not been paid in England to his determination of the general law of double refraction, his formula for determining the quantity of light reflected obliquely from transparent bodies, and the discovery of circular polarization, he adds :—

"If I should succeed in demonstrating to M. Herschel, Dr.

[a] See Dr. Young's Works, vol. i. p. 400.

Wollaston, and other English men of science who are attached to the system of Newton, that the undulatory theory merits the preference, they would not fail to say that it is entirely due to your labours that we owe the subversion of the system of emission and the progress of the theory of waves. If, disabusing your *savans* on the subject of moveable polarization, I made them adopt the explanation which I have given of the colours of crystalline plates, and those general methods by means of which one may calculate the tints in all crystals when one knows the double refraction of each species of ray, they would say that the explanation of these phenomena is due to you. They would equally attribute to you that of the complicated phenomena of diffraction."

"It appears to me (if my self-love does not blind me), that what you had left me to do in these different parts of optics was as difficult as what you had done. You have gathered the flowers; may I be allowed to say, with English modesty, I have dug down laboriously to discover the roots?"

"I am far from pretending to what belongs to you, as you may see in what I have written. I have publicly confessed, with sufficiently good grace, on several occasions, the anteriority of your discoveries, of your observations, and even of your hypotheses. Nevertheless, between ourselves, I am not persuaded of the justice of the ingenious expression (*mot spirituel*), in which you would-compare yourself to the tree, and me to the apple which that tree has produced. I have the inward conviction that the apple would have (*poussé*) budded and put forth branches without the tree; for the first explanations which I gave to myself of the phenomena of diffraction and of coloured rings, of the laws of reflection and refraction, were drawn from my own resources, before I had seen your work or that of Huygens. I had myself remarked that the difference of the paths of the ordinary and extraordinary ray upon issuing from a crystalline plate was equal to that of the rays reflected from the first and second surface of the plate of air which gives the same tint in the coloured rings. It was when I had communicated this observation to M. Arago, that he told me for the first time of the note which you had published two years before on the same subject, but which he had not before that sufficiently understood. This, however, does not give me the right of sharing with you, sir, the merit of your discoveries, which belong to you exclusively by right of priority. Likewise, I have judged it useless to inform the public of all that I have found out by myself independently, though after you ; and if I speak of them, it is merely to justify my paradoxical proposition, *that the apple would have come without the tree.* I have long wished, sir, to speak to you on these subjects with open heart, and to show you cordially the whole extent of my pretensions."

After speaking in very strong and somewhat exaggerated terms of the habitual injustice of English scientific journals, in speaking of French discoveries, he adds :—

" This letter will perhaps appear to you, sir, the outbreak (*boutade*) of an invalid tormented by the bile, whose self-love was hurt at the little attention which has been paid to his labours in your country. I am far from denying the value which I would attach to the praises of English men of science, or to pretend that they would not have flattered my pride. But for a long time, that sensibility or that vanity which is called the love of glory has been greatly sobered in me. I work less to attract the suffrages of the public than to obtain that inward approbation which has ever been the sweetest recompense of my efforts. Without doubt I have often needed the spur of vanity to stimulate me to pursue my researches in moments of disgust and discouragement ; but all the compliments which I have received from Arago, La Place, or Biot, have never given me so much pleasure as the discovery of a theoretical truth, or the confirmation of my calculations by experiment. The little eagerness which I have shown to publish my Memoirs, of which extracts only have appeared, shows that I am not tormented with the thirst for fame, and that I have sufficient philosophy not to attach too much importance to the enjoyments of vanity. But it is useless to say more on this subject in writing to a man too superior to be a stranger to this philosophy, and who will easily both comprehend me and believe me."

It would appear, from a second letter which Fresnel wrote in the month of January following, that Dr.

Young, in his reply to the first, had endeavoured, and not without success, to soothe the somewhat troubled spirit of the invalid, by showing, from the terms in which his observations and theories had been noticed both by himself and his countrymen, that there never existed any just grounds for charging them with reluctance to do full justice to his claims. It would, in fact, be difficult to refer to any other example in the history of the sciences, where the combined efforts of men of science of different countries have brought about some great discovery, where national jealousies have been less offensively displayed, and where the verdict of their contemporaries has been so generally and so promptly confirmed by that of their successors.

In the year 1825, Fresnel was elected one of the fifty foreign members of the Royal Society; and two years afterwards, the medal which Count Rumford had founded, to be given biennially to the author of the most important discovery relating to light and heat, was unanimously voted to him by the Council. The proposition for this purpose was made by Sir John Herschel. "I was obliged to be *silent*," says Young, "from being too much interested in the subject; but in fact there was no opposition." In communicating this intelligence to Fresnel, in his capacity of Foreign Secretary of the Royal Society, and forwarding to him the medal and a sum of money which followed the award, he adds a hope that he will never again have occasion to complain of the neglect which his labours had experienced in this country.

" I also," says he, "should claim some right to participate in the compliment which is tacitly paid to myself in common with you by this adjudication ; but considering that more than a quarter of a century is past since my principal experiments were made, I can only feel it a sort of anticipation of *posthumous* fame, which I have never particularly coveted."[a]

Six weeks afterwards, the same letter which gave him the intelligence of his own election as one of the eight foreign members of the Institute, announced also the death of the eminent man whom the Royal Society had so recently honoured :—

" You have doubtless heard," says Arago, " of the cruel loss which the sciences have recently experienced. Poor Fresnel was already half dead when I gave him your medals. His death has plunged in the deepest grief all those who are worthy of appreciating the union of fine talents with a fine character."[b]

He died in the fortieth year of his age.

Almost exactly a quarter of a century before, the same medal, adjudicated on the same grounds, reached Malus on his deathbed. He was the precursor of the great series of discoveries which had reached their culminating point by the labours of Fresnel. Like Fresnel, also, he died in the flower of his age; like Fresnel, also, he was lamented by the lovers of science in all countries, who measured the magnitude of the loss they had sustained by the standard of what he had done.

[a] Works, vol. i. p. 409.   [b] Works, vol. i. p. 410.

CHAPTER XIII.

RESEARCHES ON THE VALUE OF LIFE AND LIFE ASSURANCE.

THE years 1824 and 1825 were memorable for one of those great disturbances of the financial and mercantile world, which occur at intervals of ten or twelve years with a regularity, which seems to point them out as constitutional paroxysms of great commercial communities, and which are probably not without their advantages as periodical warnings to impress upon them those great lessons of prudence and good sense, which are as necessary for the welfare of nations as of individuals. It is recorded that out of 624 schemes which were projected during the first outburst of this fever of speculation, not more than one in five survived the cold stage of reaction which succeeded it, and of these not a few were seriously, if not irreparably, crippled, by the ruined or damaged fortunes of many of their founders.

Though the Palladium Insurance Company had its origin in the general excitement of this period, its projectors gave the best proof that could be afforded of their desire that its affairs should be conducted upon just principles, by selecting a man of Dr. Young's scientific eminence as their Inspector of calculations and medical referee.[a] The most liberal terms were

[a] The following is a copy of the resolution of the Directors appointing him, " 30th March, 1824—Resolved, that Dr. Young, F.R.S., be requested

offered to him, and, in addition to his salary, the directors placed at his disposal a considerable number of reserved shares, which then bore a high price in the market; an arrangement which was equivalent to the gift of the whole of the premium upon them. With characteristic forbearance, however, he refused to reap where he had not sown, and declined to accept the offer. In the same spirit, he afterwards voluntarily proposed and accepted a reduced salary of 400l. per annum, as soon as he had ascertained that the duties of his office occupied a much smaller portion of his time than he had at first anticipated; a rare example of conscientiousness in the administration of such institutions, which are not unfrequently less designed by their founders for the benefit of the general body of shareholders and insurers, than of the officers who conduct them.

It was not the practice of Dr. Young to content himself with the performance of the merely routine duties of any office which he undertook, but to make important questions which arose out of them, the occasion of elaborate investigations. He had many years before proposed an empirical formula, adjusted to the results of observation, for expressing the value of life, and had founded upon it a method for calculating the value of any number of joint lives, which was more expeditious, if not more correct, than any which had been previously made use of:[a] and he was naturally invited, by the subjects which were now brought so frequently under his notice, to a renewed consideration not merely of his former speculations,

to undertake the situation of Inspector of Calculations, at a salary of 500l. per annum, to commence from the establishment of the Society; and that he be permitted to hold the appointment of Physician at the same time."

[a] Works, vol. ii. p. 359.

but also of many other questions of considerable interest connected with reversionary payments and annuities.

The proper value of the expectation of life, an element of political science affecting so many moral and material interests, is capable, even under the most favourable circumstances, of an approximate solution only. It is different for different classes of society, for different localities, for different nations. It has been materially increased by the protective effects of vaccination, by improvements in the practice of medicine and surgery, by the increased temperance and better social habits both of the rich and the poor; and there exists a moral certainty that it will continue to increase with every improvement in the application of science and art to the business of life, and most of all by the general adoption of those better sanitary arrangements for our towns and villages which are now in the course of introduction, and which it is the duty of a wise and provident government, not merely to encourage, but to enforce.

Three quarters of a century ago, Dr. Price, the real founder of correct views both of the theory and practice of Life Insurance, called attention to the fact that the duration of life was much less in large towns than in the open country. Out of every 1000 inhabitants, there died annually at that period, 52 in Stockholm, 48 in London, and 37 in Northampton. The town population of Manchester was 27,000, and the mortality 36 in 1000, indicating a degree of salubrity which in those days was somewhat unusual in large towns; but in the rural parts of the same parish, with a population of 13,000, one generation of the inhabitants, lived as long as two in the town, the annual mortality not exceeding 18 in the 1000. Similar results, though not always of so striking a character, were elsewhere observable—so great was the sacrifice of life which was occasioned by the unwholesome dwellings of our crowded cities and by the debased habits of the inhabitants which were to a great extent consequent upon them.

There is no other proof of the improved comforts and moral habits of all classes, and more especially of the poor, which is equally remarkable with the general reduction which has everywhere taken place, during the last century, in the rate of mortality, and the rapid increase of the population which has resulted from it. The millesimal mortality of London has been reduced, since the time that Dr. Price made his first observations, from 48 to 27   The tables which were constructed by him from observations at Northampton, and which were conceived to represent, as they probably did at the time they were made, the mean mortality of the kingdom, now afford a mean value of life, reckoned from the moment of birth, in the very locality for which they were framed, which is too small by one-third.[a] Even a millesimal mortality of 23 is now reckoned so much beyond what is considered to be consistent with adequate sanitary arrangements, that it has wisely been made, by an Act of the Legislature, a sufficient ground for compelling the inhabitants to adopt them.   Even in our rural districts, the improvement in the condition

---

[a] This table was constructed by Dr. Price from observations made at Northampton between the years 1735 and 1780.   It was long almost exclusively used, and has been made the foundation upon which the premiums of nearly all the Insurance Companies of London have been calculated ; it is, however, so erroneous, even for the middle of life, that it can hardly be resorted to except for purposes of deception and fraud.   In a recent and very important instance, its use has been forbidden by the legislature.

of the people, though less marked than in our towns, is considerable; and it has been sufficiently shown, by the marvellous effects which have been produced in particular localities, even in the midst of our most crowded cities, by perfect sewerage, by the abundant supply of pure water, and by good ventilation, that the rate of mortality, more especially in middle life, admits of a diminution so considerable, as to justify the most strenuous efforts of all friends of humanity to secure it.

When we consider how different are the conditions which determine the value of life in different places and at different times, it would seem to be hardly practicable to include them in any single general formula, even supposing the constant numbers which it includes to be adjusted by special observations. Many such hypotheses, or the equivalent formulæ, into which they are translateable, have been proposed; and Dr. Young has added several to their number. But, though many of them are applicable to some periods of life, none of them can be considered of much value when extended to all ages. The most celebrated, and much the most useful of such formulæ, is that founded upon the arithmetical hypothesis proposed by De Moivre more than a century ago. It assumed that out of 86 persons born, 1 died annually—an hypothesis entirely inapplicable to infancy and old age, but showing a very remarkable accordance with some tables of mortality—more especially with the Northampton tables— during the whole middle period of life, when interpreted as indicating the same number of deaths among successive bodies of survivors. Thus, by the last-named tables, it would appear that out of 1000 persons living at the age of 20, about 14½ would die annually for the next 50 years, without presenting any remarkable breach of the continuity of this law at any intervening period.[a] As these tables were formerly accepted very generally as correctly representing the law of mortality, and as this law afforded formulæ of great comparative simplicity for the calculation of the values of annuities, they became the basis of nearly all the tables for that purpose which were used in the vast multitude of important transactions connected with them, until they were partially superseded in recent times by more correct principles and more accurate observations.

We have before referred to Young's formula for expressing the value of life which he contributed to the Philosophical Magazine in 1816. In the Philosophical Transactions for 1826 we find another Essay[b] on the same subject, where a second formula of extremely complicated structure is proposed for expressing it, formed with a view of exhibiting a law of mortality which gave a mean of the results of the best authorities.[c] He was disposed to justify his predilection for empirical formulæ, when carefully constructed and adjusted to observation, as calculated to exhibit the steady progression which is characteristic of all natural

[a] In the Carlisle tables, constructed by Mr. Mylne, from observations made at Carlisle between the years 1779 and 1787, the annual mortality under the same circumstances would be about 9 instead of 14½, for the 30 years, which succeed the age of 25; at the critical age of 55, it rapidly increases from 9 to 17, and attains the maximum value of 25 or 26 at the age of 73.

[b] Works, vol. ii. p. 366. A Formula for expressing the Decrement of Life, in a letter addressed to Sir Edward Hyde East.

[c] Such, besides the Northampton and Carlisle tables, were those founded upon the French tontine, beginning in 1695, which had been tabulated by De Parcieux; the English tontines and government annuitants, beginning in 1800, which had been computed by Mr. Finlaison; the results of 30 years' experience of the Equitable Society, which had been analyzed and somewhat variously interpreted by Mr. Morgan, Mr. Babbage and Mr. Davies; and some others.

laws and to avoid those somewhat violent transitions in the value of life, which are exhibited by some of the most popular of our tables and which thus afford manifest indications of their being deduced from imperfect observations. But it should always be kept in mind that the correctness of such formulæ must be in all cases brought to the test of the most carefully constructed tables, and when discrepancies are observed in the results which they afford, it is the authority of the latter which must always be allowed to prevail. The extreme uncertainty which exists in the statistics of life in large towns and even in entire kingdoms, not merely from natural causes which no legislation can control, but also from the influence of good or bad government upon the condition of the people, must continually tend to derange not merely the constants of such formulæ, but even the algebraical connection of the variable elements which enter into them.

It was another serious objection to the formula proposed by Young, that its extreme complexity made it altogether inapplicable—unlike the simple formula which symbolized the arithmetical hypothesis of Demoivre—to the calculation of annuities. He was induced by a sense of this defect to enter, at a subsequent period, upon a Practical Comparison of the different Tables of Mortality,[a] with a view of testing the correctness, during certain periods of life, of some other hypotheses, of a simple nature, respecting the law of mortality, as well as their use in the calculation of annuities. One of these, to which he has given the name of the *quadratic hypothesis*, supposes that out of

---

[a] In 1828, in a letter to Sir Edward Hyde East, published in Brande's Journal, for 1828. See Works, vol. ii. p. 389.

86 persons born, the number of survivors at the end of any number of years will not be expressed, as in the arithmetical hypothesis, by the excess of 86 above the given age, but by dividing by 86 the excess of the square of 86 above the square of the age. He has pursued the results of this hypothesis through all its consequences, in the calculation of the expectation of life, of the probabilities of survivorship and of the value of annuities both on single and joint lives : but though they are found to be supported by some of the best tables during certain periods of life, they are less simple, and lead to conclusions not generally entitled to greater confidence than those which are furnished by the hypothesis which it was designed to supersede.

It was in the course of these investigations that he called attention, somewhat conspicuously, to a very simple and elegant theorem, as a consequence of Demoivre's hypothesis, for expressing the probability of survivorship of the younger of two given lives, which appeared to him to be original. The volume of Brande's Journal which contained this Essay had not been published more than a few days, before Young found out that he had been anticipated in the discovery of his theorem by Mr. Baily, who had enunciated it in a note to his well-known work on Annuities. An apologetic letter was instantly addressed by Dr. Young to Mr. Baily, acknowledging his oversight.[a] His brother actuaries, however, who resented with a truly professional instinct the intrusion of a stranger into a province which they claimed as their own, and some of whom had been not a little offended by the tone of superiority which he assumed in criticizing the productions of some of their number, were not slow to notice what they termed an attempt to " deck himself in borrowed plumes, and then to hold them so high that the slightest breath would blow them away." It was with a view of silencing these foolish slanders, and of placing himself in a right position, that he inserted in the next number of Brande's Journal a letter to Mr. Baily, candidly acknowledging his error, and calling the attention of his readers to what he considered the primary object of his Essay, which was to establish " the superior convenience of a good formula over all tables founded upon a limited observation for all ordinary cases of the valuation of annuities between the ages of ten and seventy years; and also to show that a uniformly increasing decrement of survivors, such as his quadratic hypothesis affords, will give a value of mortality sufficiently near the results of tables, even the most discordant among themselves, provided that the rate of increase be properly adjusted to the table."

The experience of the London Life Offices, of which seventeen had been established a sufficient length of time in 1843 to afford materials for discussion, has afforded a table of the expectation of life from the age of 20 upwards, so nearly in accordance with the results of the Carlisle Tables, as to leave no doubt of its correctly representing the rate of mortality, for the middle of life, of a past generation, amongst that class of persons who are concerned with insurances on lives: but the question may reasonably be asked, whether it is equally competent to furnish the value of this expectation for future generations as well as for the past?

Though the progress of sanitary reform and the
more general diffusion of the comforts and conveniences
of life affect the longevity of the lower much more
than of the higher classes, yet they are not without
their influence upon the latter. It has been asserted
by one of the best informed and most profound of our
actuaries, in a Report addressed to the House of
Commons,[a] that "the duration of existence now
compared with what it was one hundred years ago
is as four to three in round numbers;" a conclusion
which is probably true of the great mass of our
population, though Dr. Young has given very good
reasons for doubting the correctness of some of the
special grounds upon which it was founded, by shewing
that the annuitants upon the French and English
Tontines, the first at the close of the seventeenth
century and the other a century later, were almost
equally long-lived: but it is very possible that a more
careful selection of lives at one period may have
operated as a compensation to the general increase
of the value of life at the other. The fact, however,
of a steady diminution in the rate of mortality
amongst the rich as well as amongst the poor, is
indisputable; and there are few questions of greater
political and economical interest than to define the
influence of good legislation and improved social
habits upon the progress of the population, as well
as upon all the other elements of national prosperity.

In one of his Essays, Dr. Young pointed out what
he conceived to be *an error of Dr. Price and his
followers,* in the estimation of the values of annuities
when paid half yearly or quarterly instead of yearly.
The term *followers* referred principally to Mr. Morgan,

[a] Works, vol. ii. p. 367.

one of whose statements, which was an obvious oversight or error of the press, he had noticed in the same
Essay in a manner which was calculated to give
offence. Mr. Morgan was the nephew of the celebrated Dr. Price, whose memory he idolized, and by
whose influence he had been appointed actuary of the
Equitable Society, which he continued to manage,
with greater prudence than equity, for more than half
a century. He was a laborious and useful, though a
very obscure and inelegant, writer on the subject of
annuities and life insurances, and having been for many
years regarded as the highest authority on all such
subjects, he was prompt to resent any imputations
upon the correctness of his own views, and resisted
with characteristic obstinacy any observations dero-
gatory of the celebrated Northampton Table, which
his uncle had framed, and his predilection for which
he persevered in retaining, in defiance of the results
which the experience of his own office was daily
furnishing him. He lost no time, therefore, in reply-
ing to Dr. Young, and at the close of a vindication
of Dr. Price and his followers, whilst retaliating, not
without effect, upon his opponent, he did not neglect
the opportunity of expressing his discontent at the
progress of these new opinions :—

" The public," says he, " have lately been overwhelmed with
tables of the decrements of human life, framed either by
amalgamating all the old tables into one heterogeneous mass
and thus giving the true probabilites of life in no place whatever, or by interpolating some of the decrements in one table
into those of another ; for which purpose a vast variety has been
given of complicated and useless formulæ. But little or no
advance has been made in determining more correctly the probabilities and duration of human life. The tables published in
the Report of the Committee of the House of Commons, are, in

general, so incorrect and some of them even so absurd, as to be unfit for use, and serve only to encourage the popular delusion of the improved healthiness and greater longevity of the people of this kingdom."

There can be little doubt that the tables which are used in calculating annuities and reversions should be adapted, not merely to the general chances of life of the classes for whom they are intended, but also to the motives of those who make use of them. One class of tables might be suited to life insurers for considerable sums, who usually belong to the upper classes, whose healthy condition is made the subject of previous investigation; a second, to benefit societies, composed of artisans in our large towns, exposed to all the influences of unhealthy occupations and still more unhealthy dwellings; a third, to the purchasers of government annuities for themselves or others, who have the strongest inducement to select the most healthy lives, and whose selection is not subject to challenge. In these and in all other cases there would be also one table for males and another for females; but if the object of research was the general progress of the population, in calculations which have no reference to special classes or special localities, then an amalgamated table, such as that which Dr. Young attempted to deduce from his general formula, would properly come into operation. For such a purpose special tables like those above mentioned, or others, would be as inapplicable, as the experience of a country town, like that of Northampton or Carlisle, to cases altogether disconnected with the population of those places, unless the results which they gave were verified by experience.

Dr. Young proposed several methods [a] for calculat-

<hr />

[a] Works, vol. ii. pp. 361, 401, and 410.

ing annuities on single and joint lives which are founded
upon empirical formulæ for expressing the value of
life, some of which are remarkable not merely for
brevity and facility of application, but also for the
near approximation of the results which they afford
to those which are given by the ordinary and much
more laborious processes.   Such empirical methods,
however, when they do not involve some novel and
important principle of calculation, which is capable of
much larger application, are of very little value, more
especially where the results of the calculation, as in
all cases relating to annuities, are of such importance
as to justify the labour of constructing tables, which
are not approximatory merely, but correct.   It is well
known that there is no result of experience in whatever manner acquired, having a positive bearing upon
such questions, which is not promptly tabulated,
whatever be the labour which its calculation involves.

CHAPTER XIV.

MISCELLANEOUS MEMOIRS.

WE propose, in the present chapter, to call the attention of our readers to some of the more remarkable Memoirs, or Philosophical Essays, of Dr. Young, which have not elsewhere been noticed; selecting those which are distinguished by the importance of the subjects of which they treat, or of the conclusions to which they lead, or which are otherwise calculated to show the extraordinary capacity which he possessed of solving the most difficult problems in the applications of mathematics to natural philosophy, by processes apparently the most inadequate to the purpose. He never confined himself to the beaten track of a systematic investigation. We find in his writings no symmetrical formulæ or analytical refinements. There is no seeking after generalities, when the particular question which he has in hand does not require them; whilst every expedient is freely resorted to, however irregular and unusual, if it serves the purpose which he has in view. Important and difficult steps are passed over as manifest, terms are neglected as insignificant, analogies take the place of proofs, and we are surprised to find ourselves at the end of an investigation, even within the limits of space which would commonly be deemed hardly sufficient to master the difficulties which meet us at the beginning. But his rare sagacity hardly ever deserts him; and though he has occasionally been led to hasty and premature conclusions, or committed mistakes in numerical calculations, from the brevity and rapidity of his processes, yet nothing can be more surprising than the general soundness of his views of mechanical principles and their applications, and the correctness both of his philosophical and numerical results.

We shall consider these Memoirs generally in the chronological order in which they were written.

A Memoir on Hydraulics, printed in the Philosophical Transactions for 1808, was introductory to another in the same Collection for the following year, on the Functions of the Heart and Arteries. The connection between these subjects was considered by him, as we have before observed,[a] sufficiently close to give them both a professional character, and thus to exempt them from the restriction which he had imposed upon the class of publications which alone should be allowed to appear under his own name.

The motion of water in rivers and canals, both straight and crooked, and in tubes with different diameters and under various circumstances, had been made a special subject of investigation by a long succession of eminent Italian, and by several French, writers, but by very few of our own. The questions which it involves are extremely interesting from their important practical bearings; but, like all those connected with the motions of fluids, the conclusions to which they lead are extremely unsatisfactory, being expressed generally by empirical formulæ only, constructed chiefly with a view of representing the results of experiment, and with little reference to physical

* Supra, p. 212.

grounds, which were too difficult to investigate, and too little understood to afford a secure basis upon which they could be founded. The important element of friction alone, which enters so largely into all these questions, has never yet been, and probably never will be, brought completely within the control of an accurate analysis.

It was the formulæ proposed by Du Buat, one of the most laborious and most successful of the French writers on Hydraulics, which were tested by Dr. Young, when preparing his Lectures for the Royal Institution, by an extensive series of experiments, and which received at his hands several amendments of their form, in order to adjust them more nearly to the results which those experiments gave. He was at that time ignorant of a nearly contemporary work [a] on this subject by Prony, who had availed himself of a happy application which another French engineer, Gerard, had made of Coulomb's theory of friction to the estimation of the resistance of water in pipes and canals, and who had been enabled, by means of the assistance which it gave him, to construct a formula not only much more simple than those of Du Buat or Young, but also much more conformable to experiment. This formula failed, however, in correctly giving the discharge of water through very narrow— and much less through elastic—tubes ; and it was therefore not available for the physiological researches for which Young's investigations were chiefly designed to be subservient.

As a basis for these ulterior inquiries, Young makes a series of hypotheses with respect to the arterial and

[a] "Recherches Physico-Mathématiques sur la Théorie des Eaux Courantes." Paris, 1804.

venous systems of the human body, and the quantity of blood which they contain, which, though they assume a regularity of distribution as a foundation for calculation which anatomical examination would not altogether justify, is sufficiently accordant with truth to enable us to reason with tolerable correctness with respect to the general effects which would follow from it. The aorta being supposed to be three-fourths of an inch in diameter, and the arterial circulation to be continued through a succession of twenty-nine classes of bifurcating branches, each pair of which are about three-fourths the diameter of those from which they issue, they will end in extremely minute capillaries, not exceeding one eleven-hundredth of an inch in diameter, but sufficiently wide to transmit freely two or three particles of blood side by side, according to the estimate of their magnitudes which he had made by the aid of his Eriometer.[a] If we further assume the length of the aorta to be nine inches, and that of each successive class of arteries to be five-sixths of that preceding it,—making that of the last of the capillaries about one-twentieth of an inch only,—the weight of the whole blood required to fill such an arterial system would be about ten pounds, or nearly one-fourth part of that in the whole frame. If we should further assume the heart to pulsate seventy-five times in a minute, and at each pulsation to throw out an ounce and a half of blood, the velocity of its transmission in passing from the first to the last of this arterial series would diminish from about eight inches to one-ninetieth of an inch in a second.

It was the celebrated Dr. Hales who made the bold and singular attempt to measure the hydrostatic pres-

---

[a] Works, vol. i. p. 350.

sure propelling the blood in the arteries. He found it
to be more than nine feet in the arteries of a horse, and
five in those of a dog; and it was assumed, upon very
probable grounds, to be seven and a half feet in those
of an ordinary man, being reduced when it reaches the
veins to about six inches, leaving a balance of seven
feet in the former to continue the circulation. Dr.
Young, assuming these facts as the basis of his reasonings, then proceeds to consider how far the results to
which they lead may possibly be modified by the
antagonistic effects of the resistance from friction and
the muscular contractions of the coats of the arteries;
but arrives at the conclusion that neither of them are
so considerable as they have commonly been supposed
to be, and that they may be neglected, in our physiological reasonings upon the phenomena of the arterial
and venous circulation, without the danger of any very
material error.

If it be the business of the mathematician, aided by
the researches of the anatomist, to explain the action
of the machinery by which the circulating system of
the human frame is carried on, it is that of the physician and physiologist to trace out the various causes
which may derange it—to point out, in fact, the influences exercised by exposure to heat and to cold, by
fevers and inflammations, by bleeding from arteries or
from veins, and by various diseases and their treatment. The deviations, which may thus be produced,
from the healthy state of the circulation, are followed out
with great minuteness of detail, in connection with the
medical agents and other applications which may be best
calculated to counteract them. Few persons can be
found—and I readily confess that I am not one of their
number—with a union of acquirements so remote from

each other as to be able to prosecute an inquiry of this nature, or to judge of the correctness of the conclusions to which it leads ; but as such it was exactly suited to Dr. Young, who delighted in questions so obscure and difficult, where his various knowledge and bold spirit of speculation had full room for their exercise.

The Article Bridge, in the Supplement of the Encyclopædia Britannica, was prepared by Young with more than ordinary care and labour. The theory of bridges has usually been considered by mathematicians as one of pure geometry only, where the curve of equilibrium was to be determined under any assigned law of the distribution of the weight, with the super-added condition of such an arrangement of the outer and inner curves of the arch as would be sufficient to secure its stability within any reasonable limits of variation of the load to which it could be exposed. Little or no regard was paid in such theories to the character of the materials of which such structures were required to be composed, and they were always assumed to be absolutely inextensible and incompressible, if not crushed and disintegrated; and even the friction of their surfaces in contact was rarely taken into consideration as one of the elements of stability.

Dr. Young had already called attention, in his Lectures, to the cohesion, the elasticity, and the strength of materials, in questions of construction, and to the principles by which their mechanical effects could be estimated; and he has incorporated in this Article the ordinary theory of bridges, with the conclusions to which these principles lead; presenting the whole subject in a form which was calculated materially to assist an engineer—provided that he was capable of appreciating the import of his investigations—in combining sufficient strength and stability with a due regard to economy in the use and the choice of his materials.

In the year 1801 a plan was proposed by Messrs. Telford and Douglass—the first of whom was afterwards so well known for the construction of the Menai Bridge and other great engineering works—with a view to the improvement of the port of London, by replacing the old London Bridge by one of iron, with a single arch of the span of six hundred feet. As might have been expected, considerable doubts were expressed of the feasibility of a proposal which was at that period so novel and so bold ; and the Committee of the House of Commons, under whose consideration it came, drew up a series of twenty-one questions respecting it, which were submitted to some of the most eminent men of science and engineers of the age. Amongst them we find Dr. Maskelyne, the Astronomer Royal; Dr. Milner, of Cambridge ; Dr. Robertson, of Oxford ; Professor Playfair, of Edinburgh ; Dr. Robison, of Edinburgh ; Dr. Hutton, of Woolwich, and Mr. Atwood, of Cambridge, all of whom had written largely on the theory of arches and bridges ; the well known Mr. Watt ; General Bentham, the primary inventor of the block-machinery ; Sir John Rennie ; and several other practical engineers. The questions were very skilfully drawn up, and passed for some time under the somewhat irreverent designation of the Bridge-builders' Catechism, as expressing very briefly and clearly the principal points of inquiry which may be suggested by every considerable structure of this nature, more especially where materials are employed which are sensibly elastic and therefore compressible. The answers which were given were singularly humiliating to the pride of philosophy : they were not only altogether at vari-

ance with each other, but in every instance incomplete
and unsatisfactory. Some of them, like Dr. Milner,
were conscious that the problem presented to their
consideration was new, and that there were no recognised principles of estimating the distribution and
effects of the pressures on the different parts of a
bridge on so vast a scale, built of expansible and
compressible materials, and no experiments to be
referred to, which were competent for its solution:
others evaded the difficulties which they could not
meet; whilst the majority of the practical engineers
cut the Gordian knot, not by answering the questions,
but by proposing plans of their own. The scheme, as
is well known, was afterwards abandoned. But the
interest attached to these remarkable questions, and the
importance of the principles involved in the answers
to them, were not confined to the particular occasion
which gave rise to them ; and it was for this reason
that Young, who was attracted by a problem, which
had so completely baffled his predecessors, has given a
complete series of very careful and elaborate answers to
those queries in the Article under consideration, as
affording the best means of exemplifying his own views
of the theory of such constructions. It would be difficult to refer to any contemporary or subsequent contribution to the science of engineering which was
equally original and important.

The article Carpentry, in the former Supplement of
the Encyclopædia, had been written by Dr. Robison,
of Edinburgh, with his usual vigour and clearness of
exposition and fulness of practical detail; but it was
subject to many of the same deficiencies as had hitherto
prevailed in the theory of bridges, as well as to others
which more affect the peculiar material employed in

this art, such as the measures of its power to resist extension or compression, or of its stiffness to resist flexure or tension, or of its strength to resist pressure, or of its resilience—a term first used by Dr. Young—to resist impact. In the determinations of the measures of these powers, the modulus of elasticity becomes a most important element, which all previous works on this subject had left entirely unnoticed. We have before referred to these and other kindred investigations as really forming a new epoch in practical mechanics. It was the conviction that he alone amongst his countrymen was in possession of the key to the solution of problems of this nature, which induced him, as we have elsewhere observed, in spite of professional and other objections, to undertake the task committed to him by the Admiralty of reporting upon the changes, introduced by Sir Robert Seppings,[a] into the construction of our ships of war.

In connection with this subject we may notice two other essays, one of which he contributed to Dr. Hutton's Mathematical Dictionary [b] and the other to the Philosophical Magazine.[c] The subject of one of them was the pressure of semifluid and cohesive substances, and was chiefly founded upon principles laid down in an early essay by Coulomb,[d] to which he has himself referred, as having furnished the principles of many of his investigations. The second originated in a very serious accident which occurred in one of our great breweries in consequence of the failure of the hoops of a vat of vast size : it was entitled An Inves-

---

[a] Supra, p. 350.   Works, vol. i. p. 536.

[b] Works, vol. ii. p. 166   [c] Works, vol ii. p. 159.

[d] " Sur une application des Règles de Maximis et Minimis à quelques Problèmes de Statique, relatifs à l'Architecture."—*Mem. des Savans Étrangers*, tom. vii. p. 343. See also Dr. Young's Works, vol. ii. p. 529.

tigation of the Pressure sustained by the Fixed Supports of Flexible Substances. It is not otherwise remarkable except as shewing his great promptitude in bringing his science to bear upon any subject to which his attention was called by local or other circumstances.

It was in connection with the investigations of Captain Kater, which we have elsewhere referred to,[a] that Young addressed two papers to the Royal Society, as well as some others to scientific journals. The first Memoir was read in the year 1818, and gave a very simple demonstration of a theorem which had been previously investigated by La Place, by the aid of a very difficult and refined analysis. The convertible pendulum employed in these researches performed its oscillations on knife edges, which, mathematically considered, were more or less perfect portions of cylindrical surfaces. Was Captain Kater justified in assuming the distance of the knife edges to be the length of the convertible pendulum, or was it necessary to apply a correction to it dependent upon the radii of the rolling cylinders of which those edges were portions? The theorem in question shewed that the first assumption was correct, and it further appeared, from the same investigations, that its correctness would not be sensibly affected by slight irregularities in the form of the knife edges, which are found to be inevitable, however carefully they might be formed. The same conclusion was still more easily deduced as a corollary to a theorem of Euler, as Dr. Young shewed in an Appendix to a second Memoir published in the following year, the contents of which we shall now proceed to notice.

This Memoir embraces three subjects. The first, the estimation of the probabilities of error in physical

---

[a] Supra, 350.

observations; a question which has occupied the attention of the greatest mathematicians of modern times,—of La Place, of Legendre, of Gauss, and of Bessel. The second, the effect of pressure in augmenting the mean density of the earth through the compressibility of the substances of which it is composed. And the third, the effect produced on the direction of a plumb-line and the vibrations of a pendulum by irregularities on the earth's surface, and of masses of materials near the place of observation whose densities are different from the mean density of the crust of the earth. These several questions have little connection with each other except through their common bearing on the solution of the problem upon which Captain Kater was at that time engaged.

We are accustomed to accept it as a fact that the mean of several measurements and observations is likely to be more accurate and trustworthy than one of a smaller number, and that the combination of a multitude of independent sources of error, whether they be confined between given limits or not, has a tendency to diminish the aggregate variation of their joint effect. Thus, the ratio of male to female births, so variable in a small number of families, becomes nearly, if not absolutely, constant for the whole kingdom : and however much the number of dead letters which pass through a country post-office may vary, those which reach the Metropolis will be found to bear, from year to year, a nearly constant ratio to the whole number sent. Such circumstances are apt to present to an unprepared mind an appearance of mysterious fatality, whilst even to a practised mathematician their explanation involves considerations of no ordinary difficulty and refinement.

The solution of this class of problems which Young

has proposed, is not the least remarkable of the many attempts which he has made, and with so much success, to evade the more elaborate processes which other analysts have felt it necessary to employ: his conclusions also are reduced, as is usual with him, to forms which are easily adapted to calculation, and are exemplified by their application to questions of great interest, both in history and literature, to some of which we have elsewhere had occasion to refer.[a]

It is in the determination of unknown elements in philosophical inquiries—and more especially in astronomy—from a great number of observations, that the question perpetually arises of so adjusting their errors or discrepancies as to obtain the most probable result. Such observations may furnish equations of condition much more numerous than the unknown quantities to be deduced from them. How are these equations to be treated, in order that the values of the elements obtained from the joint consideration of the whole of them may be invested with the highest authority which the observations can give? The method of least squares which is commonly employed for this purpose is undoubtedly one of the most valuable contributions which analysis has made to astronomy; but there are many cases where the formula which has been proposed by Dr. Young will serve to effect the same object with equal certainty, and with much greater rapidity. The application, however, of such methods should in all cases be made with great caution; for when the observations which we are discussing are made by one instrument or by one observer, and in all cases when the essential condition of absolute *fortuity* is wanting, the most refined applications of analysis for the determination of the minimum or the limits, of error, may become altogether nugatory. Such was the opinion expressed by Bessel in a letter to Dr. Young, with reference to this Memoir; but whilst we venture to deprecate the dogmatic assertion of extreme accuracy in many astronomical and other determinations to which the occasional abuse of these methods has given rise, we readily allow that their judicious use has been the real foundation of the increased accuracy which they are daily attaining.

The subject of the second part of this Memoir is equally interesting to the geologist and the astronomer. It has been sufficiently ascertained that the mean density of the earth bears to that of its crust a proportion of not less than three to two; and assuming that this density increases uniformly, or according to any other law, in passing from the surface to the centre, it may be asked, to what cause is this increase owing? The usual reply which was given to this question referred it to the increased proportion of metallic and heavier materials the farther we recede from the surface. Dr. Young was enabled, by an easy investigation, to show that this result might be explained by the compressibility of the ordinary substances of which the earth is composed, and that a modulus of elasticity equal to half the earth's radius, or about twelve million feet—which exceeds that of the hardest and most elastic material with which we are acquainted—would be more than sufficient for the purpose. A sphere of water, with a modulus of elasticity such as the experiments of Canton assigned to it, would give a much higher ratio between the superficial and mean density than is known to exist, whilst the disproportion would have been enormous if water had been replaced by air;—sufficiently great, in fact, even if extended to the much smaller globe of the moon, to afford a plausible explanation of the much agitated question of the disappearance of her atmosphere, by its absorption within those vast volcanic cavities by which it has been imagined that she is penetrated.

These researches of Dr. Young were very favourably noticed by La Place, in a Memoir on the Figure of the Earth, which appeared in the *Connaissance des Tems* for the following year. "Until now," says he, "mathematicians have not included in their researches the effect resulting from the compression of the strata. Dr. Young has called their attention to this subject by the ingenious remark that we may thus explain the increase of the density of the strata of the terrestrial spheroid." Young[a] when noticing, on another occasion, these and other remarks of this great analyst·on the density of the earth, proceeds to combat an opinion which he had expressed that the law of elasticity of solid bodies increased much more rapidly than their density, and to show that a modulus of ten million feet, acting according to his original assumption, would produce a spheroid with an ellipticity and distribution of density sufficiently conformable to the various observations which have been resorted to for the purpose of determining it, as well as to the effects which it produces on precession and nutation and the motions of the moon.

The investigations contained in the third and last part of this Memoir, pointed out, amongst other conclusions of importance, a considerable error in the correction usually applied in connection with experiments

[a] Works, vol. ii. p. 78. Remarks on La Place's latest computation of the Density of the Earth.

for determining the length of the seconds pendulum, for elevation above the level of the sea. The correction which Kater had applied in the first reduction of his experiments in the preceding year was shown to be too great by nearly one-third, and the error was recognised by him in a subsequent Memoir.[a] The final result of this and other theoretical corrections, applied to his first determination, increased the length of the pendulum by about seven ten-thousandths of an inch —a quantity considerably beyond the limits of error which were likely to occur in the measurement of the distances between the knife edges.

The propriety of this correction was at first doubted by La Place, but it has since been generally admitted. Young subsequently gave, in a short article in Brande's Journal,[b] a masterly vindication of the correctness of his conclusion.

The effect produced by the resistance of the air, and the law which it follows, could hardly escape the attention of one who was so much engaged with the theory of the reduction of pendulum experiments, at a period when they were made with so much diligence. There will be found in his works[c] a short Memoir on this subject, where the effects of some different laws of resistance are considered, more especially of such as are simply proportional to the velocity, which was indicated in some of Captain Kater's observations[d] at a later period.   Bessel[e] called attention to the necessity of introducing corrections for the inertia of the air put in motion by the pendulum, as well as for its buoyancy ;

---

[a] Philosophical Transactions for 1819, p. 353.
[b] Works, vol. ii. p. 99. Brande's Journal for 1826.
[c] Works, vol. ii. p. 93. Brande's Journal for 1823, vol. xx.
[d] Philosophical Transactions for 1819, p. 337.
[e] Berlin Memoirs for 1826. Astronomische Nachrichten, No. 128.

and very important experiments were instituted by
Colonel Sabine,[a] both in vacuo and in airs of different
densities, and in some of the gases, for determining both
the necessity and the amount of this correction. The
difficulty of eliminating all the sources of error in such
experiments seemed to be increased rather than diminished by the elaborate researches on the subject which
were instituted by the late Mr. F. Baily.[b] Their whole
theory has received an admirable discussion by Professor Stokes, in the Cambridge Transactions[c] for 1851;
by whom also we are promised a series of experiments
on the vibrations of pendulums in gaseous atmos-
pheres, which can hardly fail to lead to results of no
ordinary importance.

There were few subjects of public interest, where
investigations involving a difficult application of mechanical principles were concerned, in which Young's
assistance was not required ; and when required it was
rarely withheld. It is recorded in his Journals, that
when he was a medical student· in London, in his
twenty-first year, a Mr. Churchman, the author of a
Magnetic Atlas, proposed to him a problem for determining the dip of a magnetic needle, in case it was
attracted to two magnetic poles any where situated on
the surface of the earth. After making the question
the subject of his night thoughts, he produced in the
morning a correct and not inelegant solution of it, upon
three different suppositions : first, when the attractions
were equal; secondly and thirdly, when they varied
inversely as the distance or its square. The results

---

[a] Philosophical Transactions, 1829.
[b] Philosophical Transactions, 1832.
[c] Vol. ix., part 2. On the Effect of the Internal Friction of Fluids on
the Motion of Pendulums, p. 8.

of any of these hypotheses, as might have been anticipated, would only approach to a very rude representation of the phenomena of the dip and variation of the needle; and the modifications of them which are suggested, rather than proposed, in his Lectures, are sufficient to show how little these phenomena had at that period been made the subject of accurate observation.

The observation of the movements of the magnetic needle in high latitudes, and the possible determination of the position of one of the magnetic poles, was one of the chief objects proposed by the first Arctic expedition under Sir John Ross and Captain Parry; and we must look to the results of the observations which were made by Colonel Sabine in the course of that expedition as having given the first great impulse to the systematic study of the phenomena of terrestrial magnetism; and it is to the same distinguished observer that we are chiefly indebted for the organization of the vast system of magnetic observatories which have been established in later times, and for the complete discussion of the observations which they have afforded, and which have totally changed the whole aspect of the science. It appeared from the statement which he communicated to the Royal Society upon his return,[a] that the directive force of the horizontal needle in the Arctic regions was so much reduced by the greatness of the dip, that the best suspended compasses not only traversed with great difficulty, but were so much dominated by the magnetism of the masses of iron, whether induced or permanent, of the ships themselves, that their indications became utterly useless. The attention of Dr. Young was naturally called not only to the general inferences with respect to the

[a] Philosophical Transactions for 1819.

distribution and variation of intensity of the earth's magnetism which followed from these important observations, but also in a more especial manner, from his connection with nautical astronomy, as Editor of the Nautical Almanac, to the practical expedients then recently proposed in their first form by Mr. Barlow, for neutralising, under ordinary circumstances, the disturbing action of the magnetism of the ship. The short Memoir[a] which he wrote upon this subject—though its value has been superseded by later investigations—is remarkable for the thorough mastery which it shows of the subject, both in its theoretical and practical bearings; he gives a table of corrections for clearing the compass of the regular effect of the ship's permanent attraction for different values of the dip, and for all angular distances of the magnetic North from the line joining two neutral points or positions of no disturbance in the ship: pointing out also some disturbances in these corrections which do not vary with the dip, and which he attributes to the temporary or induced magnetism of portions of soft iron in the ship. He then proceeds to some observations, characterised by his usual acuteness, on the theory of Mr. Barlow's sphere, and on the circumstances which may limit the sufficiency of the correction which it affords.

It has been generally observed that the advances of science go hand in hand with its useful applications to the business of life. It was the careful study of the theory and phenomena of magnetism with a view to their action on the needle which enabled Mr. Barlow, to his lasting honour, to make the first great step towards protecting its movements from the effects

[a] Works, vol. ii. p. 102.

of local disturbances. It was the same union of
theory and practice which guided the Astronomer
Royal in the application of his compensating mag-
nets in ships constructed of iron plates strongly
magnetised by the processes of hammering and rolling
which they have undergone; an application which
must ever be regarded as one of the most valuable
gifts which abstract science has made to navigation,
notwithstanding the doubts which have been thrown
upon its permanent efficiency, in certain cases, by some
recent observations of Dr. Scoresby.

When Young was first appointed secretary to the
Board of Longitude, he proposed to compile, or super-
intend the compilation of, a Corpus Astronomiæ, in a
series of treatises, comprehending all that was known,
or rather all that was required to be known, of practical, plane, and physical astronomy. The only part
of this scheme that was ever executed, was a small
octavo volume, entitled Elementary Illustrations of
the Celestial Mechanics of La Place, which was published in 1821. It embraces the laws of equilibrium
and motion, both of solid bodies and fluids, and includes among the latter several of the most important
propositions on the theory of the oscillations of the
sea and the atmosphere, exhibited in a much more
simple form than that which they assume in the great
work from which they are taken. This Treatise presents a somewhat mosaic character, being preceded by
the Rudiments of Mathematics as given in his Lectures, whilst the propositions transferred from the Mécanique Céleste are intermixed throughout with demonstrations and remarks founded upon his own views
on the elementary doctrines of motion and other
subjects, which, though often original and extremely

valuable, are altogether out of harmony, both in character and form, with the singularly systematic treatment which they have received in the original.

We have elsewhere had occasion to call attention to the valuable Appendix which is added to this Treatise, on the Cohesion of Fluids.[a]

Dr. Young was accustomed to regard his Theory of the Tides as nearly the most original and successful of his physico-mathematical investigations. The substance of it was stated with great clearness and precision in his Lectures;[b] but it was first presented, of course anonymously, in its completely developed form, in Nicholson's Journal for 1813;[c] as, however, it was probably little read and still less understood, it passed into entire obscurity and was never noticed.

At a later period, he revised his theory in the Article Tides, printed in the Supplement to the Encyclopædia Britannica,[d] when his more matured study of the works of La Place and of the processes of modern analysis, enabled him to give to his investigations a more complete development; and. he subsequently gave, in the Royal Institution Journal,[e] a popular exposition,—as far as so difficult a subject admitted of being made so, —of the results which he had obtained, a considerable part of which had previously appeared in the Quarterly Review.[f] So little, however, had public attention been called to these researches, notwithstanding the celebrity which had long been attached to his name, that when the present Astronomer Royal was preparing his well-known Article on Waves and Tides for the Encyclopædia Metropolitana, he was ignorant of their existence. "You ask my opinion," says he, in a letter

[a] Works, vol. i. p. 485.
[b] Lecture xlvii. p. 576.
[c] Works, vol. ii. p. 262.
[d] Works, vol. ii. p. 291.
[e] Works, vol. ii. p. 336.
[f] For October, 1811.

addressed to me, "of Dr. Young's Researches on Tides. As far as they go, they are capital; when I was writing my Article, I totally forgot Dr. Young, although I well knew that in writing on *any* physical subject it is but ordinary prudence to look at him first." [a]

It is well known that Newton pointed out and assigned generally, not only the nature and the magnitude of the periodical forces which are concerned in producing the tides, but likewise indicated their true character as undulations, in one very remarkable proposition,[b] as well as in a special explanation of the phenomena presented by the tides of the Port of Batsha [c] The equilibrium theory of Daniel Bernoulli[d] adopted the first part of Newton's views, but altogether neglected the second.

It had been shown that if the earth was a spherical body covered with water, and if both the earth and moon were at rest, the water would assume the form of a spheroid of equilibrium, of extremely small eccentricity, such as would be due to the disturbing action of the moon's forces.   A similar but less eccentric spheroid would be formed beneath the sun.   Under such circumstances the joint effect of the elevations or depressions of the two spheroids would produce the elevation or depression of the water, or the tide.   The theory *further assumes that the same effects would follow if the earth revolved round her axis and the earth and*

  [a] Works, vol. ii. p. 262.   Note
  [b] Principia, lib. i. prop. 66, cor. 19.
  [c] Principia, lib. iii. prop. 24, *ad finem.*
  [d] Traité sur le Flux et Réflux de la Mer.   An Essay written in 1740, for the prize offered by the Académie des Sciences at Paris.   Euler and Maclaurin were also competitors for and sharers of the prize.   All these Treatises are given in the edition of Newton's Principia by the Jesuits Le Seur and Jacquier.

moon in their orbits, and that no effect was produced by the spontaneous oscillations of the sea. Totally false as are the principal assumptions upon which this theory is founded, it is extremely remarkable that it not only sufficiently separates from each other the principal movements of the tides, but represents generally the law and order of succession of the periodical phenomena which they present. " The greatest mathematicians and the most laborious observers of the present day," says Professor Airy, "including Sir John Lubbock and Dr. Whewell among the number, have agreed equally in rejecting the *foundation* of this theory, and comparing all their observations with its results."

The same eminent authority has pronounced the theory proposed by La Place in the Mécanique Céleste, —if viewed with reference to the boldness and comprehensive character of its design rather than to the success of its execution—" as one of the most splendid works of the greatest mathematician of the past age." The problem, however, was not considered by him in the most general form which it is capable of receiving. He assumed the earth to be entirely covered by water, and its depth to be uniform, at least throughout the same parallel of latitude, and he neglected the resistance both of the particles of the fluid amongst each other, and of that which arises from the irregular surfaces in the channels over which the tide is transmitted. He was consequently obliged to omit the consideration of the tides in canals, rivers, and narrow seas, which constitute some of the most interesting, and by no means the most unmanageable, of the problems which later, and even in some respects more simple, investigations of the oscillations of the sea have brought within the control of analysis. Imperfect, however, as the results of this theory were as it came from the hand of its author, their importance cannot easily be estimated too highly. Dr. Young adopted the general principles which they involved, though he has subjected them to a totally different treatment; and Professor Airy, who has materially simplified the investigations which it contains, by rejecting some conditions which they included, such as the density of the sea, by which they were made needlessly difficult and complicated, has not only verified the more remarkable of the conclusions at which La Place arrived, but has also made important use of his methods in his own theory of waves and tides, which is by far the most complete and comprehensive that has ever yet appeared.

There is one result of a very unexpected kind, which La Place regarded as one of the happiest of his discoveries,—it is the entire evanescence, if the sea be of uniform depth, of the diurnal tide in elevation, but not in horizontal motion. At the equator, under such circumstances, the water moves north and south, resting for a moment at the change of motion. At the poles the motion is transverse to the meridian passing through the luminary. At all other points on the earth's surface it is perpetually changing. Few persons have attempted to follow the mazes of the difficult analysis by which this great mathematician has arrived at this conclusion, which has been verified by the Astronomer Royal.[a] Its correctness, however, has been disputed by Dr. Young,[b] who contends that the diurnal tide will not disappear, unless the depth of the sea be not merely uniform, but evanescent.

Though Dr. Young was not disposed to give his

[a] Tides and Waves, § 102, Encyclopædia Metropolitana.
[b] Works, vol. ii. p. 357.

assent to the results of an extremely difficult analysis,
—which few persons of his age could venture to follow,
and which might appear to those who could not trace
them through the long train of consequences which
connected them with the principles from which they
were deduced, to be either paradoxical or contradictory
to the first principles of mechanics—he was sufficiently
prepared to seize the general purport of other parts of
this comprehensive theory; and by divesting it of the
unnecessary generalizations by which it was encum-
bered, not only to bring its principles to bear immediately upon the ordinary phenomena of the tides, but
to apply it to cases which it was otherwise incompetent
to reach. Such were the tides of narrow seas and
rivers, and the modifications which those tides undergo
from the effects of the resistance of the particles of
water upon each other, or upon the channels through
which they are propagated. The same questions have
been made the principal subject of the investigations
of the Astronomer Royal, in his Article on Tides
and Waves, in the Encyclopædia Metropolitana, where
they have been treated with that rare combination
of mathematical skill and clearness and completeness of exposition for which all his writings are so
remarkable. It will be found, however, that there are
not many of his results which Young had not already
attained, though in a much less definite form, by
methods which are, it is true, much less regular and
systematic, but which are not less distinguished for
the sagacity and philosophical power which they display.

There are two principal species of waves which the
theory of the tides requires us to consider. The first
are the great waves of the ocean, produced by the ac-

tion of the moon and sun, such as are alone considered
in the equilibrium theory, where they are assumed
immediately to obey the action of the forces, with
whose periods also—for all such forces are periodic—
they entirely coincide. Such waves are called *forced*
waves, as being compulsory and not spontaneous. The
second class are those which are primarily produced by
the disturbing action of the periodical forces, but which
follow spontaneously the laws of oscillation of water.
If the length of such waves be great, but less than one
thousand times the depth of the water, the velocity of
their propagation is sensibly dependent upon that depth
only, being equal to the velocity which a free body
would acquire by the action of gravity[a] if it fell
through a space equal to one half of it. If the length
of the waves be not greater than the depth of the
water, their velocity will be proportional to the square
roots of their length.[b] For intermediate relative
values of the lengths of the waves and of the depths of
the water, the velocity is dependent upon both these
elements, by a somewhat complicated law. It is the
first of these classes of free or spontaneous waves only,
which have hitherto been considered in the theory of
the tides.

There are two classes of *forced* waves, produced
respectively by the lunar and solar forces acting upon
every particle of the sea; the first of which is more
than twice as great as the second. They form one great
wave by their interference, producing the two tides of
each tidal day of about twenty-four hours and fifty minutes; when the solar and lunar tides entirely corroborate each other, they tend to form the spring tide, and

---

[a] Encyclopædia Metropolitana, Tides and Waves, § 171.
[b] This is Newton's proposition. Principia, book ii. prop. 45.

the neap tide when they oppose each other. But these effects are materially modified in their magnitudes, and in some degree also in the time of their occurrence, by other waves which also interfere with them, as well as by the resistances which they experience.

In fact, the same forces which agitate the whole mass of the water, to produce the *forced* waves, produce also spontaneous or *free* waves, whose natural period of undulation, as we have seen, is determined by the depth of the sea. If this depth was about thirteen miles or fourteen miles, the free wave would move with nearly the same velocity as the solar wave at the equator in one case, or as the lunar wave in the other. In such cases the free wave would synchronise with the solar or lunar tide, and produce by its corroboration a maximum effect. If the depths of the sea were greater or less than is required to produce synchronous oscillations, the free would precede the forced wave in one case and lag behind it in the other; but their periods of oscillation would be sooner or later compelled to synchronise with those of the periodical forces; the forced waves would be increased by them in the first case and diminished in the second,—the first being called a *direct* or *positive*, and the second an *indirect* or *negative* wave.

Young assimilated these effects to those which would be exhibited by a compound pendulum under the following circumstances. Let there be two pendulums one of which naturally vibrates in the period of the forces, whether of the sun or moon, and the other in that of the spontaneous oscillations of the sea; let the first pendulum be supposed to vibrate round a fixed centre, and let its extremity carry the second; then whatever be the initial condition of the pendulums, they will sooner or later arrive at a state of permanence, and the period of vibration of the second pendulum with a moveable centre of suspension will become identical with that of the first, but its motion will be in the same or in opposite directions to that of its centre, according as the time of this compulsory vibration is greater or less than that of its natural oscillations; and inasmuch as these vibrations ultimately become symmetrical with respect to each other, passing their middle points at the same time, it will follow that the maximum effect of the second pendulum, representing that of the free oscillations of the sea, will corroborate the forced oscillations due to the periodical forces for direct waves, and oppose it on the other. It will follow, therefore, generally, that the time of *high* water will coincide with the passage of the luminary over the meridian in the first case and with that of *low* water in the other.

The theorem for determining the laws of vibration of a pendulum with a moveable centre of suspension in a medium, whether absolutely non-resisting or where the resistance varies according to the simple power of the velocity or its square, were investigated by Young in his first published Essay on Tides, partly by the aid of simple and elegant geometrical constructions and partly by other expedients, which display in an extraordinary degree his great resources in dealing with problems which were beyond the legitimate powers of the machinery which was brought to bear upon them : it was like the capture of a fortified town by open assault, without resorting to the more regular and slow, but therefore more certain approaches which the rules of war prescribe. In the revised and amplified form of this

Essay, which is given in the Supplement to the Encyclopædia Britannica, the same problems are solved by analytical processes which, though greatly deficient in symmetry and elegance, are not only complete but also in a form immediately adapted to the deduction of the inferences which the phenomena of the tides should present in conformity with the refined conception by which the causes which produce them were thus brought into immediate connection with each other.

There exists no method of determining from observation the effects which resistances produce upon the time of high water, or the law according to which they vary. La Place had neglected the consideration of them as being altogether inconsiderable; but Young, relying upon some calculations and experiments of Du Buat, which he has noticed in his Memoir on Hydraulics and elsewhere, had arrived at a very different conclusion. Assuming such resistances to vary according to the simple power of the velocity, they would be found not to disturb the regularity of the oscillations concerned, only retarding them when direct and accelerating them when inverted by a quantity which admits of a definite expression. For an equal resistance varying as the square of the velocity, the displacement of the time of high water would not be very materially different; but if we pass from general to particular effects, such a resistance would serve to explain some peculiar circumstances in the phenomena of the tides which have caused considerable difficulty and embarrassment: thus the proportion of the lunar to the solar forces which has been deduced from the heights of the spring and neap tides,—being assumed as proportional to their sum in one case and to their difference in the other,—has been found to be much greater than other and more trustworthy results furnished by the lunar theory would warrant; and La Place, who found this proportion, as deduced from the tides of Brest, to be three to one, instead of about five to two as it should have been, was obliged to resort to some local peculiarities to account for a discrepancy so considerable. Young, however, was enabled to give at least a plausible explanation of this anomaly, by shewing that the proportion of the effects of resistance upon the lunar and solar tides would approach more nearly to that of the periods than of the magnitudes of the forces which produce them, and that consequently the residual tides, when those effects are abstracted, would no longer furnish the means of determining, unless the effects of the resistances were given, the proportion of the forces of the sun and moon. Another anomaly, of a still more embarrassing description, namely, the retardation of the time of the highest tides, by intervals varying from half a day to a day and a half, behind the time of new and full moon, has been shown by Young, upon very probable grounds, to be referable to a similar cause.

Dr. Young has applied his theory with great success to the tides of canals or narrow seas, making any angle with the meridian: if such seas coincide or nearly coincide in direction with the meridian, the periodical forces vanish; if they extend east and west to a great length, the phenomena which they present will approximate to those of the open sea; if that extent be comparatively limited, and the tides be reflected from the terminating shores, there will be no tide but a great horizontal motion at the middle, and it will be high water at the west when it is low water at the east, and conversely. If such a sea or lake be not more than about eight degrees across from east to west, the waves would be direct, if its depth exceeded two hundred yards; if the depth was not less than one mile the waves would be of a similar character, if its length was not less than twenty-five degrees; whilst for a sea like the Atlantic, whose breadth across varies from fifty to sixty degrees, it would require a depth of four miles to produce direct waves : and as there is reason to conclude that the waves of this sea are not direct but inverted, we have a limit of average depth which it cannot exceed;—it is probably considerably less than four miles.

The same principles of calculation are applicable to the explanation of the tides of the atmosphere : they will be very small at the poles, of moderate amount at the equator, but about the latitude of 42°, where the rotatory velocity of the earth is nearly equal to that with which any impression is transmitted by the atmosphere, the height of the oscillations will only be limited by the resistances, the greatest elevation occurring about one hour after the transit of the luminary. It is unfortunate that no sufficient observations have been made upon atmospheric waves to enable us to bring them to the test of this or any other theory.

Though Dr. Young has indicated the general cause of the rapid rise of river tides compared with their slower fall, he has not pursued the application of his theory to the detailed examination of the phenomena which they exhibit. The theory of such tides and the effects of friction upon them, have been very fully investigated by the Astronomer Royal ; and it would be difficult to refer to any physical essay which has appeared in later times where an extremely difficult analysis has been so successfully brought to bear upon the explanation of so great a number of curious and apparently anomalous facts of observation. The method which he has adopted in the treatment of this and every other department of this theory is extremely different from that which has been followed by Dr. Young ; and whilst we admire the straightforward and systematic march of the investigations which is pursued by the one, and his lucid and vigorous interpretation of the results which he obtains, we cannot fail to do justice to the rare sagacity by which the other was enabled to explain the machinery of the tides by a conception so novel and ingenious, and to deduce from it a series of results which had evaded the laborious researches of the greatest of modern writers on the mechanism of the universe.

CHAPTER XV.

MISCELLANEOUS EVENTS IN LATER LIFE.   HIS DEATH.

WE have had occasion to mention, in our account of Dr. Young's literary and scientific labours, those events of his later life which were especially connected with them, leaving, as might be expected, very few others sufficiently important to be noticed. Few, however, and unimportant as they are, some reference to them is more or less necessary to give some degree of continuity to our narrative; and it may be urged as an additional reason for noticing them that it is usually considered as one of the privileges of those who have deserved well of mankind that more or less of interest is always attached to every detail which tends to make us familiar with their habits and characters.

His course of life, considered apart from the variety of his occupations, was remarkably uniform. He resided in London from November to June, and at Worthing from July to the end of October. His professional engagements restricted his visits elsewhere within very narrow limits; though we find him occasionally at Sunninghill, with Mr. George Ellis, or with Mr. Gurney in Norfolk. But he had really no taste for life in the country; he was one of those who thought that no one who was able to live in London would be content to live elsewhere. He loved occupation, and was never embarrassed by the variety of forms under which it presented itself. In writing to a friend, who complained of *ennui* and a want of resolution to employ himself, he says:—

" About this time last year,"—the letter is dated December, 1820,—" I was giving myself a holiday of a few weeks, and I fell into a sort of fidgetty languor, and fancied I was growing old. It wore off very soon, however; and I am convinced there is no remedy so effectual for this and other intellectual diseases as plenty of employment, without over fatigue and anxiety. This autumn I have been, in fact, going on with a work which I was then almost frightened at having undertaken, and am already printing the first part of it,[a] being only a translation with a commentary; it will do better without my name than with it. I am also writing over again my Article on Languages in the Quarterly Review, with many additions,[b] for the next Supplement of the Encyclopædia Britannica; and a Biographical Memoir on Lagrange will be almost as long, requiring a list of one hundred different papers on the most abstruse parts of the mathematics.[c] I have then the business of the Board of Longitude to manage, and some of the Royal Society. The Arctic expedition is now settled; but we are fitting out our astronomer for the Cape with all his books and instruments.[d] Then there is a Committee of Elegant Extracts to consider the tonnage of ships, appointed by the Royal Society, the Admiralty, the Board of Trade, and the Treasury—which will not take long, but I shall have the onus. Then there is my hospital—to speak nothing of my private patients, who are very discreet at this time of the year. Then I must not forget that I must shortly do a little more to the hieroglyphics; and after one

---

[a] Elementary Illustrations of the Celestial Mechanics of La Place, published in 1821.

[b] Works, vol. iii. p. 478.

[c] Works, vol. ii. p. 557.

[d] The late Rev. Fearon Fallows, the contemporary of myself and Sir John Herschel at Cambridge: an excellent mathematician, and a very zealous and skilful practical astronomer, who lost his life in attempting to carry on the business of the observatory, whilst labouring under the effects of a severe attack of fever. His observations at the Cape have been published, at the expense of the Admiralty, by the Astronomer Royal.

number more I shall be able to judge if the thing is worth continuing or not. I suppose the Review of Belzoni will give the subject some popularity.

" I have not seen the Article, but I suppose my friend Barrow will feel less remorse in exposing my infidelity to my professional consort than I have generally done myself. Certainly, if a man that is married to a profession cannot avoid keeping a mistress or two, he ought not to be the first to blazon to the world the liberties he takes."

At the conclusion of a letter full of lively observations, he adds—

" I do not believe that you are much the older for anything that occurred when you were a boy ; nor do I think that I should have been the worse *in health* if I had been less rigid in my regimen. It is well for me that I have not to live over again : I doubt if I should have made so good a use of my time as mere accident has compelled me to do. Many things I could certainly mend, and spare myself both time and trouble ; but, on the whole, if I had done very differently from what I have, I dare say I should have repented more than I now do of any thing ; and this is a tolerable retrospect of forty years of one's life. I have learned more or less perfectly a tolerable variety of things in this world ; but there are two things that I have never yet learned, and I suppose never shall—to get up and to go to bed. It is now past twelve o'clock, but I must write for an hour longer."

The Arctic Expedition under the command of Captain Parry had returned in the autumn of this year, and it was the duty of Young, as Secretary to the Board of Longitude, to examine the officers engaged in it, with a view of ascertaining whether they had reached a sufficiently high northern latitude to entitle them to a portion of the reward which had been offered by Parliament. In a letter on the subject of it he says :—

" And here is the *polar expedition* arrived, whom I am to examine on their oaths, to get them their five thousand pounds, which it seems will be well spent in lowering the price of oil by the information they have given the whalers. I imagine also they have set the practical question of the passage at rest, as it is obvious that there would be no reasonable chance of getting to Behrings' Straits in the short arctic summer of six weeks, even if there is a passage, which seems by no means improbable—though Barrow's ' Polar Bason,' is certainly nothing but a rock of ice—for they found that it was only near land that there was anything like a possibility of navigating, the mean annual temperature of the year being 0^0 on the islands, which is 30^0 lower than would be inferred from the analogy of the inhabited world. I should not, however, be surprised if the *curiosity* of the Admiralty prompted them to continue the research, and I have no objection to curiosity in others, though it is a great many years since I was scolded for that quality myself."

The same able and energetic writer who had first stimulated the public and the Admiralty to undertake these expeditions, was enabled, nearly a quarter of a century later, to rekindle it; and melancholy as the result of that renewed experiment is now known to have been, we venture to hope that the time is far distant when either dangers or failures will extinguish the spirit of daring enterprise which has ever been the great characteristic of our seamen, and the existence of which is the surest safeguard of our national greatness.

It was in writing to the same friend about three years before this time—in October, 1817—that he intimated his intention of establishing an Egyptian Society.

" I have done little in hieroglyphics," says he, " since I saw you; but I can never get to the end of them as long as there

are materials which exist unexamined and uncopied. I suppose
they might furnish employment to an academy of forty members
for half a century, and it will be enough for me to have discovered a mine by which others may enrich themselves. But I
do mean to make out more ; and in a year or two I shall publish what I have done—still anonymously, as far as the form
goes ; and then I intend to set about establishing something
between a society and a subscription for getting all the hieroglyphics in existence collected and published, with any explanations and comments which may be proposed in a separate
series—and perhaps for employing some poor Italian or Maltese
to scramble over Egypt in search of more. All this might be
done under the name of an Egyptian Society, without becoming
too prominent individually."

A year or two afterwards, this scheme was carried
into effect. Dr. Young became the Egyptian Society,
without colleague or assistant. The principal sub-
scribers to it were Mr. Gurney, Lord Montnorris,
Lord Aberdeen, Sir Joseph Banks, Sir W. Rouse
Boughton, Mr. William Hamilton, Mr. Marsden,
Mr. Taylor Combe, Mr. George Ellis, Dr. Butler, Mr.
Lloyd, and Mr. Drury, of Harrow. Two fasciculi were
published, containing about thirty plates, the last
fasciculus of the two being devoted entirely to the
Rosetta inscription, with a comparative index. The
costs of the engravings, however, were found to exceed
considerably the amount of the subscriptions—notwithstanding a large contribution from one of his friends
—and the publication was upon the point of being
abandoned, when it was proposed by some members of
the Royal Society of Literature, which had recently
been established and munificently endowed by the
Prince Regent, that the Society should adopt it as
their own. After some negociations, Dr. Young
agreed to the proposal, and continued, as before, to
edit the work, being allowed to exercise his own dis-

cretion with respect to documents which should be engraved. The papyri found by Mr. Grey, the inscriptions copied by Sir Gardner Wilkinson, and documents from other sources, supplied him with abundant materials. But the rich treasures collected by Mr. Bankes and his agents were withheld, with a somewhat unbecoming jealousy, from the publication, being reserved for a separate work which unhappily never appeared.

The appearance of Belzoni's Travels had excited more than common interest, not merely on account of his extraordinary discoveries and the courage and perseverance he had displayed in making them, but from the beautiful exhibition of the scenes in the Royal Tomb which he had discovered and opened at Thebes, where the fine alabaster sarcophagus was found which is now in the museum of Sir John Soane. Young had furnished Belzoni with some remarks on his plates, and also with an argument to show that the tomb was that of Psammes the son of Necho, and that the inscriptions upon it, as far as their purport could then be made out, would agree sufficiently well with the historical notices relating to the father which are found in Herodotus and in the Second Book of Chronicles. These observations were preceded by copious extracts from the Article Egypt, in the Encyclopædia, the whole designed to call public attention to those researches, and to furnish Barrow, who reviewed the book, with an opportunity of noticing and popularizing them, as he had undertaken to do. The result of all these preparations was very unsatisfactory to Young; for, in the first place, some very cogent arguments urged by Mr. Bankes, as well as other considerations, induced him to think that he had been mistaken in his identification of the names of the kings; and, in the second place, Barrow not only failed in his promise to make the Review a vehicle for an analysis of his researches, but he spoke of him in terms which rather recognized his diligence than his sagacity.

" You know," says he, in writing to Mr. Gurney, "how little I undervalue the praise of diligence, believing, as you are aware I do, that there is little else that distinguishes man from man. But surely something might have been said of sagacity, if not of talent, where the subject was such as to render mere *diligence* almost a negative merit. But no matter ; I know myself what he ought to have said, and that is the true satisfaction after all."

The summer and autumn of 1820 were the last which he passed at Worthing. His connection with the Board of Longitude had made his professional emoluments less important to him than they once were, and he had long contemplated a tour in Italy, to which he proposed devoting the following summer.[a] In the execution of this project, he started, in company with Mrs. Young, in the middle of June, 1821, and reached Paris in sufficient time to attend a meeting of the Institute, where he met La Place, Cuvier, Arago, Humboldt, and some of the other great men, who made it, at that period, by far the most illustrious scientific body in Europe. Though his optical theories had already been made known by the able advocacy of Arago, and had recently received in the bosom of the Institute itself a striking confirmation and extension

[a] Mr. Hodgkin, the companion of his studies at Youngsbury, when informed of his projected tour, had asked him, in the words of the poet—

Et quæ tanta fuit Romam tibi causa videndi ?

when his prompt reply—

Libertas, quæ sera tamen, respexit inertem,

expressed the somewhat buoyant feeling of pleasure at his emancipation, not from his usual, but his compulsory, labours.

by Fresnel's well-known Memoir on Diffraction, they had hitherto made few converts ; whilst his hieroglyphical researches had not yet become a popular topic of discussion, Champollion having only lately left his retirement at Grenoble, and not having yet emerged from obscurity. Though cordially welcomed by Arago and Humboldt, his reception was not such as he experienced at his subsequent visits, when other circumstances had directed public attention both to his literary and scientific discoveries.

He took the usual route through Lyons and Chambery, over Mount Cenis, to Turin ; and, like all travellers, he was delighted with the first aspect of the greater Alpine scenery :—

" We were delighted," says he, " beyond measure with Savoy, a country which seems too little known to travellers in comparison with Switzerland, at least it far exceeds any idea which I had formed of Switzerland without having seen it.   Turin is a most magnificent city, and deserving of a better fate than to be betrayed into a demonstration of independence by the imbecility of its sovereign, and then to have its most respectable inhabitants imprisoned for the acceptance of the very constitution which he offered to them."

Historians however will probably be disposed to touch lightly upon the untoward events which discredited the opening of the reign of this unhappy sovereign, when they are also required to record the courage and self-sacrifice which marked its conclusion.

The great Egyptian Museum, of which the collection formed by Drovetti was the basis, and which furnished so many valuable materials to the researches of Champollion and Lepsius, was not yet established.

At Genoa he renewed the acquaintance which he had formed at Gotha, on his German tour, with the Baron de Zach—an astronomer, a scholar, an antiquary and the most indefatigable of correspondents—who, during nearly half a century, continued to retail, in the most agreeable form, the gossip of the astronomical world.

" He lives," says Young, "with the Duchess of Gotha, complaining bitterly that he has no intercourse with civilized society, though he publishes every month a volume of astronomical correspondence—and still a little out of humour with the courts which have made the Queen of Etruria unable to pay for the instruments which she has ordered, through him, for the new Observatory at Lucca, so that he has had to pay for them himself."

This was, in fact, the dominant age of the Holy Alliance, when every act of those who had been connected with the family of Napoleon, even when designed exclusively for the public benefit, was repudiated, and when every indication of a tendency to opinions in favour of a constitutional government was promptly and sternly repressed.[a]

Having recrossed the Apennines, he proceeded by Pesaro, Foligno, and Terni to Rome, where he passed the last half of July and the first week in August, before the season of fevers had set in : but they found them very general upon their return about the end of the same month : the period at which they begin is greatly dependent upon the range of the temperature. Mr. Dodwell, whom he had known at Cambridge, acted as their guide to the more remarkable monuments of antiquity and art. He was an artist and a scholar, and the author of Travels in Greece, which

---

[a] Mr. De Morgan has called my attention to a curious example of this spirit, which is noticed in a letter addressed by Zach to Mr. F. Baily. In the course of a criticism on the advantages which arise from different observers comparing their methods together, he had added a quotation from Montaigne—" *Un esprit doit se frotter contre un autre.*" This was struck out by the *censure.*

were magnificently illustrated : he was domiciliated
at Rome, where he had married a Roman lady celebrated for her beauty and accomplishments. At Naples
he found Sir William Gell, who was contemplating
a visit to Egypt, though he never accomplished it.
He also had addressed, in the preceding February,
inquiries to Dr. Young respecting his Hieroglyphical
Dictionary and his Article Egypt, which he knew
were in the hands of Mr. Bankes, and copies of which
had been presented, through Mr. Dodwell, to the
Vatican Library. He afterwards maintained a lively
and interesting correspondence with him, which is
printed in the third volume of his works.

" Naples," says Young, " delighted us extremely ; and our
expedition to Pæstum repaid us better than I had expected ;
but much more by the beauty of the scenery about Salerno
than by the magnificent copies of the cork models which we
had seen in London, for the ruins seem to be perfect imitations of pieces of cork on a large scale. Gell says there is a
deplorable want of literary society at Naples. We fell into a
good deal of society at Rome, chiefly among the diplomatic
people."

Young's route on his return from Rome was through
Sienna to Pisa and Leghorn, and thence to Florence :—

" Pisa amply repaid us for taking this circuitous route ;
Leghorn, if possible, still more. But what you will be better
pleased to hear (he is writing to Mr. Gurney), is the discovery
that I made of a *bilinguar stone among Drovetti's things*, which
promises to be an invaluable supplement to the Rosetta inscription, as I dare say Drovetti is well aware. There are very few
distinct hieroglyphic characters about the tablet, and the rings
for the name of the king are left blank ; but there are one or
two well-known personages of the Egyptian Pantheon whom I
shall be glad to find named in Greek, and the blank names can
be of little consequence, as they must have been some of the
dynasty of the Ptolemies, and I think there are some emblems

of Ptolemy Philopater. Under the tablet are about fifteen lines of the enchorial character, and about thirty-two in Greek, not at all distinctly legible, but nowhere totally effaced, so that I believe with care every part of the inscriptions may be legible.

" I could not get leave to take a copy, the merchant having no authority to do anything beyond the safe custody of the collection. But he has consented that I should send an experienced artist from Florence, to take two casts, or rather impressions, of the stone, one or both of which I hope Drovetti will let me have, for myself or for the Museum. on fair terms; but if he does not, I have only stipulated that whenever the collection is embarked, the copies shall remain safe at Leghorn until it has arrived safe at the place of its destination without injury from shipwreck or other accidents ; and I shall have the satisfaction of thinking that I have at least done something for the second great treasure of Egyptian literature.''

In the note which Young addressed to Drovetti's agent on the subject of this tablet, he urged, as a reason for his asking for a cast of it, that *he was the only person living who could fully appreciate its value.*[a] He justified the use of this language, which, though at that time literally true, afterwards exposed him to a charge of presumption,[b] on the ground that it was such as a mercantile man was most likely to understand as a reason for his application. The very urgency, however, with which the application was made, was probably the cause of its failure, as Drovetti very naturally concluded that the greater the importance of this inscription, the greater would be the depreciation of the value of the whole collection from its publication before it had passed from his hands. It was not until seven years afterwards that Dr. Young

[a] A copy of this letter is given in his Account of Hieroglyphical Discoveries. See Works, vol. iii. p. 287.

[b] In an Essay by Mr. Peyron, of Turin. See Dr. Young's letter respecting it, Works, vol. iii. p. 398, and Peyron's reply, p. 422.

received, from the Chevalier San Quintino, the cast which he had once been so anxious to possess.[a] It had then lost much of its value, inasmuch as other documents had been in the mean time brought to light, which furnished much of the information which it was designed to supply. The enchorial inscription also was found to be nearly, if not altogether, illegible.

The travellers, upon their arrival at Florence, found letters giving very alarming accounts of the health of Mrs. Young's mother, which induced them to hasten their departure from Italy: after visiting Venice and Milan, they proceeded by the ordinary route over the Simplon to Geneva, where they received intelligence of her death.

"Our expedition," says he, "has been extremely prosperous and, like most other things which I have done in my life, I am very glad that I have done it, though I am by no means sure that I should have the resolution to do it again. It seems like the last act of my boyhood, and the first of my old age ; on the one hand a sort of finish to my Latin and Greek, and on the other a setting at defiance all professional conveniences in a way that may be deemed very imprudent in a servant of the public. But I do not owe the public much, and I suppose I shall never be paid much of what the public owes me.

"Of the science or literature of this country I know nothing: but I cannot help fancying that Pozzo di Borgo must have been dreaming when he told me at Paris that the Italians were making great strides in the improvement of the human intellect. I do not think there are any living poets of transcendent merit: none certainly to rival some of ours: in painting they have nothing but a few good draughtsmen and copyists: in sculpture, they have Canova who probably comes next to Michael Angelo ; they have Thorwaldsen, Bartelini, and a few others, about as good as our own: their taste for music seems to be altogether exhausted, and we sought in vain for a little

[a] See Chevalier San Quintino's letter, Dr. Young's Works, vol. iii. p. 389.

harmony at St. Peter's and the Pope's Choristers. At Naples, however, their opera and their ballet is well mounted: and the theatre of San Carlo illuminated was the most magnificent spectacle I ever beheld."

From Geneva, the travellers proceeded rapidly through Switzerland to Schaffhausen, and. thence by the usual route, through the valley of the Rhine, to London, where they arrived about the end of October.

A wish had been expressed by Mr. Gurney to possess a portrait of Young, and negotiations were entered into, through Mr. Chantrey, the sculptor, to induce Sir Thomas Lawrence, who was at that time in the zenith of his reputation and overwhelmed with engagements, to paint it. In a letter, written at the end of September, 1822, he says :—

" The Maxwells intend to spend the greater part of the winter in Florence, and Mrs. Young and myself have agreed to escort them as far as Paris. I called yesterday at Chantrey's ; he is still strenuous in desiring me to make the application to Lawrence through him ; while I am absent he promises to complete the negociation, and I will let you know his success when I return. I am told that Lawrence will certainly undertake it, and even his beginning it will be the greatest—or rather the only—personal honour that I have ever received ; for which, as for sundry other particulars, I shall not forget my obligations to you. I hope, for the sake *of my friends and the. public,* that I shall not be blown up in the steam-boat before this important affair is completed, and still more before I have made another attempt at Paris to aim another blow at Drovetti and his stone of Menouf."

The portrait was not only undertaken by Lawrence, but, what was not always the case, it was finished by him. It was the original from which the engraving which forms the frontispiece of this volume was taken. It was said of this great painter, that he rarely failed

to realize whatever was most distinguished in the
intellectual expression of the face of a man, or graceful
and attractive in that of a woman ; and his portrait of
Young was no exception to the truth of this observation.

A letter addressed to Miss Caroline Maxwell, now
Countess of Buchan, on her route to Florence, refers to
some occurrences which signalized this visit to Paris,
and which have been elsewhere more particularly
noticed.[a]

"I have been extremely interested to-day at a sitting of the
Academy of Inscriptions. The principal paper that was read
belonged as much to my pursuits as the one I heard on Monday
at the Academy of Sciences—both being an extension of my
own researches, this on hieroglyphics as that was on optics ; and
its author, M. Champollion, has adopted all my interpretations,
almost without alteration ; but he has had the good fortune to
discover several important documents which were unknown to
me. . . . . . . This morning has been occupied with optical
discussions with Fresnel, who really has been very ingenious in
extending my theory of light, and who is doing himself very
great credit by his investigations. M. Ampère has come again
to talk of magnetism. Champollion is to be here on Sunday,
and Dureau de la Malle, a *bel esprit* and a poet, who brought
me a letter from Humboldt last year, is to be here on Monday."

It was Arago who introduced Champollion to Dr.
Young, who gave him—as I am informed by Mrs.
Young, who was present at the interview—the most
cordial reception, expressing the pleasure which it
afforded him to welcome a successor to his hieroglyphical studies who possessed leisure and so many qualifications to pursue them with effect. He readily promised him also whatever assistance his own collations of
the Rosetta stone and other collections could give him.

The letter of Champollion to M. Dacier, which shortly

---

[a] Supra, p. 321.

afterwards appeared, tended not a little to dissipate these flattering illusions, and rendered it necessary for him to take some measures for vindicating his own claims to discoveries which had either been ignored or misrepresented in this publication. Was he to persevere, as hitherto, in a vain attempt to preserve his anonymous character, now that his scientific celebrity was too great to be concealed, or was he, as he himself expressed it, "to throw away his cane and wig and show his bare forehead to the public, undefended and without disguise?" His more intimate friends were strenuous in urging him to adopt this second course, not merely as due to his public character, but as in reality calculated to increase rather than diminish his practice as a physician. The recent discovery also of the papyri of Mr. Grey, and the new views which they opened to him respecting the extent to which an alphabetic element was used in enchorial texts and in the expression of Egyptian as well as foreign names, supplied an additional motive for bringing them before the public, in connection with his own vindication. In a letter to Mr. Gurney, written on St. Andrew's Day, the anniversary of the Royal Society, he announced his intention of bringing forth an octavo volume, under the title of "An Account of some Recent Discoveries in Egyptian Literature and Antiquities, by Thomas Young, &c. &c." The work was published at the beginning of February in the following year, so prompt was he in the execution of whatever he had once undertaken.

Though he ceased from this time to undertake any regular hieroglyphical investigation, excepting the collection of documents and the preparation of materials, from time to time, for the publications of the

Egyptian Society and for his Enchorial Dictionary, yet we find in his correspondence frequent references to various points of the controversy between himself and Champollion, which shortly afterwards began to rage with considerable violence. Nor was Champollion the only one who was disposed to trespass upon the rights which an unquestionable priority of publication had given him. The hieroglyphical vocabulary attached to the article Egypt, had been distributed amongst Egyptologers, in Paris and elsewhere, in the year 1818, and the article itself appeared in the early part of the following year. Some months afterwards, Jomard, one of the principal editors of the great French work on Egypt, read a memoir at the Académie des Inscriptions, announcing the discovery of the hieroglyphical numerals, which were conspicuously noticed in the Hieroglyphical Vocabulary, a copy of which, given to him by Young, had long been in his possession. A plagiarism so gross and so manifest was instantly and indignantly denounced, both at the Académie and in the Moniteur, by Humboldt,[a] who had studied both the Article and the vocabulary with the interest and admiration which was due to a work at once so learned and so original. M. Jomard, in a letter[b] to Young, endeavoured to slur over the appropriation of his discovery by asserting that he had made it out ten years before. It seemed to be the fate of Dr. Young, in every thing relating to his hieroglyphical researches, to be plundered, misrepresented or misunderstood.

The celebrated mummy case of Petemen, discovered by Cailliaud—which, as we have elsewhere shown,[c]

---

[a] See his letter, Dr. Young's Works, vol. iii. p. 208.
[b] See the letter, with Mr. Leitch's note, Works, vol. iii. p. 207.
[c] Supra. p. 332.

furnished the first decisive proof of the use of phonetic
hieroglyphics to express Egyptian as well as foreign
names, and served also to show that the ring which inclosed them was *not* used as a mark of phonetization—
exhibited upon the exterior of its lid a representation
of a zodiac, resembling in many of its characters the
zodiacs of Denderah and Esne, which some writers on
Egyptian antiquities had attempted to raise to an extreme antiquity. The Greek inscription[a] on this case,
which was extremely mutilated, was restored by Letronne, an eminent archæological scholar, in an Essay
on this and other Egyptian zodiacs, who appealed to
its date, near the close of the reign of Trajan, as
affording a very plausible argument, that other zodiacs
which resembled it were not nearly so ancient as they
had been generally assumed to be. He then proceeded to show, with no inconsiderable display of learning and ingenuity, that this zodiac of Petemen was
an astrological scheme of his nativity ; that similar
representations were by no means uncommon on monumental records of various kinds, and that there was
abundant historical evidence to show that astrological
ideas were very prevalent amongst the Egyptians about
the age to which those zodiacs were referred. This
Essay, soon after its publication, was communicated to
Dr. Young, who, in a postscript to a letter which he
had written to Arago on optical subjects, requested
him, whilst he thanked the author for his present, to
remind him that nearly every part of his theory had
been anticipated in the Article Egypt, where, in

---

[a] The translation of the restored inscription was—" Petemen, called also
Ammonius, whose father was Soter, the son of Cornelius Pollius, and
mother Cleopatra, the daughter of Ammonius, died at the age of twenty-
one years, four months, and twenty-two days, in the nineteenth year of
Trajan the lord, on the eighth of Payni."

an admirable chapter on the Egyptian Calendar, Young
has given very sufficient reasons for considering the
zodiac of Denderah as a mythological scheme, relating
to the birth of Isis :—

"The beetle which appears at the beginning of the series of
signs is the symbol of generation, where he is represented as
depositing his globe. On the opposite side is the head of Isis,
with her name as newly born. The two long female figures
are appropriate representations of the mother, whilst the zodiac
which is interposed between them, expresses the 'revolving
year' which elapsed between the two periods. This explanation
is completely confirmed by a similar representation of two
female figures on the ceiling of a tomb of the kings at Byban
el Molouk—one with the beetle, the other with the name of the
personage just born ; between them, instead of the zodiac, are
two tablets, divided into two hundred and seventy squares, corresponding to the number of days in nine Egyptian months ;
with ten circles placed at equal distances, probably intended to
represent full moons, and relating to the ten imperfect lunations
to which these days must belong. The number two hundred
and seventy is too remarkable to be supposed to have been introduced by mere accident ; and when the argument is considered in connection with the evidence, in itself sufficiently
convincing, the whole must be allowed to be fully conclusive."[a]

An extremely candid letter of apology from Letronne[b]
was the immediate result of the communication which
had been made to him ; he pleaded ignorance of the
precise purport of Young's theory, and as he was a
man of high character, there is no sufficient reason to
doubt the truth of his explanation.

In the summer of 1824, he paid a visit for a couple
of months to Spa, with Mrs. Young and some other
members of her family, and before returning home, he
made also a short tour in Holland. In writing to Mr.
Gurney, who was at that time in Italy, he says :—

[a] Works, vol. iii. p. 124.   [b] Works, vol. iii. p. 378.

" I have lounged away a summer in the Belgian dominions with very tolerable comfort in a state of torpidity. The old Belgians are a kind, good-natured people. They complain of their new masters as they did of their old—probably not without some reason. The poor are wretchedly poor—not, as it seems, from the want of civilization, but from the excess of it for the moment, the introduction of machinery having thrown thousands out of employment; but I suppose for a few generations only. The Dutch seem sufficiently prosperous, though the people are still Dutch, phlegmatic and avaricious, as far as appears to a traveller; but the government seems to be enlightened, and to be very laudably bent on the encouragement of the arts and general instruction. At Spa we had rather a paucity of interesting characters; the standing patrons were the Binnings and the Lovaines; the flying visits of Lady Davy, the Huskissons, Sir J. Mackintosh, and the Somervilles, were the more appreciated as there was otherwise some scarcity of intellectual enjoyment. We staid there till the end of September, and returning by Antwerp, we left our carriage there, and went through Holland either in the boats, which are nearly as good as gondolas, or in hired carriages, which are also comfortable enough. From Antwerp we went by Breda to Utrecht, thence by water to Amsterdam and Haarlem; from Haarlem by Leyden to the Hague and Rotterdam, whence the river brought us back in eleven hours and a half through the mazes of the river to Antwerp. We were greatly interested, on our return, with some pictures and churches at Bruges and Ghent. To me the voyage back from Calais was rather memorable, as I was the only one of our party that did not suffer from the motion. My companions have found wonderful benefit from their season at the Well; but their saddles were probably as much concerned in their amendment as their glasses."

Dr. Young was not altogether exempt from the weakness of occasionally appearing to affect to merge the character of a man of science in that of a man of the world. He had studied, from an early period of life, to adapt his habits to those of cultivated and refined society, and found a greater relief from his severer studies in the lively conversation and elegant amusements of accomplished women than in the graver discussions of those who are brought into contact with each other by a community of scientific, literary or political interests. In such society, his manner sometimes assumed an appearance of flippancy and dogmatism from the peculiar precision of his knowledge and the prompt and off hand replies to which it occasionally gave rise. He alludes to the impression which this manner sometimes produced in the following extract from a letter written to Mrs. Earle:[a] it refers to a conversation which had taken place at Lord Dudley's table:—

"Miss White,[b] the other day, had made Sir Humphry (Davy) believe that Sotheby[c] considered me the most dogmatical and contradictory person in the world, because I had expressed dislike of the style of Livy in the beginning of his History. Lord Dudley said he delighted in contradiction, and if he became a sovereign he would certainly make me his lord chamberlain, that he might have the pleasure of being often contradicted; though he must say that he had never himself observed the said propensity which was imputed to me. In fact, there was nothing contradictory to Sotheby's expressed opinions in my remark; and if I had happened to say that I did not like turtle soup or hock, he might think it want of good taste in me, but he could not feel it as personally disrespectful, as it would be to call in question a matter of fact or even of judgment. I believe our conversation last year began upon Schiller's Thirty Years' War, which I thought full of odious affectation of language and in Livy's worst style of poetical prose; I did not say that Sotheby's prose was poetical or that his poetry was prosaic; but it certainly did appear to me when I read Livy that he began his history upon stilts, and that it

---

[a] November 20, 1824.

[b] A lady of extremely popular manners, who was accustomed to assemble at her house the most distinguished society of London.

[c] The translator of the Georgics of Virgil, &c. &c.

was not until he had worn his stilts down that he began to write like a gentleman.

"Lord Dudley could not agree with me; and he is much more familiar with Livy than I am, and he is certainly an admirable prose writer; but the distinction between the different parts of Livy's History could not well have been an invention of my own fancy. It seems, however, impossible that all persons should agree in their taste respecting beauty of style, even if they were equally capable of feeling and judging correctly; for certainly the taste is formed very much by the established habits of reading, and a person who has read as much Latin as English and a great deal of French and Italian, must have acquired a different susceptibility of the impressions made even by the style of an English author from a person who has read nothing, for instance, but English and German. I was expressing, one day, the gratification that I derived from the style of Robertson the historian; it was remarked, I think by Hallam, that it wanted *idiom:* I said that I *hated* idiom. In fact, every idiom seems to me in the nature of a proverb, and to abound in idiomatical phrases seems to me a deformity of the same kind as to interlard every speech with proverbs: there is something in it like the affectation of being very fashionable, or rather like the wish of a school-boy to look knowing; at least this is the impression that idioms make on me; and I am stupid enough to take Lord Chesterfield's precept of being neither the first nor the last in the fashion, though in language I would rather be the last, because the language of a civilized and cultivated people ought not to change materially when it is once established."

Young's own style of writing, if not idiomatic, was singularly pure: he had studied very carefully the principles of grammar, and one of his earliest essays in the Leptologist[a] was in illustration of them: his sentences are usually short: he chooses the most simple words which will express his meaning: he rarely attempts to form carefully balanced periods, and never resorts to figurative expressions when those which are

[a] See supra, p. 129.

direct and immediate will answer his purpose: he was as little disposed to admire and imitate the poetical prose of Schiller in history as of Davy in philosophy, and was apt to regard them both as almost equally misplaced. It is but just to him, however, to observe that in the same criticism in which he has intimated this opinion, he willingly concedes a great latitude to diversities of taste, and allows that an ornamented and popular style of expression may stimulate the interest and command the attention of many readers who would be repelled by a more rigid exposition addressed to the understanding only, however perspicuous and philosophical it might otherwise be.

In the year 1826, he removed from his house in Welbeck Street, where he had resided for a quarter of a century, to another in Park Square, which possessed more ample accommodation, which had been built under his own directions, and which he fitted up with great elegance and taste. In noticing this change of residence in the autobiographical sketch to which we have before had occasion to refer, he adds the observation—"That he had now attained all the objects of importance for which he had hoped or wished: *non impudenter vitæ quod reliquum est, petit, cum famæ quod satis est, habet.* But, in fact, the life which he loved was little else than the pursuit of such fame as he valued, or at least of those acquirements which he thought deserving of it."

On the sixth of August of the following year, he was elected one of the eight foreign associates of the Academy of Sciences, at Paris, in the place of Volta. The other competitors named were the great astronomers Bessel and Olbers, Robert Brown the botanist, Sœmmering the anatomist, Blumenbach the naturalist, Leopold Von Buch the geologist, Dalton the chemist, and Plana the mathematician. This is the greatest honour that can be conferred on a man of science Davy and Wollaston were already members : their places, and that of Young, are now not less worthily filled by Brown, Faraday, and Brewster.

The propriety of the selection which was made by the Institute of France, of Wollaston, Davy, and Young, as the most eminent representatives of English science in that age, was disputed by very few of their contemporaries who were capable of forming a correct opinion of their merits. Wollaston, who was the oldest of the three, is less known by any striking discoveries than by the happy invention of many novel processes in chemistry and the arts—some of which he made subservient, during his lifetime, to the interests of his fortune—as well as by various essays on very different branches of philosophy, which are generally remarkable for great precision of thought and statement and by a command of the subject of which he is treating, so complete, that he was very rarely mistaken in his conclusions. He was a good geometer, a good optician, and a thorough master of mechanical principles, as far as his very limited knowledge of analysis would enable him to apply them ; but he was wanting in the courage of Young and the enthusiasm of Davy, and would rather have sacrificed the credit of the greatest discovery than expose himself to the danger or the imputation of failure ; and there is every reason to conclude that much of the credit which Dalton and Berzelius have gained from the proposition and establishment of the great principles of the atomic theory would have been appropriated by Wollaston, if his courage and enterprise had been equal to his knowledge and to the clearness of his views of the proper import of definite chemical analyses and combinations. His name is consequently not permanently connected with any great real epochal advancement in the sciences, and it is on this account that posterity is not likely to maintain the same high estimate of his powers which was made by his contemporaries.

Of Davy, it has been said that he was born a poet and became a chemist by accident. It was indeed a happy accident which gave to the sciences a man who united so many qualifications to adorn them— great skill and promptitude in performing, varying and devising, experiments; great speculative boldness tempered by the true spirit of inductive philosophy, and united to a power of exposition both as a lecturer and a writer which has rarely been equalled, unless by the eminent chemist, who, once his pupil, has since succeeded to his office and his honours. The discovery and demonstration of the law which connects the electrical affections of bodies with their chemical powers, which was speedily followed by the decomposition of the alkalis, was sufficient to change the whole face of chemical science. Having rapidly risen to honours and fortune, his character, in later life, as a man of science, became somewhat subordinate to that of a man of fashion, whose society was equally courted from his great celebrity and his remarkable powers of conversation: and we subsequently find him relaxing from those habits of active and laborious research which are more or less necessary, even for the most gifted of mankind, to maintain their leading position in the advance of the sciences. But though his productions were less numerous and his career less brilliant in later than in early life, there was no subject which he touched upon which he did not adorn; for both his

philosophical and inventive powers were of the highest
order, and the most obscure indications and analogies
which would have escaped the notice of common
minds, became with him the guides to some of his
most considerable discoveries : such was his safety-
lamp, one of the happiest practical conclusions that
was ever deduced from a philosophical fact through a
most delicate but perfectly connected net work of consequences, and his invention for protecting the copper
sheathing of ships, the failure of which, from extraneous causes, was no derogation from the merit of the
philosophical conception upon which it was founded.

The lapse of a quarter of a century, since the grave
—within the brief space of six months—closed upon the
labours of these three eminent philosophers, has somewhat changed the order in which they were classed by
their contemporaries. If Young held the lowest place
in the order of precedency then, he unquestionably
occupies the highest now. The most brilliant achieve-
ments of Davy, whether considered singly or collec-
tively, are probably surpassed in importance by the
discovery and demonstration of the interference of
light ; but whilst the first received the prompt and
unhesitating acknowledgment of the scientific world
and at once secured for their author the honours and
rewards which were due to his merits, the second, even
after emerging from a long period of misrepresentation
and neglect, had to make its way, step by step as it were,
and with various and fluctuating fortunes, against
the opposition of adverse and long established theories,
supported by the authority of the two greatest men
known to the scientific history of the past and the present
age ; and it only received a tardy and reluctant recognition—and that rather by implication than avowedly

—when near the close of his life, the Rumford medal was awarded by the Royal Society to Fresnel, who completed the structure of which Dr. Young had laid the foundations.

If we refer to his other scientific works, embracing so wide a range of subjects, and some of them—more especially his essays on the tides and the cohesion of fluids—so remarkable for the boldness and originality of their treatment, we shall find that they were rarely read and never appreciated by his contemporaries, and even now are neither sufficiently known nor adequately valued : whilst if justice was awarded more promptly and in more liberal measure by his own countrymen to his hieroglyphical labours, these also were singularly unfortunate, as far as concerned the general diffusion of his fame, by coming into collision with adverse claims which were most unfairly and unscrupulously urged in his own age, and not much less so by some distinguished writers in very recent times. The great variety also of his titles to commemoration as a classical scholar and archæologist, a medical writer, an optician, a mathematician, or a physical philosopher, increases the difficulty of judging his relative rank amongst men of celebrity, whether they were his contemporaries or not : for the position which he might not venture to claim in virtue of his contributions to any single department of human knowledge, might be readily conceded to him when his combined labours were taken into consideration.

In the summer of 1827, Sir Humphry Davy, whose health had been for some time declining, and who had been lately residing on the continent of Europe, in the hope that new scenes and occupations might tend to restore it, resigned the presidency of the Royal Society,

and Mr. Davies Gilbert, the treasurer, was elected by the
council temporary president until the anniversary meeting of the Society on St. Andrew's Day. Various
speculations were afloat respecting the selection of a
permanent president, but as somewhat costly duties of
hospitality have been customarily attached to the office,
no one could be chosen whose fortune was not adequate
to meet the expenditure. Davy was anxious that Peel
should be his successor, but that great statesman, with
his characteristic good sense, gave no encouragement
to those who made the proposition to him :- some
members were favourable to Lord Lansdowne, others
to the Duke of Somerset. There were not wanting advocates of a total change of a system which excluded
men of science from a position which, under other
circumstances, would have been the most appropriate
reward of the highest scientific merit, and, amongst
those who favoured such views, the claims of Dr.
Young could hardly be overlooked. In writing to his
sister-in-law, Mrs. Earle, who was then in Italy on
her marriage tour, he says :—

"I find there has been a pretty general conversation about
making *me* President of the Royal Society, and I really think
if I were foolish enough to wish for the office, I am at this
moment popular enough to obtain it ; but you well know that
nothing is further from my wishes.

The choice, at the anniversary of the Society, fell upon
Davies Gilbert, a man of most amiable character and possessed of very considerable scientific and general knowledge, who had taken a leading part, as a member of the
legislature, in promoting, on all occasions, the interests
of science ; but his good nature sometimes amounted
to weakness, and unfitted him to keep under due
control some members of the council or of the society

who were perpetually preferring complaints or urging reforms, and that not in very temperate language. "I told him," says Young, "that he had not quite enough of the devil in him; that Sir Joseph Bankes should have left his *eyebrows* to go with his cocked hat, if he left the Society nothing else."

We have referred before[a] to the circumstances attending his last journey to Paris and Geneva in the summer of 1828, and to the symptoms of decaying strength which were unmistakeably manifested before its conclusion. He had hitherto enjoyed a singular freedom from complaints of every kind, with the exception of the consumptive tendency which had visited him in youth, and no person appeared to give greater promise of longevity. He returned in the autumn to his residence in Park Square, to his usual occcupations, and though old age appeared to be creeping upon him, there was no relaxation of activity in the prosecution of his studies. In a letter, written soon after his return, he says :—

" As for myself I am perfectly content with the life I lead : walking on business of routine every day from eleven to two : the rest of the day sitting over my hieroglyphics or my mathematics, and conversing in my library with people beyond the Alps or the Mediterranean. I have lost all ambition for a more bustling life or more active scenes, and I believe I am as happy as a person so old in *soul* is capable of being. In mental faculties I am not yet old, and I amuse myself almost daily with some petty *bonnes fortunes* among some of the nine sisters. I hear nothing whatever from the Admiralty, and so much the better, except receiving three hundred pounds a year instead of four hundred.[b] As for Croker, I never believed a word of his

---

[a] Supra, p. 342.

[b] Supra, p. 364. The Board of Longitude, of which he was secretary, had been recently abolished, and no arrangements had yet been made for officially advising the Admiralty on matters of science.

going out, and he may remain in for ought I care and be Lord
Melville's master, if he chooses ; for the stronger of two heads
will generally direct the weaker in the long run. I am deep in
the value of life, and I really begin to think that people do live
longer than was formerly supposed, though not in the extravagant degree that was asserted." [a]

In the autumn of 1828, Dr. Wollaston was attacked
by a disease, the character of which, though it left
in the first instance his faculties unimpaired, gave him
no hopes of recovery : he consequently took measures
for communicating to the Royal Society some processes
which he had kept secret on account of the income
which they secured him, and at the same time made a
deed of gift to the Society of two thousand pounds, the
produce of which was to be applied by the Council to
the encouragement of experimental researches. This
gift was augmented by another of one thousand pounds,
from Mr. Davies Gilbert, the new president, and by
smaller benefactions from Mr. Warburton, Mr. Guille-
mard, and other members. In writing to Mr. Gurney,
in reference to these transactions, he says,

" When Gilbert had announced his benefaction, Amyot said
he had never heard me make a speech, and I summoned up
courage to take the first opportunity of muttering out : ' Mr.
President, a gentleman on my right observes that he never
heard me make a speech. Now, Sir, I cannot help remarking
of you and your magnificent donation,

Tu mutis quoque piscibus
Donatura cygni, si libeat, sonum . . .

And as I am accidentally the senior officer of the Society,
though by no means in the highest rank, I take the liberty of
thanking you and Dr. Wollaston, in the name of the Society,
for your princely liberality, and for the example you have set of

[a] Works, vol. ii. p. 389. Practical Comparison of different Tables of
Mortality.

the way in which science ought to be encouraged in this country, and not by tormenting the government to do this, that, and the other for us, but by doing what is wanted for ourselves, which is the truly dignified character of an independent English gentleman.' If I had wished to be applauded the plot was well laid, as I was unavoidably a sharer in the tremendous noise which was made for Wollaston and Gilbert. Wollaston is said to be sinking daily."[a]

The principle, advocated in this address, that science should be independent of the patronage and assistance of the government, was the basis,[b] as we have seen, of Young's opposition to any extension of the Nautical Almanac, for the sole benefit of those who were engaged in the cultivation of astronomy. It was, in fact, little more than the simple affirmation of the principle which had previously been uniformly acted upon by the legislature of this country, and it was commonly defended upon the plea that such assistance or interference would tend to paralyse private enterprise and defeat the very purposes it was designed to serve, and that it was consequently safest to trust to things as they were and to the effects produced by the natural progress of the arts and of knowledge, which had hitherto been found sufficient to secure the continued improvement of the general condition of the people. It was probably forgotten, however, by those who were accustomed to rely on such arguments, that many material, social and moral evils were in the mean time apt to increase much more rapidly than the natural remedies by which they were assumed to be counteracted : that whilst our great towns increased in wealth and population, they became more and more completely encompassed by wretched and unwholesome suburbs, without adequate drainage and water, or any

---

[a] He died on the 22nd of December.   [b] Supra, p. 365.

other provision to protect the public health : that whilst the masses of the people were rapidly advancing in political privileges and in a sense of the power which they thus acquired, there was no corresponding advance in their education or in the acquisition of those moral and religious habits which alone could make them safe or useful members of the commonwealth : and whilst the connection between our material prosperity and even our moral welfare, with the more general diffusion of scientific and all other species of knowledge amongst the better classes of society, became daily more and more manifest, it was the legislature and not the exertions of individuals, however public spirited and liberal, which alone could maintain the just balance between the demand for instruction amongst all classes and the means of supplying it.   In later times, wiser counsels have happily prevailed, and we have already began to experience the advantages which result from a centralizing and controlling action of the government sufficiently powerful to give definite direction and support to local enterprise without interfering unduly with local administration.

In a subsequent letter, he speaks of the proposition which had been made for collecting contributions to augment the Wollaston Donation Fund sufficiently to make its produce the means of affording effective assistance in the performance of philosophical experiments : he objected to this scheme as tending to merge the gift of Dr. Wollaston in a multitude of others :—

" For my part," says he, " it is my pride and pleasure, as far as I am able, to supersede the necessity of experiments, and more especially of expensive ones.   I have just been inventing a mode of determining the figure of the earth from two points in sight of each other, without going either to Lapland or Peru;ᵃ and this must stand instead of my contribution to the Donation Fund; for, if I save expense, I do more than if I paid it."

In another part of the same letter, speaking of his Enchorial Dictionary appended to Archdeacon Tattam's Coptic Grammar, he says :—

"My Dictionary is getting into the hands of the lithographist.ᵇ I give no hieroglyphics, except as illustrations of the running hand, where they are well identified; partly to avoid discussion and partly because there is more difficulty in preserving the Enchorial words without some such work than the distinct characters, which would lead me too far."

In a postscript, after some references to the new Council of the Royal Society, which Mr. Davies Gilbert was not generally able to keep in order, he adds :—

"We had Peel last week at our new Council, and certainly he did us great service and helped us to get the business done an hour before the usual time, though he said not a word that I heard. But the consciousness that a man *respected by the public* is present has a wonderful effect in keeping triflers in awe and making people think before they speak."

There are few persons familiar with the proceedings of such meetings who will not feel the truth of the last observation.

The last letter, in the month of January following, which I find in my possession, refers to the death of

ᵃ See Appendix (B).

ᵇ In a letter written ten days before, he had said, "I-have just finished the fair copy of my little Egyptian Dictionary, except that I must copy it all over again as the lithography goes on, which will be the work of two or three months for the fingers and eyes, but little or nothing for the head. It contains little or nothing striking; but it preserves from oblivion all that I have made out of the running hand, which is no where methodically recorded. It makes about a hundred pages."

Dr. Wollaston, and the appointment of the new Committee of Longitude.

" Poor Wollaston's disease," says he, "was exactly what we
all expected : we are rather more modest than we were in
Sydenham's time, when he said, that if he once knew a disease
he could always prescribe for it. Our new Committee of Longitude is settled, at least for the present, though the radical
abuse of the Nautical Almanac is likely to continue ; but fortunately for my security, they have put the Admiralty and the
Nautical Almanac together, so that they may do their worst.
Croker has appointed Sabine and Faraday and me to constitute
a Scientific Committee to advise the Admiralty, which was all
that the Board of Longitude could do, and it is better that
things should be called by their right names."

The agitation relating to this subject, which had
previously raged with so much violence, reached its
culminating point when the appointment of this committee was made known, and led, as we have elsewhere
stated, to the presentation of a Memorial to the Duke
of Wellington, who was at that time Prime Minister,
to which Young was obliged to draw up an elaborate
reply. The labour incident to the preparation of this
Report, and the harassing effect of the personal attacks
which preceded it, exacerbated a complaint, which it
afterwards appeared must have been long in progress,
but which was now bringing him rapidly to a state of
extreme debility.

We shall avail ourselves of the account which Mr.
Gurney has appended to a short Memoir—chiefly,
though by no means entirely, founded upon an autobiographical sketch which he had himself prepared—of
the circumstances attending Dr. Young's last illness and
death, and which is in exact accordance with the representations of the same melancholy scenes which have
been made to me by Mrs. Young.

" He had from the month of February, 1829, suffered
from what he considered repeated attacks of asthma,
and though he said little of it, as unwilling to alarm
those about him, was evidently uneasy at the situation
of his health. This gradually deteriorated. He had
in the beginning of April great difficulty in breathing,
with some discharge of blood habitually from the
lungs, and was in a state of great weakness. His
friends and physicians, Doctors Nevison and Chambers,
considered that there was something extremely wrong
in the action of the heart, as well as that the lungs
were very seriously affected.

" Though thus under the pressure of severe illness,
nothing could be more striking than the entire calm-
ness and composure of his mind, or could surpass the
kindness of his affections to all around him. He said
that he had completed all the works on which he was
engaged, with the exception of the rudiments of an
Egyptian Dictionary, which he had brought near to
its completion, and which he was extremely anxious to
be able to finish. It was then in the hands of the
lithographers, and he not only continued to give directions concerning it, but laboured at it with a pencil
when, confined to his bed, he was unable to hold a
pen. To a friend who expostulated with him on the
danger of fatiguing himself, he replied it was no fatigue,
but a great amusement to him; that it was a work
which if he should live it would be a satisfaction to
him to have finished, but that if it were otherwise,
which seemed most probable, as he had never witnessed
a complaint which appeared to make more rapid progress, it would still be a great satisfaction to him never
to have spent an idle day in his life.

" His last anxiety concerning the proceedings of one

or two persons who had made him the object of reiterated attacks, in consequence of being dissatisfied with the arrangements of the Nautical Almanac, was, that nothing should go forth on his part to increase irritation, and when papers were sent him which went to enumerate and to prove the errors, into which these individuals had fallen, his desire was that they should be suppressed.

" In the very last stage of his complaint, in the last lengthened interview with the writer of the present Memoir, his perfect self-possession was displayed in the most remarkable manner. After some information concerning his affairs, and some instructions concerning the hieroglyphical papers in his hands, he said that, perfectly aware of his situation, he had taken the sacraments of the church on the day preceding ; that whether he should ever partially recover, or whether he were rapidly taken off, he could patiently and contentedly await the issue : that he thought he had exerted his faculties through life as far as they were capable of, but for the last eight years he had been careful of straining them to more than he thought they could compass without injury ; that he had settled all his concerns ; that if his health had been continued to him, he might have looked forward to the prolongation of much that was to be enjoyed; but that though he was in no other suffering than that of great oppression and weakness, still that if life were continued in the state he then was of inability to any of his accustomed employments, he could hardly wish it to be long-protracted.

" His illness continued with some slight variations, but he was gradually sinking into greater and greater weakness till the morning of the 10th of May, when he expired without a struggle, having hardly com-

pleted his fifty-sixth year. The disease proved to be
an ossification of the äorta, which must have been in
progress for many years, and every appearance indicated an advance of age, not brought on probably by
the natural course of time, nor even by constitutional
formation, but by unwearied and incessant labour of
the mind from the earliest days of infancy. His
remains were deposited in the vault of his wife's family,
in the Church of Farnborough in Kent.

"To delineate adequately the character of Dr. Young
would require an ability in some proportion to his
own, and must be ill supplied by one incompetent to
judge of the talents of a man, who as a physician, a
linguist, an antiquary, a mathematician, scholar, and
philosopher, in their most difficult and abstruse investigations, has added to almost every department of
human knowledge that which will be remembered to
aftertimes—'who,' as was justly observed by Mr.
Davies Gilbert, in his eloquent address to the Royal
Society, over which he so worthily presided, ' came
into the world with a confidence in his own talents
growing out of an expectation of excellence entertained
in common by all his friends, which expectation was
more than realized in the progress of his future life.
The multiplied objects which he pursued were carried
to such an extent, that each might have been supposed
to have exclusively occupied the full powers of his
mind; knowledge in the abstract, the most enlarged
generalizations, and the most minute and intricate
details, were equally affected by him; but he had most
pleasure in that which appeared to be most difficult of
investigation.' The president added, that ' the example is only to be followed by those of equal capacity
and equal perseverance ; and rather recommends the

concentration of research within the limits of some defined portion of science, than the endeavour to embrace the whole.'

"Dr. Young's opinion was, that it was probably most advantageous to mankind, that the researches of some inquirers should be concentrated within a given compass, but that others should pass more rapidly through a wider range—that the faculties of the mind were more exercised, and probably rendered stronger, by going beyond the rudiments, and overcoming the great elementary difficulties, of a variety of studies, than by employing the same number of hours in any one pursuit—that the doctrine of the division of labour, however applicable to material product, was not so to intellect, and that it went to reduce the dignity of man in the scale of rational existences. He thought it so impossible to foresee the capabilities of improvement in any science, so much of accident having led to the most important discoveries, that no man could say what might be the comparative advantage of any one study rather than of another; and though he would scarcely have recommended the plan of his own as the model of those of others, he still was satisfied in the course which he had pursued.

"It has been said, that the powers of imagination were the only ones of which he was destitute. From the highly poetical cast of some of his early Greek translations, this is at least doubtful. It might, perhaps, have been said more justly, that he never cultivated the talent of throwing a brilliancy on objects which he had not ascertained to belong to them. Dr. Young was emphatically a man of truth. The truth, the whole truth, and nothing but the truth, was the end at which he aimed in all his investigations, and he could not bear, in the most common conversation, the slightest degree of exaggeration, or even of colouring. Now, all exercise of what is ordinarily called imagination, is the figuring forth something which, either in kind or in degree, is not in truth existent; and whether originally gifted with this faculty, or otherwise, Dr. Young would, on principle, have abstained from its indulgence.

" To sum up the whole with that which passes all acquirement, Dr. Young was a man in all the relations of life, upright, kind-hearted, blameless. His domestic virtues were as exemplary as his talents were great. He was entirely free from either envy or jealousy, and the assistance which he gave to others engaged in the same lines of research with himself, was constant and unbounded. His morality through life had been pure, though unostentatious. His religious sentiments were by himself stated to be liberal, though orthodox. He had extensively studied the Scriptures, of which the precepts were deeply impressed upon his mind from his earliest years; and he evidenced the faith which he professed, in an unbending course of usefulness and rectitude."

Of the family of Dr. Young, two brothers, Richard and John, and two unmarried sisters, Hannah and Anne, all resident at Taunton, still survive him. His eldest brother Robert died a few years ago, leaving two sons and three daughters: his eldest son, Robert, who had long been physician and confidential agent of the Newab of Bengal, died lately at Moorshedabad; the second, Thomas, is a distinguished member of the same profession with his illustrious uncle, who took a great interest in his education and establishment in life. The eldest of the three sisters, Mary, is unmarried and lives with her relations at Taunton ; the second is married to the Rev. Charles Escott, Vicar of Sandall Magna, near Wakefield, Yorkshire ; the third, who was the wife of the Rev. A. Cridland, Incumbent of Hensall, also in Yorkshire, died two years ago, leaving three children.

It was the anxious wish of Mrs. Young to place an appropriate monument to her husband in Westminster Abbey, and a place for that purpose was kindly offered by Dr. Buckland, the Dean, as an expression of his respect for the memory of so great a man. Sir Francis Chantrey readily undertook the preparation of the bust by which it was designed to be surmounted : the cast, however, which had been taken after death, and the picture, by Sir Thomas Lawrence, represented his front face only, so that the artist, though perfectly familiar from frequent personal intercourse with the general character of his head, found himself foiled in his attempts to produce a correct representation, in consequence of some peculiarity in its form which he could not reproduce. A profile medallion was therefore substituted for the bust, of which a representation is given in the engraving which forms the frontispiece of the first volume of his works. The inscription on the slab beneath it, which is given in the following page, was written by Mr. Gurney.

SACRED TO THE MEMORY OF

THOMAS YOUNG, M.D.,

FELLOW AND FOREIGN SECRETARY OF THE ROYAL SOCIETY,

MEMBER OF THE NATIONAL INSTITUTE OF FRANCE;

A MAN ALIKE EMINENT

IN ALMOST EVERY DEPARTMENT OF HUMAN LEARNING.

PATIENT OF UNINTERMITTED LABOUR,

ENDOWED WITH THE FACULTY OF INTUITIVE PERCEPTION,

WHO, BRINGING AN EQUAL MASTERY

TO THE MOST ABSTRUSE INVESTIGATIONS

OF LETTERS AND OF SCIENCE,

FIRST ESTABLISHED THE UNDULATORY THEORY OF LIGHT,

AND FIRST PENETRATED THE OBSCURITY

WHICH HAD VEILED FOR AGES

THE HIEROGLYPHICS OF EGYPT.

ENDEARED TO HIS FRIENDS BY HIS DOMESTIC VIRTUES,

HONOURED BY THE WORLD FOR HIS UNRIVALLED ACQUIREMENTS,

HE DIED IN THE HOPES OF THE RESURRECTION OF THE JUST.

———————

BORN AT MILVERTON, IN SOMERSETSHIRE, JUNE 13TH, 1773,

DIED IN PARK SQUARE, LONDON, MAY 10TH, 1829,

IN THE 56TH YEAR OF HIS AGE.

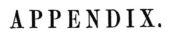

APPENDIX.

APPENDIX—A.

HERCULANENSIA;[a]

OR,

ARCHEOLOGICAL AND PHILOLOGICAL DISSERTATIONS:
CONTAINING A MANUSCRIPT FOUND AMONG
THE RUINS OF HERCULANEUM.

From the Quarterly Review for February, 1810.

THE publication of this highly interesting volume must ever be considered as a memorable event in the history of classical literature. One only of the eight hundred manuscripts, found almost fifty years ago at Herculaneum, has hitherto been printed; the remainder has been lost to the world till the present day, when we are informed that no less than eighty volumes have been rendered legible, by persons employed

[a] The article in the text, which was omitted in the selection made of Dr. Young's Philological Essays, is appended to this volume in consequence of the frequent references which are made to it in Chapter IX. It produced replies both from Mr. Hayter and Sir William Drummond. Upon the copies of these replies, found in a volume of Tracts belonging to him, Dr. Young has written a series of notes and criticisms, which are not less damaging to the character for scholarship and good sense, both of the editor of the Fragment and his commentator, than those which are contained in the Review. When I was engaged in writing the Chapter referred to, I was not aware that the Article which was there stated (page 237) to have been withdrawn from the Edinburgh Review had really made its appearance in the number for August, 1810. It is more discursive, but much less minute and critical, than that which is given in the text, but is not unworthy of the high reputation for scholarship and ability of the distinguished person to whose pen it was attributed.

under the munificent patronage of the Prince of Wales. We are confident that every lover of elegant literature in these kingdoms must feel the exertions of His Royal Highness on this occasion as a personal tie of gratitude, giving additional force to those sentiments of duty and respect which he is bound to entertain for the heir to the crown of the empire: and that so marked a demonstration of an enlightened zeal for the cultivation of learning, exhibited to the world under many difficulties, and in a distant country, cannot but add another ray of glory to the lustre of the British character.

The Herculanensia are the joint production of the Right Honourable William Drummond and Mr. Robert Walpole. We most willingly bear testimony to the profound erudition and extensive knowledge which they have displayed in their dissertations; and we thank them most sincerely, Sir W. Drummond in particular, for their co-operation in promoting the great work of rescuing these remains from oblivion. We shall proceed to give some account of the steps which have been taken for this purpose at different times, in the words of our authors.[a]

1. Of the ten dissertations contained in this work, the first relates to the size, population, and political state of the city o Herculaneum. Sir W. Drummond maintains that it was large, crowded with inhabitants, wealthy, and luxurious; and that it was rather a *colonia* than a *municipium*, though called occasionally by both names. 2. The second is an essay, by Mr. Walpole, on Campania in general, and that part of it called Felix; which last he limits to a breadth of 28 geographical miles, from the Mons Tifata to Misenum, and a length of 25 from the Pons Campanus to the Sarnus. 3. The etymology of Herculaneum Sir W. Drummond refers simply to Hercules, which he construes as a Hebrew or Phœnician compound, meaning universal fire, and alluding to the attributes of the

---

[a] There follows in the original a long extract from the Dedication to the Prince of Wales and from the Preface, containing statements respecting the circumstances which led to the publication which forms the subject of the Review, and of the various attempts to unroll the papyri, which have either lost their interest or have been otherwise sufficiently noticed in the article Herculaneum reprinted in the third volume of Dr. Young's Works.

sun. 4. He next copies and explains two Latin and two Etruscan inscriptions found at Herculaneum, and illustrates the subject by three plates of the Etruscan characters. 5. In the fifth dissertation, which is the longest of the whole, Sir W. Drummond displays much learning and ingenuity in deducing the names of places, in the Campania Felix, from the Phœnician; certainly, in the words of the manuscript, ΤΗΣ ΔΡΙΜΥΤΗΤΟΣ ΑΠΟΛΑΥΩΝ ΑΚΟΠΙΑΣΤΩΣ. He argues that Phœnicia was probably peopled from the East and from Egypt; that a Phœnician colony was established in Lydia; that the Lydians colonised Umbria and Etruria; and that their descendants became the Osci, Tyrrheni, Pelasgi, and Samnites, and retained a dialect founded on the Phœnician language, until the Romans conquered them. On p. 61 of this dissertation, we must observe, that the author appears to us to have been somewhat precipitate in his conjecture respecting the sense of a passage in the Bacchæ of Euripides : he thinks that *Io*, *O*, and *Ion* may probably have meant Lord, the common appellation of the sun; and says, that " when the Bacchants are asked whom they worship, and when they answer Σεβομεν Ω, *We worship O*,ᵃ we can scarcely be justified in understanding a simple exclamation." But, in fact, they are not asked whom they worship: Bacchus is present in person: the chorus, or perhaps rather the semi-chorus, exclaims, Dionysus is under this roof, adore ye him! The semi-chorus answers, O yes, we do adore him. The interjection ὢ is used in a similar manner in the Ion, 716. Ο'λοιτ', ὄλοιτ', ὢ, ποτνίαν ἐξαπαφὼν ἐμάν. In page 65, κατακόροις is an adjective, and not a substantive : and we are not quite satisfied with the passage of Eustathius, as here quoted and translated by our author: we should rather read it thus, Βασσάραι εἰρημέναι διὰ τὸ βάσιν ἐπ' ΑΕΡΑ ποιεῖσθαι, διὰ τὸ μανιῶδες : *they were called Bassarae, as if from walking on the air, on account of their frantic attitudes.* When Herodotus speaks of πεσσῶν, he does not mean " chess," p. 69, but backgammon. Salmasius has given a figure of the τάβλα, or tables, Hist. Aug. p. 466 ; and we learn from an epigram of Agathias, that the game was played with three dice. Chess is said to be an Eastern invention of much later date.

ᵃ The Edinburgh Reviewer concurs in this criticism.

6. The sixth is an interesting dissertation, by Mr. Walpole, on the Knowledge of the Greek Language, and on the State of the Art of Painting, among the Romans, before and about the time of the destruction of Herculaneum. He might have found some additional matter in an excellent essay on the state of painting among the ancients, published by Mr. Cooper, in the third volume of the Manchester Memoirs. 7. As the principal materials on which the ancients wrote, Sir W. Drummond enumerates tablets of stone, tablets of lead, of wood, of wax, of brass, and of ivory, skins and parchments, the bark of trees, leaves of trees, and linen books, which last he thinks consisted of cloth covered with wax.

8. The next article is a very ingenious essay by Mr. Walpole, entitled Palaeographical Observations on the Herculaneum Manuscripts, written at Palermo in the year 1807. He informs us that the whole of the manuscripts then in Sir W. Drummond's house, amounting to more than eighty, were Greek, with the exception of one fragment of a Latin poem. Of the line which he quotes from this fragment, a fac-simile has already been published in this country; *consiliis nox apta ducum, lux aptior armis;* another line, he tells us, speaking of Cleopatra, ends with *trahiturque* libidine *mortis.* The Greek manuscripts are all in capitals, without any spaces between the words, and without accents. Mr. Walpole adduces an inscription from the Pitture Antiche di Ercolano, written on a wall, in small or running characters, and accented in the common manner. He has quoted several authors, in order to prove that accents were sometimes employed in writing, at least as early as Callimachus, in the 133rd Olympiad, although their invention is commonly attributed to Aristophanes of Byzantium, who lived in the 145th; but it does not appear to us that any of the passages require to be understood, as relating to the accent employed in writing, rather than to the pronunciation only: their general tendency is however to confirm the accuracy and utility of the modern mode of accentuation. We could indeed have wished that these statements had been accompanied by a little more attention to the accents in Mr. Walpole's own quotations, and had induced his colleague not to disfigure his Greek by their total omission. "That the ancients had some method of making the accentual process harmonize with a just regard to quantity,"

is not to be doubted; but we do not see any great "difficulty" or "complication" in the subject. The modern musical notation is capable of expressing length or shortness, acuteness or gravity, and force or softness, all accurately, and independently of each other, so that every good musician may give to each of these qualities its proper expression. The length and shortness of the syllables of the ancients were correctly denoted by their quantity, so much that, among their musical characters, they required no particular marks to express the duration of the corresponding sounds. Accent in speaking was and always is distinct from quantity, though not always independent of it: with the Greeks it seems to have consisted in a combination of force with acuteness or gravity; with us it implies force, generally, but by no means universally, united with length. The French have little or no determinate accent; and although they have some distinction of quantity, yet their poetry is almost as independent of it as ours, which is governed by accent alone. There is something inconsistent in the high value which is attached, in critical researches, to prosody, and the low estimation in which rhythm is held by musicians: a single modern sonata exhibits a greater variety of prosody than the choruses of a whole Greek tragedy; and yet musicians scarcely condescend to take any notice of this subordinate department of their art, after the first elements of its notation have been explained. It is well known that the hemistich of Homer, which Mr. Walpole says Aristotle's commentator could not find, is extant almost literally in the twenty-first Iliad, v. 297; and that the memory of the great philosopher must have failed him when he referred it to another part of the poem.

9. The ninth dissertation contains the manuscript of Herculaneum, entitled 'περὶ τῶν Θεῶν,' with a commentary by Sir W. Drummond. 10. The tenth relates to some Latin inscriptions at Herculaneum, at Stabiæ, and at Pompeii, and to the paintings found at Herculaneum. Mr. Walpole observes that none of these inscriptions are accented, although some other Latin inscriptions have accentual marks, which are in general correct: it is remarkable that some of them exhibit a character resembling the small Roman letters now in use. Among these inscriptions the author has printed, by some oversight, a modern one, which relates to the restoration of the statue of a horse from its frag-

ments, by order of the King of Naples ; " REGIA CURA." In mentioning the temple of Isis, Mr. Walpole takes occasion to insert the altar of Dosiadas, with a literal translation, " for the sake particularly of observing a circumstance in it which escaped the learned Salmasius," but which *did not escape* Brunck, Anal. III. L. 95 ; and the circumstance is, that the poem is an acrostich, as Lacroix first observed. In the fifth line, Brunck's φίδοντο appears to be far preferable to " φιδοιντο." Λινοθώρηκες, page 182, are the men, and not the armour. The Latin translation of Euripides seems to have puzzled Winkelmann and Mr. Walpole very unnecessarily, by putting, besides another error, *inter*, μεταξὺ, instead of *intra*, for εἴσω. Orestes was only to enter the vacant space *within* the triglyphs, or within the walls which supported them. The last page of the work is occupied by a figure of a sun-dial at Orchomenus, taken from a drawing made by Dr. Clarke ; it must obviously have been constructed by a person very ignorant of his art.

As a specimen of the state of the manuscript, we shall exhibit its first page, which is the most defective, as nearly as possible in the form in which we suppose it to stand.[a]

<table>
<tr><td>This the Academicians read :</td><td>We are disposed to read it thus :</td></tr>
<tr><td>ΚΑΛΕΣΕΙν εις την προ-</td><td>ΚΑΛΕΙν εις την προ-</td></tr>
<tr><td>εδΡΙαν, ουτως επει</td><td>εδΡΙαν· ούτως επει</td></tr>
<tr><td>παΡαδεδονται τινες</td><td>παΡαδεδονται τινες</td></tr>
<tr><td>Μεν αγαθοι, και ευερ-</td><td>Μεν αγαθοι και ευερ-</td></tr>
<tr><td>γετΙκΟΙ κελευσειν</td><td>γετΙκΟι, κελευσειν</td></tr>
<tr><td>ΤΙΜΑν αΥτους ΘΥΣΙ-</td><td>ΤΙΜΑν αΥτους ΘΥΣΙ-</td></tr>
<tr><td>ΑΙς τοιαυταις. αυτος</td><td>ΑΙς τοιαυταις. αυτος</td></tr>
<tr><td>Δ' ουΚ ευξασθαι τοις</td><td>Δ' ουΚ ευξασθαι τοις</td></tr>
<tr><td>θεοΙΣ δωρεαν, γαρ</td><td>θεοΙΣ· ΜωρΙαν γαρ</td></tr>
<tr><td>ΕΙΝΑΙ ΜΗθεν διει-</td><td>ΑΝ ΕΙΝΑΙ, ΜΗθεν διει-</td></tr>
<tr><td>λΗΦΟτα περι αυτων</td><td>λΗΦΟτα περι αυτων,</td></tr>
<tr><td>ΘΟΡΥΒΕιν εαυτον. αλ-</td><td>ΘΟΡΥΒΕιν έαυτον· αλ-</td></tr>
<tr><td>ΛΑ ΟΙΕΤαι χρυσΙπ-</td><td>ΛΑ ΣΕΒΕΣΘαι. χρυσΙπ-</td></tr>
<tr><td>ΠΟΣ. ΤΟ Παν επιδια-</td><td>ΠΟΣ ΔΕ, ΤΟ Παν επι δια</td></tr>
</table>

[a] A page in the original Review, printed with types cast for the purpose of representing conjecturally the state of the first thirty-three lines of the Fragment, with the spaces assumed to correspond to the letters obliterated in the process of unrolling the papyrus, has been omitted : partly on account of the difficulty of reprinting it, and partly on account of its want of authenticity from not having been founded upon an actual comparison with the original.

This the Academicians read :

ΚΡΙΝΩΝ ΕΝ τω πρω-
ΤΩ ΠΕΡΙ ΘΕΩΝ διαΡρη-
ΔΗΝ ΤΗΝ ΦΡΕΝα παν-
ΤΩΝ, ΚΑΙ ΠΑντα λογον
κΑΙ ΤΗΝ του ολου ψυ-
χηΝ, ΚΑΙ τη τουτου
μΕΝ ΨΥΧΗ παντα
ΠΑΝΤΑΧΟΥ ΓΙΝΕσ-
Θαι ΘΕΟΝ, και τους λΙ-
Θους. διο και ζηνα
καλΕΣθαι δια δοτΗ-
ριον, ΑΥτον τε κοσμον των ανοσω-
Ν εμψυχον ειναι, Και
θεον Και το ηΓΕΜΟΝΙ-
κον ΕΙΝαι την οΛΟΥ
ΨΥχΗν. και ΟΥΤω
Αναλγον ευνΑΖΕΣ-
θαι τον δια, και την
κοινην παντων φυσιν.

We are disposed to read it thus :

ΑΝΑΦΕΡΩΝ, ΕΝ τω πρω-
ΤΩ ΠΕΡΙ ΘΕΩΝ, δια Φη-
ΣΙΝ ΕΙΝΑΙ ΝΟΥΝ απαν-
ΤΩΝ, ΚΑΙ ΠΑντα λογον,
κΑΙ ΤΗΝ του όλου ψυ-
χηΝ. ΚΑΙ τη τουτου
μΕΝ ΠΡΟΝΟΙΑ παντα
ΠΑΝΤΑΧΟΥ ΓΙΝΕσΘΑΙ,
Και ΤΑ ΖΩΑ και τους λΙ-
Θους. διο και ζηνα
καλΕΙΣθαι δια δοτΗ-
ριον. τον τε κοσμον σω-ᵃ
ΜΑ εμψυχον ειναι. Και
θεον ΕΙΝαι το ήΓΕΜΟΝΙ-
κον, Και την ΤΟΥ ΚοΣΜΟΥ
ΨΥχΗν. και ΟΥΤωΣ ΜΕΝ
Αναλγον ευνΑΖΕΣ-
θαι τον δια· και την
κοινην παντων ΕΙΝΑΙ φυσιν.

We also read, in p. 2, line 10, ὡs ΚΑΙ μηδε ; l. 16, ΜΗνα ;
l. 18, τεΘΕΙΣΘαι; l. 25, το ΦΩs δε ; l. 31, πλατΤεσθαι
ΑΥΤΟΥs ανθρΩΠΟΕΙΔΕΙΣ, ΚΑΘ' όν. P. 3, l. 3, τοΝ δε ;
l. 4. διὰ ; l. 19, ΜΥΘΙΚα ; l. 23, ΟΥs ; l. 26, αυτωΝ ; l. 29,
ΩΣ φησι καν ; l. 30, μηΔΕΝ. P. 4, l. 4, συνοικειΩΣΕσΙ· καν
τω περΙ αρετων ΠΡΩΤΩ, Τον δια νομον φησιΝ ειναι ; l. 9,
καΤαρχαs ; l. 15, ΣΥΝΟμΟΛΟΓΕΙ ; l. 18, πΡΩτΩ ΜΕΝ
την νΥκτα ; l. 32, και λογους εΠΑΓΕΙ .. ΟΙΣ Η ΛΟΞΑ
ΠΕΠΥΚνωται παντας. P. 5, l. 2, ζωον ; l. 16, τον ΜΕΝ ;
l. 19, περιεχειν ΔΕ ; l. 25, ΟΥΔ' ΕΙΣΔΥσειν θεΟυs ΑΛΛΟτρΙους
ΟΥδ' εισλΗΨΕΙν ; l. 28, ΕΙΝαι· τα τε του διος, το ; l. 31,
ποσειδΩΝΑ ΕΙναΙ. P. 6, l. 1, κΑΙ ΤΟΝ ΠΛΑτωνα ; l. 2,

ᵃ Mr. Hayter attacks many of the restorations proposed by Dr. Young
as not properly adjusted to the spaces in the papyrus where the original
letters are wanting. In this line, which is apparently complete in the
original, Mr. Hayter introduces eight additional letters, making twenty-
three in all, though few of the other lines contain more than seventeen :
he translates it "that the order (των ανοσων) of indefectible things is
animated," pretending that it expressed a great mystery of the stoical
philosophy, to which the fragment related. The restorations of Dr. Young
are not only much better adjusted to the deficient spaces than those of
Mr. Hayter, but have the additional recommendation of being generally
good Greek and intelligible.

ὡς εαν; l. 4, ΤΟ δ' εις τοΝ αιΘερα; l. 13, γαΡ; l. 14, μητΙν, καλειΙοθαι; l. 15, εν ΜΕΝ; l. 18, την ΑΘηνχν γεΓονενΑΙ; l. 21, φωνην ΕΙΝΑΙ εκ; l. 24, ὑποδειΞαι ΔΕ ΤΟΥΘ᾿ ὅτι ΤΗ ΤΕχνη ΣΥνεθη Η φρονησις; l. 29, ΠΑΛΛΑ δα δε, και ΤΡΙΤΟΓΕΝειzΝ. P. 7, l. 4, αυτΗΣ; l. 17, οΙ πολλους; l. 19, Καν ἐΝΑ μΟΝοΝ ΛΕΙΠΩσιν, ἀναιρΕιν; l. 21, τοις πολλοιΣ; l. 31, μεμΕΛηκασιν; l. 34, τιΝΑΣ. P. 8, l. 2, ΟΥ νομιζουσιν; l. 12, καθαπερ ΚΑΙ εν; l. 22, τΕ; l. 34, δ' ΩΣαυτωΣ. P. 9. l. 8, αΝΕλευθερΩτεροι; l. 20, ΩΣ Ενιοι; l. 28, φαινΕΣΘΑι; l. 31, Αφθαρτους. P. 10, l. 1, καΝ; l. 15, προς ἃ μεγιΣΤοις; l. 19, τα ΓΗΡΕΙΑ; l. 34, τιν' αΙεΛουρου. P. 11, l. 2, ΟΤΑν τΕ Λεγουσι; l. 11, αφεξεσθαι; l. 13, ΩΣ Μεν; l. 14, αΔικιας; l. 24, βλεπΕται δ' ουΝ ΟΤΙ καΙ; l. 32, εναργωΣ αναισθητους. P. 12, l. 2, τινες εισι θεΟΙ δΟκΟΥΝτας, or ΛεΓΟΝτας; l. 9, αυτΩν; l. 11, φιλαΡχιας; l. 19, καιρος αν εΙΗ Επι.

We do not mean to insist on every one of these corrections as certainly preferable to the text which has been printed, much less as affording us decidedly the genuine words of the author; but we imagine that the greater number will be admitted as indisputable. In several instances we have made some slight alterations of doubtful passages, in order to bring the lines as nearly as possible to a uniform length, so as to contain from fourteen to seventeen letters, or a very few more or less. We should often have been able to judge with much more confidence of the true reading, if the relative situations of the remaining letters in their respective lines had been accurately represented, and we do not see that there would have been any difficulty in doing this: even the insertion of spaces between the words, at the discretion of the copier, may often unintentionally have given rise to error. On a few passages we shall make some more particular remarks.

ᵃ Title. At the conclusion of the manuscript, the work is

ᵃ The last words of the Fragment as restored by Mr. Hayter are, καιρός ἂν ἐπὶ τὸν περὶ τῆς εὐσέβειας λόγον τῆς κατ' ἐπίκουρον αὐτὸν παραγράφειν, which he translates, "It is proper time here to subjoin to the Discourse upon Piety (a Discourse upon Piety) according to Epicurus:" making, as Dr. Young remarks, an ellipsis of the whole subject of the sentence, and leaving παραγράφειν, supposed active, without a case. Dr. Young introduces ἔιη (the ε is in the papyrus) before the ἐπὶ, and translates the passage, as in the text, "It is now time to conclude this Treatise on Piety according to the doctrines of Epicurus." Mr. Hayter objects to the use of called ΠΕΡΙ ΕΥΣΕΒΕΙΑΣ ΚΑΤ' ΕΠΙΚΟΥΡΟΝ; and there does not appear to be any authority for entitling it ΠΕΡΙ ΤΩΝ ΘΕΩΝ. Page 1. l. 26. This line, as printed, contains twenty-five letters, and is totally unintelligible: by leaving out των ανο it may be made to accord perfectly with the context. P. 2, l. 16. Πανα. We cannot find that Pan was ever identified with the moon, although she is said to have been once his mistress. Our reading Μηνα is fully supported by Strabo, who speaks of more than one ἱερὸν Μηνός. Orpheus also calls the moon θῆλύς τε καὶ ἄρσην. See Casaubon in Hist. Aug. script. p. 132; and consult the "pressmen at Oxford,"ᵃ who are supposed, by some of our contemporaries, to be extremely well acquainted with the god Lunus. It appears from this passage that Strabo could not have been the inventor of the Greek appellation Μὴν, as Casaubon seems to suppose: l. 25. The letters of the manuscript are printed τους δε τον Απολλω, και την Δημητρα γ ν, η το εν αυτη γονευμα: but, besides the redundance of the plural article, it could never have been intended that Apollo should be identified with the earth or its fruits; and το φως may easily have been corrupted into τους. P. 5, l. 29. The corrected text stands thus: το μεν εις την θαλατταν διατεταγος Ποσειδωνα, το δ' εις την γην

the verb παραγράφειν in the sense of "to conclude," but Young justifies it by the occasional use of the noun παραγραφὴ to express the conclusion of a sentence or paragraph. The Edinburgh Reviewer would read the concluding words thus, καιρὸς ἂν εἴη περὶ τῆς εὐσεβείας λόγον κατ' ἐπίκουρον αὐτὸν παραγράφειν, and translate (including the preceding sentence) thus: "So that now, this part of the subject at first proposed having been sufficiently discussed, it may be time to write, in the next place, the division which treats of Piety according to Epicurus." "For it is evident," he adds, "from the style of this fragment, that it was only one section of a larger treatise; and as this chapter treats in general περὶ θεῶν, so the next seems to have been περὶ τῆς εὐσεβείας κατ' Επίκουρον." The Reviewer seems to assume that there was some authority, beyond the character of the Fragment itself, for entitling it a treatise περὶ θεῶν, which can hardly be considered to have been the case; for the vague conjectures of Mr. Hayter, upon which he arrived at that conclusion—as is evident from his own defensive statement—are not entitled to any credit.

ᵃ The reference is to a passage in a celebrated article on the Oxford Strabo in the Edinburgh Review, vol. xiv. p. 438,—"Is it possible that even the pressmen of Oxford should be ignorant that there was at Rome a *deus Lunus* as well as a *dea Luna.*"

Δημητρα, το δ' εις τον αερα Ηραν, καθαπερ και Πλουτωνα λεγειν, ως καν πολλακις αηρ λεγη τις, ερειν Ηρα· ουδεις τον αερα Αθηναν. Now in the Cratylus of Plato we have these words, Ἴσως δὲ μετεωρολογῶν ὁ νομοθέτης τὸν ἀέρα Ἥραν ὠνόμασεν, ἐπικρυπτόμενος, θεὶς τὴν ἀρχην ἐπὶ τελευτήν. γνοίης δ' ἂν εἰ πολλάκις λέγοις τὸ τῆς Ἥρας ὄνομα : and it is remarkable that Sir W. Drummond, in his learned note on the word Pluto, which has no connection whatever with the context, should have quoted a part of this very passage of Plato, without being aware that the author of the fragment alluded to it. This is certainly a good specimen of *verbal* criticism.ᵃ Our correction, το δ' εις τον αιθερα Αθηναν, is supported by a passage of Diogenes Laertius, in his life of Zeno, 147, ΑΘΗΝΑΝ δὲ, κατὰ τὴν εἰς ΑΙΘΕΡΑ διάτασιν τοῦ ἡγεμονικοῦ αὐτοῦ. ΗΡΑΝ δὲ, κατὰ τὴν εἰς ΑΕΡΑ. The passage, as it seems to have been understood, in direct contradiction to thᵉ authority of Diodorus Siculus, as elsewhere quoted by Mr. Walpole. P. 6, l. 8. Ζευς αρρην, Ζευς θηλυς..Φρονησιν γ ἀν ειναι, διο και μητον καλεσθαι : this passage, as we have corrected it, is illustrated by the words of Orpheus in his Hymn to Minerva ; ἀγάθοις δὲ φρόνησις· ἄρσην μὲν καὶ θῆλυς ἔφυς, πολεμάτοκε ΜΗΤΙ. The corrected text continues, Χρυσιππον δ' εν τω στηθει το ηγεμονικον ειναι, κακει την φωνην αν γεγονεναι, Φρονησιν ουσαν. τω δε την φωνην εκ της κεφαλης εκκρινεσθαι λεγειν εκ της κεφαλης υποδεησαι οιειν οτι τεχνη συνεθη Φρονησις. If this passage were both coherent and grammatical,

---

ᵃ "What connection," says Mr. Hayter, "the passage in Plato has with this passage, as far as it mentions Pluto, I cannot divine, nor upon what account the words of Plato can interfere with a deity, mention of which has occurred before in this Fragment, and is, in this place, agreeable to the whole sense of the passage." To this Young appends the observation, "The passage has only a connection with this passage, as far as it does *not* mention Plato, who is not at all *agreeable* in this place. That the reading Plato should not have occurred to Mr. Hayter is not surprising, but that when it was once suggested, he could have had the slightest hesitation in adopting it, does appear to be beyond all conception." . Sir William Drummond, in his letter to Mr. Hayter, after intimating that he was at first disposed to think with the Reviewer, relapsed into his original opinion upon again consulting the Herculanensia : "but I leave you," says he, "to defend your own interpolations, and shall only state that ΠΛΟΥΤωνα still appears to me the true reading." It is hardly necessary to observe that the letters Π, Λ, Ο, Υ were introduced to replace those obliterated in the papyrus.

it would still be unconnected with the subject discussed by Diogenes: we have suggested, κακει την Αθηναν γεγονεναι, φρονησιν ουσαν. τω δε την φωνην ειναι εκ της κεφαλης, εκκρινεσθαι λεγειν εκ της κεφαλης· υποδειξαι δε τουθ" οτι τη τεχνη συνεθη ή φρονησις. In the preliminary origin of Minerva from the parent's breast, as here supposed, there may have been some allusion to the story of Jupiter's having swallowed her first mother Metis before her birth, as related by Hesiod, Theogon. 890. Immediately afterwards we find και Αθηναν μεν οιον Αθηλην αν ειρησθαι. Παρθενιδα δε και Γοργοφονειαν δια το την φρονησιν εκ τριων συνεστηκεναι λογων. There is a line quoted, if we recollect rightly, by Hephaestion, ΠΑΛΛΑΣ ΤΡΙΤΟ- ΓΕΝΕΙ', ανασσ' ΑΘΑΝΑ, which sufficiently justifies our correction of this-passage; to say nothing of the etymology of τριτογενεια, εκ τριων λογων. The learned editor observes very truly, that Minerva seems to have been known at Athens by the name of the Virgin ; but where do we find the term Παρθενις? He expresses some doubt respecting γοργοφονειαν, but does not propose a less objectionable term. P. 10, l. 19, Τα γρυ επι των ακανθιων παππων. We cannot find that γρυ was ever applied to gossamer ; it means the paring of a nail, or something nearly similar : the appropriate term is γηρειον, which is used by Aratus and by other authors : thus Nicander says in his Alexipharmaca, a poem, by the way, of which the obscurity is equalled only by the stupidity, οιά τε δη ΓΗΡΕΙΑ νεον τεθρυμμενα, παππου, ηερ' επιπλαζοντα, διαψαιρουσιν αελλαις. L. 34 ; we can scarcely imagine that the Academicians ever meant to propose so portentous a combination of letters as Τινα τε δουρ' ου βωμος επιτριψειεν αν ; the lines of Timocles are found in the seventh book of Athenæus : the alteration which our editor, in defiance of his text, has borrowed from Casaubon, Τιν' αιλυροιο, is not much less objectionable than the reading imputed to the Academicians. Dawes had proposed αιολουρου, in his remarks on the Acharnenses of Aristophanes, but Pierson, the acute commentator on Moeris, has very justly preferred αιελουρου, as better supported by the authority of grammarians as well as of manuscripts ; and it is extremely satisfactory to have found a single letter in so unquestionably ancient a manuscript as this fragment, which fully establishes his opinion. With these corrections, the sense of the whole fragment may

be understood, as we apprehend, without any material chance
of error : how the Academicians and the editors have intended
some of the passages to be construed without them, they have
not thought proper to inform us, and we are wholly at a loss to
conjecture. We shall proceed to lay before our readers such a
translation as will enable them fully to comprehend the author's
meaning ; we shall not, however, attempt to free every expression
from all appearance of embarrassment, for fear of making the
copy less faithful, in rendering it more agreeable.

" FRAGMENT OF A TREATISE ON PIETY,
ACCORDING TO EPICURUS.

"...... [As it is natural that those who are distinguished
for their virtues should] be invited to take precedence of others,
so, the Gods being described as good and beneficent, he advises
us to honour them with such sacrifices : but for himself, he has
made no vows to the Gods, thinking it a folly for one, who has no
distinct conceptions respecting them, to give himself trouble on
their account ; and regarding them with silent veneration only.
(A) But CHRYSIPPUS, referring everything to Jupiter, maintains,
in his *first book*, that Jupiter is the mind, the reason, and the soul
of all things, and that every thing in every place owes its
existence to his providence, not only animals, but even lifeless
stones : (B) and that Jove is therefore called ZHNA, as giving
existence, and that the world is as it were an animated body,
and that God is the governing power, and the soul of the whole.
And thus that Jove remains at rest, and without pain : and that
he is the same with the common Nature of all, with Fate, and
with Necessity ; and that Equity, and Justice, and Concord, and
Peace, and Venus, and the like, are all the same being. And
that the Gods are no more male and female than cities, or
virtues, but that their names only are masculine and feminine,
the substances themselves not differing, as Luna and Lunus.
And that Mars is put for war, and for the science of tactics : that
Vulcan is fire, and Saturn the continual flow of the stream of
time : Rhea the earth; Jupiter the air; the light, Apollo; and
Ceres the earth or its fruits : and that it is a mere puerile fancy
to represent them, by words, or paintings, or sculpture, under
the human form, as we do cities, and rivers, and places, and
moral qualities. And Jupiter he supposes to be the air above
the earth; that which is dark to be Pluto ; and that which per-
vades the earth and the sea Neptune. In the same manner he

adapts the other Gods to other inanimate substances; and he thinks that the Sun, the Moon, and the Stars are deities, as well as the Law; and he maintains that men also may become divinities. (C) In his *second book* he treats of the stories related of the Gods by Orpheus, and Musaeus, by Homer, Hesiod, and Euripides, and by the other poets: whom CLEANTHUS also attempts to accommodate to the opinions of the sect. According to him, the Æther, which is every thing, may be both father and son: and in his *first book* he maintains that it is not incongruous that Rhea should be both the mother of Jupiter and his daughter; making them the same by his appropriations. And in his first book on the *Virtues*, he says that Jove is the law, and that the Graces are our libations, and our acknowledgments for benefits. He also writes in a similar manner in his books *on Nature*, agreeing with Heraclitus in reducing all things to qualities. In the *first book* he says that Night is the first of the Goddesses; and in the *third*, that the World is one of the intelligent principles, governing in common with Gods and men; and that War and Jove are the same, as Heraclitus also affirms. In the *fifth book* he has introduced all the reasons by which his sect is supported in believing —that the world is animated, and rational, and sentient, and, in short, a deity. And in his work on *Providence*, he explains the same identifications of the soul of all, and accommodates the names of the Gods to his purpose, allowing full scope to his acute and indefatigable imagination. (D) DIOGENES, the Babylonian, also, in his book concerning *Minerva*, asserts that the World is the same with Jove, and that it comprehends that divinity as the body of a man does his soul: that the sun is Apollo, and the moon Diana: that Jove can neither enter into the forms of other Gods, nor receive them in his own; and that the thing is impossible. And with respect to the parts or attributes of Jove, that which extends to the sea is called Neptune, that which belongs to the earth Ceres, and to the air Juno; as Plato also observes, that if we pronounce the word AHP several times in succession, we shall say HPA; and that which belongs to the æther is named Minerva, being called ΛΘΗΝΑ, as if ΑΘΗΛΗ; making a male and female Jove. And that some of the Stoics affirm, that Minerva is the governing principle in the head; for that she is the same with intellect, and is therefore called Metis, or Wisdom: but that Chrysippus places the governing principle in the breast, and says that Minerva originated there, being identical with intellect: and since the voice is uttered from the head, therefore Minerva is supposed to

have been born from the head; which indicates the natural
union of intellect with art. And that she may have been called
Athena, as if AΘHΛH; and also Pallas; and Tritogenia, because
intellect is composed of three elements, the physical, the moral,
and the rational faculties. And in the same manner he appro-
priates very elegantly the rest of her appellations and attributes.
All the followers of ZENO, therefore, if they have left us any
Gods at all, as some of them have left none, and others have
taken away many, say that God is one; or in other words, the
universe and its soul: and those, who allow a plurality, vary in
their statements, being aware that, if they affirmed the existence
of one God only, they might be traduced before the multitude as
destroying the Gods, by allowing only one universal Deity, and
not several, much less all those who are generally held in estimation: while we assert the existence not only of the Gods
worshiped by the Greeks, but also of many more. Besides,
they have not thought fit to leave even those, respecting whom
they agree with us, in a form like that in which they are
universally worshiped: for they admit no Gods in the resemblance of men, but only the air, and the winds, and the
æther: so that I should confidently assert that they are more reprehensible than even DIAGORAS: for he has treated the Gods with
levity at most, but has not directly attacked them, as Aristoxenus
has observed in the Customs of the Mantineans; and in his
poetry, he remarks, Diagoras has adhered to the truth, introducing nothing like impiety in any of his verses; but in the
capacity of a poet, speaking with reverence of the Deity; as,
besides many other passages, is evinced by one which is addressed to Arianthes of Argos:

> ' The Deity's all perfect mind
> Directs each action of mankind :'

And, again, to Nicodorus of Bithynia, he says,

> ' Frail man, for each adventure's end,
> On God and Fortune must depend.'

And the Encomium of the Mantineans contains other similar
expressions. But these philosophers, although they insert the
names of the Gods in their writings, annihilate them in reality
by their reasoning: being deliberately more illiberal than
Philippus and others, who have simply denied their existence.
In the next place we must censure them as affirming, that the
Gods are not, as some say, the causes of injuries and evils to

men, with the view of inducing them to abstain from unjust
actions: in these positions we agree with some of their sect: but
the greatest and best existences, if they establish their notions
respecting the nature of the Deities, must appear to be secondary
in their origin, and perishable : but we, with uniform consistency,
maintain that the Gods are eternal and incorruptible. As to
what follows, therefore, leaving the rest to be discussed on a
future occasion, if they declare that the Gods do sometimes
injure or benefit us, it shall be shown that this second opinion is
also inconsistent with their principles. For it must be evident
to every one, that no man ever abstains out of fear of the
air, or the æther, or the universe, from doing the slightest
injustice, much less from those things to which he is incited by
the strongest desires ; any more than he would regard a heap of
sand, or the down on the feather of a thistle, which he evidently
perceives to be insensible. It seems to me, therefore, that we
may apply to these philosophers what was said by Timocles, in
his comedy of Egypt, respecting the Gods of that country :

‘ While even the Gods, whose power all nations own,
The crimes of impious men but slowly punish.
What perjured wretch shall dread Grimalkin’s altars ? ’

And when they speak of the Gods from conceiving them such as
their arrogance has represented them, while each man must consider himself as at liberty to do ill at his pleasure, wherever he
has an opportunity, can we suppose that he will abstain from
any of the greatest crimes for fear of the Air ? And if this is the
principal check for repressing injustice, they may be very fairly
reproached with transferring to mankind the habits of wild
beasts; especially if they disregard, as they profess to do, the
clamour of the multitude on this account. It appears, therefore,
even on the grounds that have been advanced by all those
who have undertaken their cause, that no man would ever be
deterred from injustice by the fear of those beings, who are
utterly unable to approach him, or are even manifestly insensible ;
nor upon the principles of those who say that we are ignorant,
who, or what, the Gods are; nor of those who either openly
declare that they do not exist, or merely allow them an existence, in order to deprive them of all active properties; nor of
others who, if they were permitted, would be urged by their
ambition to wage an eternal war with all the Gods: so that,
having sufficiently discussed this part of the division of our
subject which was laid down in the beginning, it is now time

to conclude this Treatise on Piety according to the doctrines of Epicurus."

One of the principal points which Sir W. Drummond has endeavoured to establish in his dissertation on this manuscript, is this,—that the work was employed by Cicero in compiling his treatise De Natura Deorum, and that the commencement of the fragment " seems to have been the prototype of a considerable part of the speech of Velleius ;" observing that " it would be idle to suppose that the Greek author was *the plagiarist.*" Now, that Cicero, writing upon the doctrines of the Greeks, must have borrowed his matter from some Greek authors, is too obvious to admit of dispute ; and that he did sometimes borrow more than the mere matter, is evident from his own statements, in many of his works. If therefore Sir W. Drummond had even made good his charge, the offence would certainly not have amounted to the guilt of *plagiarism,* for which no writer had ever less occasion than Cicero. But in fact, he appears to us to have failed altogether in rendering it probable, that Cicero had ever seen this important fragment: the passages in which there is any resemblance, relating, without exception, to what each author is reporting of the doctrines of certain older philosophers, as expressed in their works ; and the reports are not by any means so precisely similar as to induce us to suppose that Cicero had even taken the very justifiable liberty of saving himself some little trouble, by making use of another author's abstract from Chrysippus, and from Diogenes the Babylonian.　There is often a resemblance between our anonymous author and Diogenes Laertius ; but they had both, of necessity, the same things to relate, and therefore very naturally sometimes used almost the same terms.　We shall translate the passages of Cicero which Sir W. Drummond quotes, referring by letters to the corresponding parts of the fragment.

" (A) Chrysippus asserts, that the divine power consists in reason, and in the soul and mind of the universe : and that God is the world itself, and the mind diffused through it : and the government of all things, depending on mind and reason; and the common nature of things, containing all things ; and the concatenated order and necessity of future things : besides this, that the same being is fire, and the æther : and also identical with the fluid elements, as water; and with the earth, and the air, the sun, the moon, the stars, and the universe which contains them all; and with those men who have become immortal. (B) He also insists, that the æther is the same with Jupiter; and the air which flows on the sea, Neptune; and the earth Ceres : and in the same manner he goes through the names of the other Gods. (C) All this we find in the first book on the Nature of the Gods : and in the second he attempts to accommodate the fables of Orpheus, of Musæus, of Hesiod, and of Homer, to what he had said respecting the immortal Gods in his first book : so that even the oldest of the poets must have been Stoic philosophers, without knowing any thing of the matter. (D) And his follower, Diogenes the Babylonian, in his book entitled De Minerva, explains the history of the pregnancy of Jupiter, and the birth of the Virgin, in a physical sense, and annihilates altogether its mythological signification."

The attention which we have bestowed on this fragment, we presume, will entitle us to the indulgence of our readers, if we venture to offer our opinion on the most eligible mode of proceeding, with respect to those manuscripts which remain in the possession of the Prince of Wales ; and we sincerely wish that our sentiments may obtain an impartial consideration from those who are likely to influence his Royal Highness on the occasion. Almost forty years were spent in preparing for the press one work of Philodemus, which had been completely unrolled in 1755, and was only published in 1793 : when we consider this, and reflect on the shortness of human life, and on our own grey hairs, we tremble to think how little chance there is of our being benefited by any great proportion of the eighty manuscripts still unpublished ; especially if some of the most learned of our commentators are to hang whole pages of notes, on words which have even been erroneously inserted, or are to copy whole poems, for the sake of repeating remarks, which are to be found almost in our school books. The public of Great Britain too, we apprehend, has some pretensions to be considered : besides the liberal patronage of his Royal Highness the Prince of Wales, some expenses have been defrayed by the community ; of these every enlightened individual will most cheerfully contribute his share ; but trifling as they are in this point of view, some complimentary retribution ought perhaps to be conceded to the public; and this can in no way be done so effectually, as by allowing the collectors of books to acquire the whole of these treasures at an easy rate, without filling their shelves with eighty large volumes of commentaries.

There was indeed a man, whom the nation might, consistently with its own dignity, have invited, by the offer of a liberal remuneration, to undertake the employment of editing and illustrating these monuments, in a manner that must every way have been conducive to the advancement of literature. But our prophet is no more; and where shall we find his mantle? Where shall we look for his critical acumen, for his rapid perception, for his unerring sagacity, for his inexhaustible memory, and for his solid judgment? And had we even a Porson to undertake such an office, it would still be highly desirable that the simple text should be published somewhat more expeditiously than would be compatible with an elaborate discussion of every point requiring investigation or illustration.

Even without so good a reason for delay, the tardiness of our academical printers and publishers is sometimes truly disheartening. We remember that about twenty years ago a subscription was raised for the publication of a most valuable work of Hoogeveen, in the form of a Dictionary of the terminations of Greek words, which, even in the task of correcting a mutilated manuscript, would have rendered us the most material assistance: it was certainly sent, not long after, to the press at Cambridge; but some unlucky stagnation of the alacrity which, as we suppose, is usually felt within the walls of a college, has hitherto prevented its appearance.[a]

We should therefore earnestly recommend that the simple text of the manuscripts should appear at once, in all the pristine dignity of an EDITIO PRINCEPS, unsullied by the addition of any extraneous matter. The editors of Philodemus are universally allowed to have succeeded admirably in their attempts to restore the genuine text of their author; but we are very sorry to observe how lamentably the modern Academicians of Portici appear to have fallen short of their predecessors: and we believe that their labours have hitherto been extended to a small part only of the manuscripts which have been unrolled.

[a] The hint thus given was attended to, and the work of Hoogeveen was shortly afterwards published.

At the same time, their suggestions may certainly render occasional assistance to a reader, and even the greater facility afforded to a modern eye, merely by the separation of the words, would be a sufficient advantage to justify the reprinting of the text on an opposite page, with the insertion of such letters or words only as are obviously pointed out by the context. The characters of the Alexandrian manuscript are not materially different from those of the work of Philodemus, which has been published, and they probably approach still nearer to those of some of the other manuscripts. As a specimen of the mode which we think might be adopted with great propriety, we have printed the first page of the fragment, with some types which were obligingly cast, at a very short notice, by Mr. Fry. In this form, two or three octavo volumes would contain everything that is really wanted by the literary world ; although we are informed, from good authority, that the bulk of the manuscript copies which have been· brought to this country is by no means inconsiderable, and that many of the pages exhibit but very few deficiencies.

In the work before us no mention whatever is made of those specimens of the charred volumes, which, as we have understood, were sent over by the court of Naples in the first instance as a present to his Royal Highness the Prince of Wales. The caution which· is said to have been adopted with respect to these valuable relics deserves to be highly applauded. Four of them, we believe, are still altogether untouched : the other two were first submitted to the examination of some persons high in office in the Royal Society and in the British Museum, and of several other literary men ; and such experiments were made as were thought to afford the best prospect of leading to a method of unrolling them : but none of these attempts appear to have succeeded : the external parts of the rolls, as far as they have been penetrated, being almost uniformly conglutinated into one mass by so strong an adhesion that nothing could separate them, without destroying the brittle substance of the charcoal. The machine employed in Italy must have been totally inapplicable in such cases, since it afforded no means whatever of overcoming any considerable adhesions ; and it is probable that the outside of such manuscripts has always hitherto been destroyed ; the fragment on Piety appearing, for instance, to consist of only a small portion of the central parts of a roll. After some time, these two manuscripts were placed, at the recommendation of a person every way well qualified to give an opinion on the subject, in the hands of a medical gentleman* who was known to have formerly employed himself in minute anatomy, and to be familiar with the processes of mechanics and the operations of chemistry, in hopes that he would be able to discover some means of detaching the conglutinated surfaces from each other. At first, as it often happens in such cases, he appeared to be very confident of ultimate success; but difficulties afterwards occurred, and he did not continue his experiments long enough to overcome them, or even very materially to lessen them: his professional engagements interfered; much of his time had already been sacrificed; and the intelligence, that Sir W. Drummond had succeeded in obtaining possession of the whole collection of the works which had been unrolled made his own attempts appear comparatively too insignificant to deserve immediate prosecution.

We understand, however, that one mode of treating the papyri occurred to this gentleman, which appeared to him to promise a decided advantage to such as might hereafter proceed in the operation. This was the employment of the anatomical blowpipe, an instrument which he had many years before been in the habit of using for delicate purposes, in the place of a dissecting knife. The blowpipe served him, like the ςῖς Κάστορος in the epigram, for a knife and a forceps; for the gum, the goldbeater's skin, and the threads of the Italians. No instrument can be so soft in its pressure as the air, for holding a thin fragment by suction, without danger of injuring it: no edge nor point can be so sharp as to be capable of insinuating itself into all the crevices which the air freely enters. But the humidity of the breath he found to add much to the utility of the instrument: the slight degree of moisture communicated to the under or inner surface of a fold, made it curl up and separate from the parts beneath where the adhesion was not too strong; while dry air from a bladder was perfectly incapable of detaching it. But the process of separating every leaf in this manner was always tedious and laborious, where there was much adhesion, and sometimes

* Dr. Young.

altogether impracticable. Chemical agents of all kinds he tried without the least advantage; and even maceration for six months in water, applied at first with very great caution, was unable to weaken the adhesion. It is remarkable that the characters were not effaced by this operation, so that the gum which had fixed them on the paper must have wholly lost its solubility, and the rest of its original properties.[a]

It has indeed been supposed by some travellers that the manuscripts were in reality never charred, the ashes, thrown out by the volcano, having been probably incapable of communicating to them a sufficient degree of heat for producing this effect. In fact it is said that some of the spices found in an embalmed body retained a considerable portion of their aromatic smell. But there is no doubt whatever that the papyri are now complete charcoal, such as is formed by heat only : a small fragment of their substance burns readily, like common charcoal, with a creeping combustion, without flame and with a slight vegetable smell: fresh papyrus burns with a bright flame ; and almost all mineral coal, which may possibly have been formed from vegetable substances without the operation of heat, flames abundantly ; Bovey coal, for example, which retains much of the appearance of wood, exhibits a considerable flame. It is highly probable that many of the adhesions have been formed by the oily and smoky vapours distilled off from the hottest parts, and irregularly condensed in the colder : and so far as this conjecture may be true, it would perhaps be advisable to try the effects of a longer maceration in alcohol and in ether, than has hitherto been employed. The " spear of Achilles " might also be applied with very reasonable hopes of success : a repetition of the exposure to heat, kept up more equably and more powerfully, might very probably expel the adhesive substances, without injuring the texture of the charcoal ; proper care being taken to preclude completely the access both of air and of water, which might be done first by means of the air-pump, and then by the insertion of a little potassium, together with the roll, in a vessel hermetically sealed. But the adhesions appear sometimes to be of a mere

---

[a] The farther progress of the attempts to unroll these papyri is detailed in the article 'Herculaneum,' from the Supplement of the Encyclopædia Britannica, which is reprinted in the third volume of Dr. Young's Works, p. 560.

mechanical nature, being derived from the irregular folds into which the manuscripts have been pressed, or from some roughnesses of the contiguous surfaces.

Until the manuscripts already unrolled shall have been published there can be little inducement to bestow much labour on the few that have been brought to this country in their entire state : but at a future time, we think that some attempt to unrol them ought to be made, even with such means as we have at present in our power, without however sacrificing any part of their substance. The outer parts might be separated into as many portions as possible, without breaking through the adhesions, so that the characters on the internal surface of each piece might remain legible ; and we should probably find that the internal parts would be capable of being much more completely unrolled : the adhering portions might be kept in proper order, until the discovery of some more effectual means of separating their component parts.

We are informed that the gentleman to whom we allude had gone so far as to ascertain that the two manuscripts entrusted to his care appeared to be in prose, and that their subjects were probably of a philosophical or critical nature. They were certainly not the *delicatissimi versus* which Philodemus, as Cicero informs us, had addressed to Piso, not in order to enforce the genuine Epicurean precepts of temperance and frugality, but in compliance with his pupil's predilection for that school, which has put a more popular construction on the dogmas of the philosopher. But whatever may have been the moral value of these poems, they would certainly be far more esteemed, by the genuine votaries of Greek literature, than a thousand grave essays on the Metaphysics of Music, or on the Piety of Atheism. If we calculate upon the doctrine of chances, we fear that there is little probability of the discovery of any works of a class very superior to those which have already been rendered ligible ; although, on the other hand, it appears to be scarcely possible that the library of the Pisos should retain no traces of the elegant genius and poetical talent of the *Græcus facilis et valde venustus,* who had been so intimately connected with their ancestor : nor is it very probable that many more performances will be found in the collection relating to subjects so totally unattractive as those which have already been published.

APPENDIX—B.[a]

DETERMINATION OF THE

FIGURE OF THE EARTH

FROM A SINGLE TANGENT.

HAVING observed the latitudes and any two azimuths obliquely situated in the same horizontal plane, touching the earth's surface at the first point, take the tangent of the difference of azimuths, and divide it by the sine of the latitude of the first point : the quotient will be the tangent of the difference of longitude, as is easily shewn from the elementary principles of plane trigonometry.

The first azimuth being α and the second α', considered as angles of the same triangle, then the tangent of the difference[b] of azimuths will be, $\tan (\alpha+\alpha')$ and $\frac{\tan. (\alpha+\alpha')}{\sin. \text{lat.}}$ will be the tangent of Δ, the difference of longitudes. (1.)

If we call the distance of the points unity, the linear tangent of the difference of latitudes will be $\frac{\sin. \frac{1}{2} (\alpha-\alpha')}{\cos. \frac{1}{2} (\alpha+\alpha')}$: and the chords

---

[a] The investigation, which forms the subject of this Appendix, was never published. A rough copy of it was found amongst Dr. Young's papers, written upon a small sheet of note paper a few months before his death, as appears from a reference to it in a letter to Mr. Gurney, which is noticed in page 477. The preliminary propositions are involved in the method proposed by Dalby for determining arcs of parallel, which was used in the English and Indian surveys ; the special application in the text is novel and ingenious, and well deserving of notice.

[b] By azimuth here is meant the angular distance of the observed station from the meridian.

of the parallels of latitude, as measured in the tangent plane, will be $\dfrac{\sin. \; \alpha}{\cos.\frac{1}{2}(\alpha+\alpha')}$ and $\dfrac{\sin. \; \alpha'}{\cos. \; \frac{1}{2}(\alpha+\alpha')}$, the mean, when reduced in the ratio of the radius to the cosine of half the difference of latitudes $\dfrac{\delta}{2}$, becoming the double tangent of half the difference of longitudes; and while the angles are small, the same mean may be considered as simply equal to the tangent of the difference of longitudes or $\dfrac{\sin. \; \alpha+\sin. \; \alpha'}{2 \cos. \; \frac{1}{2}(\alpha+\alpha')} = r \tan. \; \Delta$, the linear tangent of Δ, r being the radius of the parallel; while $\varrho \tan. \; \delta$ is the linear tangent of the difference of latitudes, ϱ being the radius of curvature of the meridian and $\varrho \tan. \; \delta = \dfrac{\sin. \; \frac{1}{2}(\alpha-\alpha')}{\cos. \; \frac{1}{2}(\alpha+\alpha')}$.

Hence $\dfrac{\varrho}{r} = \dfrac{\tan. \; \Delta}{\tan. \; \delta} \dfrac{2 \sin. \; \frac{1}{2}(\alpha-\alpha')}{\sin. \; \alpha+\sin. \; \alpha'} = n.$ (2.)

Now when the diameters of an ellipsis are c and d, the radius $\varrho = \left\{ \dfrac{c^2 d^2 + (c^2 - d^2)(4cx - 4x^2)}{2c^4 d} \right\}^{\frac{3}{2}}$ (Simpson, art. 71); and this becomes, when we substitute r for $c-x$, and write $2a$ and $2b$ for c and d, $\varrho = \left\{ \dfrac{a^2 b^2 + (a^2 - b^2)(a^2 - r^2)}{a^4 b} \right\}^{\frac{3}{2}} = \dfrac{b^2}{a} \left\{ \dfrac{a^2}{b^2} - r^2 \left(\dfrac{1}{b^2} - \dfrac{1}{a^2} \right) \right\}^{\frac{3}{2}}$

$= \dfrac{a^2}{b}\left(1 - \dfrac{e^2 r^2}{a^2}\right)^{\frac{3}{2}}$, if we put $e^2 = 1 - \dfrac{b^2}{a^2}$: (3): but if we neglect the higher powers of e^2, this expression becomes $\varrho = a \left\{ 1 + e^2 \left(\frac{1}{2} - \dfrac{3r^2}{2a^2}\right) \right\}$ and $n = \dfrac{\varrho}{r} = \dfrac{a}{r}\left\{ 1 + e^2\left(\frac{1}{2} - \dfrac{3r^2}{2a^2}\right) \right\}$ (4).

But the latitude being φ, we have $\dfrac{r}{a} = \dfrac{\cos. \; \phi}{\sqrt{(1 - e^2 \sin. \;^2 \phi)}} = \cos. \; \varphi$ $\left(1 + \dfrac{e^2}{2} \sin.^2 \varphi\right)$ nearly: and equation (4) becomes $n = \dfrac{1}{\cos. \; \phi}$ $\left(1 - \dfrac{e^2}{2} \sin.^2 \varphi\right)\left\{ 1 + e^2 \left(\frac{1}{2} - \dfrac{3r^2}{2a^2}\right) \right\} = \dfrac{1}{\cos. \; \phi}\left(1 - \dfrac{e^2}{2}(\sin.^2 \varphi - 1 + \dfrac{3r^2}{a^2}\right) = \dfrac{1}{\cos. \; \phi}(1 + e^2(\cos.^2 \varphi - 3 \cos.^2 \varphi) = \dfrac{1}{\cos. \; \phi}(1 - 2e^2 \cos.^2 \varphi)$: consequently $n \cos. \; \varphi = 1 - 2e^2 \cos.^2 \varphi$ and $e^2 = \dfrac{1 - n \cos. \; \phi}{2 \cos.^2 \phi} = \dfrac{\sec. \; \phi - n}{2 \cos. \; \phi}$ (5).

It remains to be proved whether there is any error in this reasoning, or whether, even if the thing is accurate, the method is capable of practical application with advantage. The only theoretical imperfection appears to be the taking the angular change of latitude from the radius of curvature appropriate to the middle of the arc: and this might be avoided, if it were necessary, by computing the exact length of the elliptic arc of the meridian between the two latitudes. But in very small triangles we may simplify the computation still more, and use the arcs indifferently for the tangents, and use the tangent of the mean azimuth for $\frac{2\sin.\frac{1}{2}(\alpha-\alpha')}{\sin.\ \alpha+\sin.\ \alpha'}$ and the latitude of the middle of an arc reduced to the horizon for that of the first point here considered.

Taking for an example Captain Kater's Observations at Crowborough and at Fairlight,[a] we have $\alpha = 121° \ 4' \ 58\cdot36''$, $\alpha' = 58° \ 33' \ 26\cdot14''$, $\varphi = 50° \ 57' \ 57\cdot59''$ and $\delta = 10' \ 41\cdot42''$; the calculation will stand thús:—

Log. tan. diff. az: $21' \ 35\cdot1''$ - - 7·7930179
Sin. $\varphi \ 50° \ 57' \ 57\cdot59''$- - - 9·8902938

Tan. Δ, $27' \ 47\cdot8''$ - - - $\overline{7}$·9077241
Other methods give $27' \ 47''$ or $27' \ 53''$

Log. tan. δ, $10' \ 41\cdot42''$ - - - 7·4927043

Log. $\frac{\text{tan. } \Delta}{\text{tan. } \delta}$ - - - - ·4150198
Log. tan. $31° \ 15' \ 46''$ - - - 9·7832744
Log. n - - - - - ·1982947
Log. cos. φ, $50° \ 57' \ 57\cdot59''$ - - 9·7991896

Log. ·994224 - - - - $\overline{1}$·9974843
Log. 005776 $= 1 - n$ cos. φ - - 7·7616272
Log. cos. $^{2}\varphi$ - - - - 9·5983792

Log. $2e^{2}$ ·01456 $= \overline{2}$, 1632480.

Hence $c^{2} = $ ·00728, and $\frac{a}{b} - 1 = $ 00364 $= \frac{1}{275}$, the ellipticity for the county of Sussex.

[a] See Captain Kater's 'Account of Trigonometrical Operations in the years 1821, 1822, and 1823, for determining the difference of Longitude between the Royal Observatories of Paris and Greenwich,' in the Philosophical Transactions for 1828, pp. 153 and 185.

It will be found that a difference of 001 in the ellipticity, for example between 003 and 004, would in this example cause a change of $3''\cdot4$ in the difference of the azimuths : and an error of this magnitude could scarcely occur in the mean of a large number of observations, so that it appears perfectly possible to employ the method in practical surveying and to determine the figure of the earth with sufficient accuracy for the correction of parallaxes, by means of the angles observed at two stations only within sight of each other.

The operation may be continued from station to station in the same parallels of latitude across a whole continent, and the true azimuth only will require to be derived from celestial observations at the extreme stations, and by these means the effects of any local change of curvature may be compensated. Thus from Falmouth to Seeberg the latitude varies but little, and by computing the difference of longitude separately for each triangle employed, the whole difference will be obtained with extreme accuracy, and the mean value of the proportion of the radii of curvature, compared with the mean latitude, will give the eccentricity with little or no sensible error : and the longitude of Falmouth with regard to Greenwich, which is of importance for the regulation of chronometers, may be deduced at once from the triangles employed in the survey without the introduction of any heterogeneous elements of uncertain magnitude.

LONDON · PRINTED BY W. CLOWES AND SONS, STAMFORD STREET AND CHARING CROSS.